JN435975

Modern Oriental Phytotherapy in Sexual Medicine

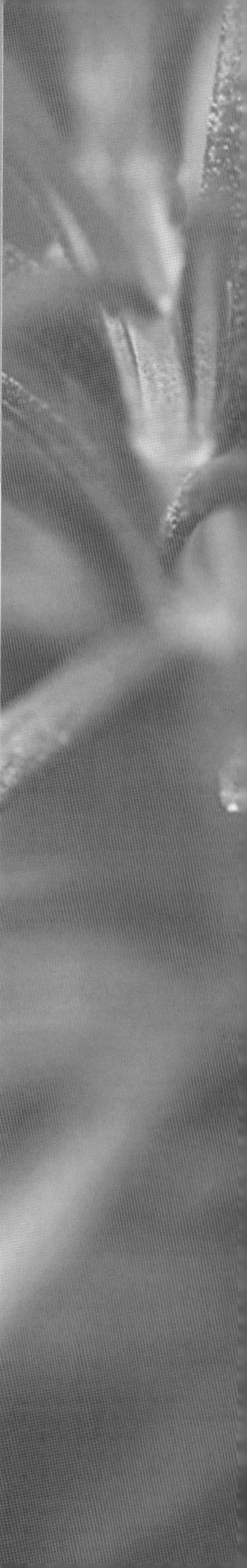

Edited by

Nam Cheol Park
Akihiko Okuyama
Zhong-cheng Xin
Jong Hee Park
Carolyn Earle
P. Ganesan Adaikan

KOON JA PUBLISHING INC.

KOON JA PUBLISHING INC.
6F Dongwon B/D 112-1,
Inui-dong Jongno-gu,
Seoul, Korea 110-717

Modern Oriental Phytotherapy in Sexual Medicine

Edited by Nam Cheol Park et al.

Copyright © 2010 by Koonja Publishing, Inc.
ALL RIGHTS RESERVED. No part of this publication may be reproduced or transmitted in any form or by any means, electronic, or mechanical, including photocopying, recording, or any information storage and retrieval system-without permission in writing from the publisher.

The publication of this book was partially supported by the APSSM budget from 2009 ISSM Fund.

For permission to use material from this text or product, contact us by
Tel (822) 762-9194
Fax (822) 764-0209
admin@koonja.co.kr
www.Koonja.co.kr

Printed in Republic of Korea.
ISBN 978-89-6278-304-9

"For Continuing Challenge
from Oriental Seed, Root, Leaf and Bark to Modern Global Pill"

and

"Special Thanks to Consistent Support of Contributors,
Koonja Publishing, Inc. and International Society for Sexual Medicine"

Contributors

Akihiko Okuyama, M.D., Ph.D.
President of Aizenbashi Hospital, Osaka, Japan

Apichat Kongkanand, M.D., FACS.
Department of Urology, Bumrungrad Hospital, Bangkok, Thailand

Balasubramanian Srilatha, M.D., Ph.D.
Department of Obstetrics & Gynaecology, Yong Loo Lin School of Medicine, National University Hospital, National University of Singapore, Singapore

Benny Tan K.H., M.D., Ph.D.
Associate Professor of Department of Pharmacology, Yong Loo Lin School of Medicine, National University of Singapore, Singapore

Carolyn Earle, B.Sc., P.Grad.Dip.Hlth.Sci
Sexologist, Subiaco, Western Australia, Australia

Chun-Hou Liao, M.D.
Department of Urology, Cardinal Tien Hospital, Taipei, Taiwan, Republic of China

FX Arif Adimoelja, M.D., Ph.D.
Andrology Sub Department, "Dr. Ramelan" Naval Teaching Hospital / Reproductive Health Unit School of Medicine, Hang Tuah University, Surabaya, Indonesia

Han-Sun Chiang, M.D., Ph.D.
College of Medicine, Fu Jen Catholic University, Taipei, Taiwan, Republic of China

Hyun Jun Park, M.D., Ph.D.
Assistant Professor of Department of Urology, Pusan National University School of Medicine, Busan, Korea

Je Jong Kim, M.D., Ph.D.
Professor of Department of Urology, Korea University Hospital, Seoul, Korea

Jihong Liu, M.D., Ph.D.
Professor and Vice Chairman, Department of Urology, Tongji Hospital, Tongji Medical College
Huazhong University of Science and Technology, Wuhan 430030, P. R. China

Johannes Soedjono, M.D.
Andrology Sub Department, "Dr. Ramelan" Naval Teaching Hospital / Reproductive Health Unit School of Medicine, Hang Tuah University, Surabaya, Indonesia

Jong Hee Park, Ph.D.
Professor of College of Pharmacy, Pusan National University, Busan, Korea

Jong Kwan Park, M.D., Ph.D.
Professor of Department of Urology, Medical School, Chonbuk National University, Jeonju, Korea

K Swayam Prakash, M.D.
Chief Consultant, S.V. Clinic & Research Center, Hyderabad, India

Kavirach Tantiwongse, M.D.
Department of Surgery, Chulalongkorn hospital, Bangkok, Thailand

Kwangsung Park, M.D., Ph.D.
Professor of Department of Urology, Chonnam National University Medical School, Gwangju, Korea

Lang Chu Lau, B.Sc. (Hons)., M.Sc.
Department of Obstetrics & Gynaecology, Yong Loo Lin School of Medicine, National University Hospital, National University of Singapore, Singapore

Mikio Namiki, M.D., Ph.D.
Professor of Department of Integrative Cancer Therapy and Urology, Kanazawa University Graduate School of Medical Science, Kanazawa, Japan

Nam Cheol Park, M.D., Ph.D.
Professor of Department of Urology, Pusan National University School of Medicine, Busan, Korea

Narisa Nakpairat
Executive Secretary, Thai Urological Association, Bangkok, Thailand

P. Ganesan Adaikan, Ph.D., D.Sc.
Professor of Department of Obstetrics & Gynaecology, Yong Loo Lin School of Medicine, National University Hospital, National University of Singapore, Singapore

Peter Lim H.C, M.D., Ph.D.
Professor of Andrology, Urology & Continence Center, Gleneagles Hospital, Singapore

Sae Woong Kim, M.D., Ph.D.
Professor of Department of Urology, Catholic University Medical College, Seoul, Korea

Sudhakar Krishnamurti, M.D.
Andrologist, Microsurgeon & Director Andromeda Andrology Center, Hyderabad, India

Sung Won Lee, M.D., Ph.D.
Professor of Department of Urology, Sungkyunkwan University School of Medicine, Samsung Medical Center, Seoul, Korea

Sung-Yeoun Hwang, O.M.D., Ph.D.
Chairman of Institute of Traditional Korea Food Globalization, Seoul, Korea

Victor Ong Y.C., M.D.
Vivo Health, LLP. Centre for Integrative Weight-Healthcare, North Bridge Centre, Singapore

Won Chul Lee, O.M.D., Ph.D.
Professor of Department of Internal Medicine, Pusan National University School of Korean Medicine, Busan, Korea

Yasushi Miyagawa, M.D., Ph.D.
Department of Urology, Osaka University Graduate School of Medicine, Osaka, Japan

Zhao Chen, M.D.
Department of Urology, Medical School, Chonbuk National University, Jeonju, Korea

Zhong-cheng Xin, M.D., Ph.D.
Professor of Andrology Center, Peking University First Hospital, Peking University, Beijing, China

Preface

Oriental Herbal Phytotherapy for Sexual Medicine

Herbal medicine, a natural therapeutic method using medical plants, is greatly differentiated from the pharmacological treatment for which various substances are made into drugs. Herbal phytotherapy is a natural therapy to prevent or treat diseases by analyzing the medical actions of certain plants and using the ingredients excellent in medical effect. Regardless of east or west, the herbal medicine has been used to keep health and cure diseases for a very long time through traditional and classical principles on life and environment. Such natural treatment began with the history of mankind: The vestiges of herb medicine are seen in the Neanderthals' tombs constructed about sixty thousand years; the medical actions of approximately 1,200 medicines are recorded in a medical lexicon published in the age of ancient Aztec Indians. China, a front-runner of Oriental medicine, has accumulated a vast amount of knowledge and clinical experience on herb medicines during the past 5,000 years. For example, Chinese Shen Nong first published a record on traditional Oriental medicinal herbs. In Korea, Heo Jun published an encyclopedia Dongeuibogam in 1613, which is composed of 25 volumes and introduces standard herb medicine prescription for each disease. This historical background allowed Asians to strongly trust in herb medicine treatment, which is much more weakly seen in Europeans and Americans. Accordingly, herb therapy was used as an important means to treat diseases as folk therapy as well.

In spite of the remarkable development of modern medicine, the majority of Asians and Africans are still favorably disposed toward herb medicines due to the aggressive treatment ways and the toxicity and tolerance of drugs shown by western medicine. Also, now is the time when it is required to develop natural remedies using the medicinal herbs that are helpful for preventing and treating the chronic diseases increased by life expectancy increase, diet change, hereditary factors, insufficient exercise, stress, environment pollution, etc. Besides, WHO data shows that while the rest follow complementary alternative medicine, only 30-40% of medical markets follow conventional western medicine, making it impossible to overlook the importance of herbal medicine. In economic terms, the herb medicine market has drastically expanded to that of billions of dollars throughout the world. These days, religious, sociocultural, or socioeconomic background or trust in traditional medicine makes various attempts to prevent diseases or to develop the drugs without side effect using the active substances extracted from herbs with a view to overcoming the problems or limitations of modern medicine.

Specifically, the natural treatment using medicinal herbs uses biological products, the same organic matters as those of human somatic cells. The medicinal herbs biologically activated make active substances similar in structure or energies exchanged between the molecules of the herbs and the metabolic substances of human cells. Indeed, it cannot be confirmed that no toxicity or side effect is included in the drugs using medicinal herbs, but herb medicines can minimize side effects by not accumulating toxic substances in human body, unlike artificial synthetic substances. Additionally, the universal use of herb remedies has an expected economic effect of laying groundwork for introducing the treatment of low cost and high efficiency and thus overcoming vast medical expenses.

Herb medicines use the various parts, i.e. leaves, fruits, roots, peels, rhizomes, etc of herb plants. The development of herbal medicine preferentially requires developing the herb medicines that can be used for natural treatment and collecting and analyzing the information, such as the geographical distribution, ingredients, production amount, and effective empirical remedies.

In sexual medicine, many clinicians have got increasingly more curious about the natural treatment of sexual dysfunction using medicinal herbs or extracted natural substances, and there has been an increase in clinical demand using herbs, like other medical fields. Currently, there are a limited number of drugs whose effects are determined by scientific verification among those extracted from medicinal herbs. The herbs known to be effective for sexual improvement or erectile dysfunction treatment are ginseng, onion, garlic, Cornelian Cherry, acanthopanax senticossus, black raspberries, Epimedium koreanum, Pleuropterus multflorus, Polygonatum, Aconitum carmichaeli, etc. They are used for traditional herb medicine as extracts, herb teas, or topical gents, and for modern western medicine that tries to produce drugs by separating active ingredients within natural substances or synthesizing active ingredients chemically. Many natural substances used for treatment by natives in Asia, Africa, or Americas have become major ideas for the development of new drugs in terms of western medicine. In practice, it seems that a series of development processes, such as separation of active ingredients from natural substances, animal study, research in vitro and clinical experiment play roles of infinite ideas for bioscience, lay groundwork for the fusion between western and oriental medicines, and provide clinical doctors with a wider variety of remedies.

The wide use of herb medicines for treatment preferentially requires the scientific verification by modern medicine analysis on treatment methods and effects and the establishment of standard clinical test directions for such verification. Additionally, it requires the understanding of country-specific foods or medicine-related laws and the analysis and evaluation of country-specific legal applications.

It is expected that this publication of "Modern Oriental Phytotherapy in Sexual Medicine" will be a touchstone for the study of herb medicines in the field of sexual medicine by settling the questions of sexual medicine researchers or doctors about oriental herbs, and will help sexual medical scientists select and use herb medicines by introducing the drugs on the market.

Editor-in-Chief
Nam Cheol Park, MD., Ph.D.
Busan, Korea

Contents

Part I

The Current Situation and the Clinical Experience in Sexual Medicine with the Oriental Herbs of Asia-Pacific Countries

Chapter 1

Australian Perspective

Phytotherapy Agents for Male and Female Sexual Dysfunction

Carolyn Earle

I. Background

1. Introduction

In this chapter we look at the current situation and clinical use of phytotherapy (herbal medicine) in Australia. We explore the use of both oriental and western therapies in sexual medicine in males and females and examine the products that are commercially available.

Australia is a multicultural society and welcomes immigrants from many nationalities to its shores. According to the most recent Australian census, the Australian population consists of 8.1% Australians defined as "Asian Australian"[1]. An Asian Australian is defined as a person of Asian continental origin or ancestry who was born in or is an immigrant to Australia. Asian Australians include Central and Southern Asians, South-East Asians and North-East Asians.[1].

In Australia both oriental and western phytotherapy products are available as complimentary medicines but most sales in Australia are of the western type, not surprising as 85% of Australians are of European descent[1].

2. History

The sources available for understanding the history of medicinal plant use are archaeological and written documents[2]. The traditions of Greece, Japan, India and China were documented in

---

Carolyn Earle, B.Sc., P.Grad.Dip.Hlth.Sci
Subiaco ,Western Australia 6008, Australia, Tel: +61-8-93814684, E-mail: c.earle@bigpond.com

many early manuscripts and books but no written records are available for Australia either because they were never produced or were lost or destroyed[2].

The earliest form of phytotherapy practiced in Australia was the medical treatment regime of indigenous Australians, (the aborigines), who it is said have existed on this continent for more than 50,000 years[3]. As indigenous Australians do not have a written language, it follows there are no written records. They rely on oral traditions and drawings to record and perpetuate their history and culture[3].

Today, many indigenous Australians still practice traditional medicine[4], however Aboriginal elders are reluctant to impart their age-old healing and health knowledge outside of their family for fear of it being misused or misappropriated. Their constant worry is that it would be taken off them and commercialized by modern medical practitioners and pharmaceutical companies.

While some academics have gone to great lengths to record the bush medicine knowledge of some aboriginal regions with the support of local families, there are other areas where this is not able to be done. At this stage, no aboriginal phytotherapy products are commercially available so they will not be discussed in this chapter.

3. Today

In recent years there has been a growing trend towards the production and use of complementary medicines in Australia, including vitamin, mineral, plant or herbal, naturopathic and/or homeopathic preparations and nutritional supplements. At the retail level, sales of Over The Counter (OTC) complementary goods are now thought to be approaching AUD 3 billion. It is not known what percentage of this AUD 3 billion is spent on sexual medicine products[5].

Low funding is limiting the research into these areas in Australia[6].

4. Future trends

At present 60% of the 22 million Australians are thought to consume complementary medicines. As acceptance of these products continues to increase, this proportion is forecast to rise[5]. There are no published trend figures for the use of phytotherapy for sexual medicine.

Revenue for the total pharmaceutical manufacturing industry in Australia is forecast to increase from an estimated AUD 8.65 billion in 2008-09 to AUD 10.125 billion in 2013-2014, representing an average growth rate of 3.2% per annum. Relatively strong economic conditions, an ageing population and changing community attitudes to health care are expected to influence the continued growth of this area. Continued product development and innovation (including the "lifestyle drug" phenomena) and the development of new products in various therapeutic areas have also fueled growth, including erectile dysfunction therapies[5].

5. Prevalence of sexual dysfunction in Australia

1) Male sexual dysfunction

Erectile Dysfunction (ED) is the inability of a man to achieve and/or maintain an erection that allows for sexual activity with penetration. Research in Australia[7, 8] shows that at least a third of men over the age of 50 have ED and about a fifth of those have complete absence of erections.

In Chew' s 2,000 study of adult males attending General Practitioners it was found that 39.4% of participants reported experiencing ED and 18.6% reported experiencing ED "all the time", yet only 11.6% of these men had received any form of treatment[9]. There have been no published prevalence studies on the Australian population for other male sexual dysfunctions such as low libido and late onset hypogonadism[10].

2) Female sexual dysfunction

Female sexual dysfunction covers a broad range of conditions such as Hypoactive Sexual Desire Disorder (HSDD), Sexual Arousal Disorder (SAD) and Orgasmic Disorder. The few studies that have been done in Australia show prevalence of between 32-58% for HSDD, 16-32% for SAD and 16-33% for Orgasmic Disorder. The wide variation is related to the different measuring instruments used[11]. Another Australian study showed that up to 19.7% of women report having multiple sexual dysfunctions[10].

II. Phytotherapy in Australia

1. The industry

In Australia, herbal medicines fall into the category of complementary medicines. Complementary medicines account for over 30% of the total Australian pharmaceutical market[5]. There is no data on what percentage of complementary medicine sales relate directly to sexual medicine.

While mainstream medicines still outsell complementary medicines by 2 to 1[5], there is a growing acceptance across the broad Australian community of non-mainstream medicines. This has occurred because of better consumer education, product promotion and availability of a broad range of non-mainstream options.

Phytotherapy sexual medicine products for men and women are openly displayed in pharmacies and health product shops and are widely advertised in national newspapers and magazines.

Growth in demand for phytotherapy sexual medicine products has also been influenced by the increased number of complementary medicine practitioners in Australia. Although there has not been an increase in the teaching of complementary medicines in the mainstream medical and pharmacy schools, there seems to be an increasing trend for medical practitioners to include complementary medicines in their treatment regimes. This may be related to consumers themselves being more aware of this type of medication as it is promoted more in the media.

2. Regulations

All therapeutic goods supplied in, manufactured in, imported into or exported from Australia must be included on the Australian Register of Therapeutic Goods (ARTG) administered by the Therapeutic Goods Administration (TGA). Medicines may be either registered (higher risk) or listed (lower risk) on the ARTG depending on factors such as the ingredients they contain and the claims made for them.

Registered medicines are higher risk preparations such as prescription and over-the-counter medicines, and are individually evaluated by the TGA for quality, safety and effectiveness. Listed medicines are lower risk preparations and may only contain ingredients that have been approved by the TGA as being of low risk and making certain therapeutic claims. The majority of complementary medicines such as vitamin/mineral supplements and herbal medicines are listed (lower risk) medicines.

Although listed medicines are assessed for quality and safety, they are not individually evaluated by the TGA for effectiveness prior to inclusion on the ARTG. However sponsors of listed medicines are required to hold appropriate evidence to support the indications and claims made for their products and must make this evidence available to the TGA upon request.

Consistent with their low risk, listed medicines may only carry claims for health maintenance and health enhancement and refer to non-serious, self-limiting conditions. They may not refer to serious forms of diseases, disorders or conditions and generally must not indicate that they are for the treatment, management, cure or prevention of any condition or disease. The TGA does not "approve" or "endorse" indications, particularly in relation to a specific ingredient.

Claims related to erectile dysfunction, hypogonadism, HSDD, SAD and Orgasmic Disorder are not permitted for listed medicines. However, claims related to supporting/assisting sexual function or libido are permitted. Indications and claims made for listed medicines can be based on evidence of traditional use of a substance or product, and/or on scientific evidence. The TGA has developed guidelines to assist in determining the level of evidence required to support indications and claims made for complementary medicines.

In the face of rising acceptance and usage levels for complementary medicines, the Australian government recently introduced the Complementary Medicines Reform Package which saw the establishment of the Office of Complementary Medicines (OCM), The Complementary Medicines Evaluation Committee (CMEC) and the Complementary Healthcare Consultative Forum (CHCF) within the TGA. The reform package hopes to shift the regulatory focus from pre-market clearance to post market vigilance for low-risk "listable" goods[5].

Other industry bodies include the Australian Self Medication Industry (ASMI), the Australian Complementary Health Association (ACHA) and the Complementary Healthcare Council (CHC). There is also the Pharmaceutical Industry Working Group (PIWG), an industry-government consultative forum designed to examine key issues affecting the industry. In June 2006 a new body, the Pharmaceuticals Industry Council (PIC) was established. It represents the innovative generic and biotechnology sectors of the industry. It also represents the peak body of three peak industry associations - Medicines Australia, the Generics Medicines Industry Association and AusBiotech. The PIC is to take forward the work of the Pharmaceutical Industry Action Agenda[5].

3. Sources of supply

There are three primary avenues open to Australians to procure phytotherapy products for sexual medicine.

1) Practitioners

Western phytotherapy is practiced by naturopaths and oriental and western herbalists, who may recommend packaged over the counter products. However most provide their own made-to-order treatments and practitioner-only products[12]. The ratio between packaged OTC and made-to-order products is unknown. It is not necessary to consult a practitioner prior to purchasing OTC products.

It is recommended practice by therapists to address sexual issues concurrently with the understanding and treating causes of the condition[12].

2) Retail shops

Most pharmacies, supermarkets and health shops sell phytotherapy products for sexual medicine. Pharmacists and health shop proprietors may offer advice on these products however purchases from supermarkets are on a self-service/no advice basis. As shelf space in supermarkets is limited, their range is restricted to the major selling products. Pharmacies and health shops generally stock a wider range of products.

3) Internet

Many phytotherapy product manufacturers and distributors have websites through which their products can be purchased. These websites provide basic product details, pricing and shopping cart facilities and orders are subsequently delivered by mail. There are also several internet pharmacy sites that carry a comprehensive range of products for retail sale/mail delivery.

III. The Products

There are 151 products listed on the ARTG, using search criteria terms including erectile dysfunction, impotence, libido, arousal, hypogonadism, gingko, horny, tribulus, panax, desire, ginseng, sexual function, sexual dysfunction, damiana, deer velvet, natural performance and maca.

Several other herbs are available that make sexual claims but they have not been included in this chapter as they are not listed on the ARTG.

Of the 151 listed products, 37 are manufactured in Australia and these will be profiled in Part II of this chapter. Products that are not manufactured in Australia will not be discussed.

IV. Clinical Experience with Phytotherapy in Sexual Medicine

Because of the increasing popularity of phytotherapy treatments, it is important for both the health practitioner and the consumer to understand if there is any evidence based support for the treatment of sexual problems. Numerous and extensive claims have been made about the sexual health benefits of plant-derived substances, yet often these claims have been based upon folklore or hearsay rather than rigorous scientific investigation[13].

Although folk remedies can provide important suggestions for phytotherapy products to treat sexual dysfunctions, the experimental evidence supporting claims of effective treatment is in many cases non-existent or at best in its infancy[13].

As many of these substances put users at risk and, equally importantly, have the potential to interact with over-the-counter and prescription medications[14-16], practitioners and consumers alike need to recognize both their potential efficacies and liabilities so they can make informed decisions regarding their use.

A recent review of herbal remedies and their relationship to male and female sexual dysfunction[17] concluded limited effectiveness for several specific botanicals and cited sporadic evidence for effectiveness in others. Evidence for the use of five botanicals in the treatment of erectile dysfunction concluded that the evidence to support natural agents for the management of ED is minimal[18]. This was further compounded by another report into five botanicals which mentioned problems with design and power, along with methodological problems rendering much of the data as unhelpful[19].

There are 28 male, 6 female and 3 unisex phytotherapy products for the treatment of sexual medicine manufactured in Australia that are registered with the TGA on the ARTG. These products account for only a small proportion of the total number of phytotherapy products now available. Whilst the majority of these products are targeted towards men, there is increasing interest in the phytotherapy market for women. Many of the ingredients in mens products are also found in womens products.

The main herbs used in sexual health products in Australia are tribulus terrestris, panax ginseng and horny goat weed. However complementary medicine practitioners in Australia also promote the use of panax ginseng, tribulus terrestris, gingko bilbo and to a lesser extent, damiana[12].

Although review articles for complementary medicine, erectile dysfunction[20] and libido[21] have been written in Australia, as far as can be investigated there are no published randomized clinical trials in the area of complementary medicine and sexual function. The evidence cited is from outside Australia.

In recent years, tribulus has gained a reputation as a "natural Viagra"[22]. There is one study from Australia that claims the Bulgarian tribulus product is superior to other tribulus products [23] that are produced in China and India. The active components of this tribulus herb are steroidal saponins, mainly the furostanol saponins and especially protodioscin[22].

It is claimed the best form of tribulus for treatment of sexual dysfunction is the leaf [22]. It seems that most preparations available on the Australian market do not have the right plant part and/or the right level of activity. MediHerb is one of the few Australian companies selling a product that is equivalent to Bulgarian tribulus, recognized as the best available[22].

Yohimbine provides the strongest effect for sexual function but is not available as a manufactured product in Australia so will not be addressed.

A small body of evidence suggests that gingko and ginseng might be worthy of further investigation, however these reviews indicate weak scientific evidence for other botanicals such as maca, damiana, muira puama, and tribulus terrestris, despite positive claims made for the latter[13].

Many of the ingredients in the mens products are also found in the womens products. Presumably it is those that might exert mild increases in androgens or that have the potential to increase smooth muscle relaxation and vascular perfusion to the genital region[13].

It seems that over the past 5 years the major ingredients of phytotherapy products have changed significantly which could be perceived as testimony to the lack of empirical evidence supporting the use of any specific herbal products for sexual medicine[13].

Consumers and health care professionals must make a decision about the use of phytotherapy for sexual health without the benefit of a body of supporting evidence of efficacy, certification of purity, guarantee of safety, or well-documented adverse effects. Even though most botanicals for sexual health have mild side effects and some may even promote general health, the lack of such evidence becomes a matter of concern when users of these products may be on medications for other reasons and have not informed their physicians of their phytotherapy treatment. The ultimate challenge will be not only to demonstrate the efficacy of specific herbal ingredients and to differentiate them from ineffective ingredients, but to also create an economic and medical climate that values serious investigation into such remedies[13].

The National Health and Medical Research Council (NH and MRC) has taken a leadership role in initiating new approaches to supporting research and the provision of evidence-based advice in complementary medicine, including identification in their 2007-2009 strategic plan. The NH and MRC have committed to funding the best and most relevant research and to facilitate the translation of the findings of that research into improved health outcomes, both among individuals and more systematically through the Australian healthcare system. There is also an expectation that improved investment in health and medical research will contribute to growth of an innovative industry sector[24].

V. Summary

Herbal medicine in Australia has reached a high degree of development. It is widely recognized that the standard of practitioner training in Australia is far better than in many other areas of the world. This is complemented by a high degree of freedom as practitioners. In many countries throughout the world, the practice of herbal medicine by herbalists is discouraged, and there is often a complete lack of government support. However here in Australia, practitioners of herbal medicine are recognized and given certain privileges under the Therapeutic Goods Administration and discussions are underway between the government and the profession to form a system of registration for natural therapists, especially herbalists.

The peak body in Australia, the National Herbalists Association of Australia (NHAA) was formed in 1920 and is the oldest natural therapy association in Australia. It has a long and distinguished history supporting herbal medicine and herbalists in this country and leads the way in creating standards of both practice and regulation.

REFERENCES

1. Australian Bureau of Statistics - Census 8th August 2006.
2. M Heinrich JB, S Gibbons, E M Williamson, ed. *Fundamentals of Pharmacognosy and Phytotherapy*. Churchill Livingstone, Edinburgh, 2004.
3. Flood J. *The Original Australians-story of the aboriginal people*; 2006.
4. Maher P. A review of 'traditional' aboriginal health beliefs. *Aust J Rural Health*. 1999;7:229-36.
5. IBISWorld I-R. Pharmaceutical Product Manufacturing in Australia : C2543. 16 September 2008.
6. Braun L. Executive Director - National Herbalists Association of Australia. 2008.
7. Pinnock CB, Stapleton AM, Marshall VR. Erectile dysfunction in the community: a prevalence study. *Med J Aust*. 1999;171:353-7.
8. Chew KK, Stuckey B, Bremner A, Earle CM, Jamrozik K. Male erectile dysfunction: its prevalence in Western Australia and associated sociodemographic factors. *J Sex Med*. 2008;5:60-9.
9. Chew KK, Earle, CM, Stuckey, B.G.A, Jamrozik,K. and Keogh E.J. Erectile Dysfunction in general medicine practice: prevalence and clinical correlates. *International Journal of Impotence Research*. 2000;12:41-45.
10. Najman JM, Dunne MP, Boyle FM, Cook MD, Purdie DM. Sexual dysfunction in the Australian population. *Aust Fam Physician*. 2003;32:951-4.
11. Hayes RD, Dennerstein L, Bennett CM, Fairley CK. What is the "true" prevalence of female sexual dysfunctions and does the way we assess these conditions have an impact? *J Sex Med*. 2008;5:777-87.
12. David M. Naturopath and Medical Herbalist (Western Australia). 2008.
13. Rowland DL BM. Plant-Derivatives and Herbs used for the Promotion of sexual health and the treatment of sexual problems. *Annual Review of sex research*;2007:225-57.
14. Abebe W. Herbal medication: potential for adverse interactions with analgesic drugs. *J Clin Pharm Ther*. 2002;27:391-401.
15. Bressler R. Herb-drug interactions. Interactions between saw palmetto and prescription medications. *Geriatrics*. 2005;60:32,34.
16. Ciocon JO, Ciocon DG, Galindo DJ. Dietary supplements in primary care. Botanicals can affect surgical outcomes and follow-up. *Geriatrics*. 2004;59:20-4.
17. Aung HH, Dey L, Rand V, Yuan CS. Alternative therapies for male and female sexual dysfunction. *Am J Chin Med*. 2004;32:161-73.
18. Mackay D. Nutrients and botanicals for erectile dysfunction : examing the evidence. *Alternative Medicine Review*. 2004;9:4-16.
19. Moyad MA, Barada JH, Lue TF, Mulhall JP, Goldstein I, Fawzy A. Prevention and treatment of erectile dysfunction using lifestyle changes and dietary supplements: what works and what is worthless, part II. *Urol Clin North Am*. 2004;31:259-73.
20. Allen R. Erectile Dysfunction. *Journal of Complementary Medicine*. 2004:24-30.
21. Kron J. Low Libido. *Journal of Complementary Medicine*. 2006:96-101.
22. Bone PK. Director of Research and Development, Mediherb Pty Ltd, Australia. 2008.
23. Lehman RP. *Revista de Fitoterapia*. 2002;2(S1):Abstract B006 page217.
24. Anderson W. Building an evidence base for complementary medicine. *Journal of Complementary Medicine*. 2007:7.

Chapter 2

Chinese Perspective

Traditional Chinese Medicine and its Clinical Application in Sexual Medicine

Zhong-cheng Xin

I. Introduction

Traditional Chinese Medicine (TCM) was developed by ancient Chinese using medicinal plants, herbs or acupuncture needles to prevent or cure diseases, and to improve the general health condition of the human body. Plants have been used as a natural medicine for therapy and health care in China for thousands of years, and the ancient Chinese have accumulated a great deal of information and experience, both in the efficacy and toxicity of TCM. Nowadays, TCM has become more and more popular for patient care as an alternative or complementary medicine, including for those who are suffering from sexual dysfunction throughout the world(NHA,1997).

TCM involves not only a health care system but also medical techniques including acupuncture for the treatment of pain; moxibustion which is the use of smouldering herbs to warm acupuncture points; herbal medicine; and massage. All of these methods play an integral role in the traditional treatment of a broad spectrum of disease and nowadays it is being improved with modern life.

With greater acceptance by the public, western scientists and researchers have begun to take an interest in evaluating and applying TCM in clinical practice. In 1979, the National Institute of Health (NIH) released a consensus statement which indicated that acupuncture was a promising modality for improving a wide range of conditions and the scientific evidence was powerful enough to bring acupuncture into conventional medicine.

Zhong-cheng Xin, M.D., Ph.D.
Andrology Centre, Peking University First Hospital, Peking University, No.A59, Dianmen West Street, Xicheng District, Beijing, China, 100009, Tel: +13701305597, E-mail: xinzc@bjmu.edu.cn, xinzc08@gmail.com

TCM is not based on modern western medical concepts in diagnosis and treatment, but its own philosophy that human physiology and pathophysiology is the reflection of the phenomena observed from nature. In the language of TCM, natural metaphors are widely used to explain the biological processes in the human body. For example, according to TCM philosophy the symptoms of red eyes and flushed face can be explained in terms of heat rising from fire in the body. The therapy strategy might then be to cool the fire by employing techniques to nourish the water of the body as water can be used to put out a fire in nature.

In TCM philosophy "Yin" and "Yang" are a pair of opposite forces which are used to identify symptoms and pathophysiology and even to develop a therapy strategy. For example, Yin represents cold, consolidation, and the quality of being at rest, while Yang represents heat, expansion, and activity. From the western perspective, Yin and Yang in the body might be understood as two sides of the internal balance between anabolism and catabolism. The homeostasis may be regarded as a perfect balance between Yin and Yang. According to TCM philosophy, disease could be regarded as the results of disharmony or disorder of the internal balance. Although TCM therapy philosophy is more complex than what we think, the ultimate therapeutic goal is to recover and keep the balance between Yin and Yang in the body.

According to TCM philosophy, "Jing" (Vital essence), "QI" (Vital energy) and "Shen" (Vital spirit) are the three active elements in the human body. Qi has such functions as warming the body, protecting it from external pathogens and producing and distributing fluids and blood.

TCM works on the treatment of various male diseases and the treatment of disease is focused on the kidney in TCM. Although such organ systems as the liver, spleen ,bladder and heart are involved the kidney is the point of the problem. Each organ has two types of Qi whose functions coincide with our modern western understanding of organ function. From a TCM perspective however an organ represents a theoretical construct of physiological patterns that may involve multiple organ systems from a western perspective.

In TCM, the two primary organs closely related to the sexual function are the kidneys and liver. According to TCM philosophy, the kidneys store the essence Qi, which is similar to male gametes in our modern concept. The liver stores blood, which is closely related to reproductive essence. Both essence QI and blood belong to Yin in nature, thus it is said that the liver and the kidney are from the same source. Weakness in one organ often leads to an imbalance in others. In addition, the liver's function is to make Qi move smoothly through all organs and keep all bodily processes in control. If the liver malfunctions, disease or dysfunction may occur in other affected organs.

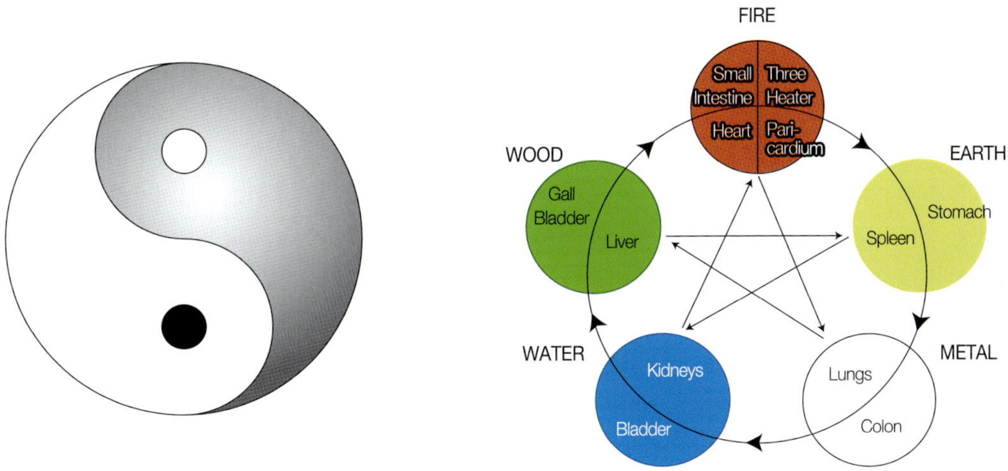

Figure 1. Ying and Yang in TCM philosophy

II. Pattern Diagnosis in TCM

Modern diagnostic thinking tends to follow a linear process of isolating structural or biochemical causes at the root of a chief complaint. A symptom is often reduced to an organ, an organ reduced to a tissue and a tissue to a pathological biochemical process. The tissue may be excised or a drug prescribed to correct, compensate for, or mask a chemical imbalance. A thorough modern intake involves asking the patient many questions but the intent is usually to allow the physician to narrow his or her focus of the problem. In contrast, the questions asked by TCM physicians tend to expand on the chief complaint and derive a broader understanding of the context in which the disease process originated.[1]

TCM diagnosis revolves around identifying patterns of disharmony. The diagnostician must gather as much information through observing, interviewing and palpating the patient. The TCM physician considers the organ correspondences for the various pieces of information gathered. Eventually, an organ or a number of organs begin to emerge as components of the disease or disharmony. The physician must then unravel the relationship between the organs that is leading to the imbalance. Each organ tends to damage or over-control another organ if its function is allowed to become excessive or replete. Each organ is also associated with another organ, which it nourishes. This is the case for the kidney and liver. If the kidney is vacuous, the liver will tend to suffer from lack of nourishment.

There are many common patterns of disharmony. Sometimes a patient will present with a clinical picture closely matching a classically recognized pattern but the majority of cases usually require a sophisticated process of gathering seemingly unrelated data and synthesizing it into a consistent picture of the patient's health. Diagnosis generally involves asking a series of questions concerning the overall state of the patient's health. Based on the knowledge of organ[1] correspondences, the physician organizes the presenting symptoms into an individualized TCM pattern. The observed signs and the reported symptoms are pieces of a puzzle. A single piece alone rarely means anything. Lumping all the pieces of the puzzle together into one disorganized pile only makes the clinical picture more confusing. The art of TCM involves the skillful synthesis of all the clinical data into a comprehensive picture of the patient's disease pattern. Once this is accomplished, the proper course of treatment to bring the body back into harmony emerges.

In general, there are no simple correspondences between TCM diagnoses and modern diagnoses. A single modern diagnosis may be explained by a number of TCM patterns. The following tables give a rough indication of what patterns may be involved in specific modern diagnoses of ED and infertility. These tables are presented not as a tools for diagnosis but to illustrate the depth and breadth of TCM diagnosis and its applicability to the full range of diagnoses recognized by the modern understanding of ED and infertility.

Table 1. Causes of ED in modern and TCM[1]

Modern		TCM
Psychogenic		Fear and Fright Damaging the Kidneys
		Heart and Gall Bladder Qi Vacuity Binding
		Depression of Liver Qi
Organic		
	Hormonal	Debility of the Life Gate Fire
		Kidney Yin Vacuity
		Kidney Yang Vacuity
	Vascular	Liver Channel Damp-Heat Pouring Downward
		Phlegmand Damp Obstructing NetworkVessels
		Stasis Obstructing Essence Vessel
	Neurogenic	
	Iatrogenic	Stasis Obstructing Essence Vessel
Mixed		
	Aging	Debility of the Life Gate Fire
		Kidney Yin Vacuity
		Kidney Yang Vacuity

III. Patterns of Sexual Dysfunction in TCM

A complete discussion of the patterns listed above is beyond the scope of this chapter. Even if a patient's condition closely matches a classical pattern, there will be nuances which can only be properly addressed by a complete diagnosis. Specific patterns are usually part of a larger disharmony. In particular, since the kidney and liver are closely related, sexual dysfunction commonly involves combinations of kidney and liver patterns. From a TCM perspective, all contributing elements of a pattern must be addressed in order to effect a lasting change in the patient's health. The following discussion focuses on a few common patterns and is presented to illustrate the rationale behind TCM diagnosis and treatment;

1. Vacuity of kidney yang

There is a Yang component inherent in the process of achieving and maintaining an erection. This is reflected in the functional and circulatory activity required as well as the heat and warmth produced in an erection. A vacuity of kidney Yang is a possible pattern that may result in various degrees of ED.

2. Vacuity of kidney yin

In cases of vacuous kidney Yin, the kidney Yang will tend to be in relative repletion. This repletion Yang manifests as heat, which may cause reckless movement in the orderly flow of the essence. The result of this heat agitation may manifest as premature ejaculation.

3. Fear and fright damaging the kidney

The dominant emotion associated with the kidney is fear. This correspondence is perhaps most graphically illustrated by the incontinence experienced during a frightening experience. The functions of the kidneys are also impaired when a certain degree of fear is associated with sexual activity. This is a relevant concern in situations where a man is overly concerned about his sexual performance or fearful about causing pregnancy or contracting a sexually transmitted disease. There is generally no problem achieving and maintaining an erection outside of a situation involving sexual contact.

4. Liver channel damp-heat pouring downward

Due to the same processes mentioned under Dampness in the Liver Channel, fluids may stagnate into dampness and obstruct the vessels of the penis resulting in the inability to achieve erection due to a physical obstruction. Accumulated dampness tends to engender heat. This condition is commonly related to emotional frustration or constraint as mentioned above. Additionally, there may be signs of heat in this pattern including itchiness and possibly rash of the scrotum, reddish urine, and dysuria. From a modern perspective, if there are prominent signs of heat in the genital region, infertility due to increased temperature of the testes may be a concern.[1]

IV. TCM Therapy

The traditional viewpoint pays much attention to the prevention of diseases. Herbs are used to recover and keep the internal balance of body. In China, there are more than 3200 herbal medicines and more than 400 formulas are used for medical care. TCM implies a cocktail of many herbs are used as an integrity to patients. It consists of different components in different forms such as powder, capsules, tinctures, or syrups. Among all the herbs in the cocktail, one or two herbs work on the major aspects of the problem to be treated and the others work on the minor aspects or help the major herbs to work more effectively. Differing from western medicine, all the interactive elements and individual components are looked as integrity and individual therapy is looked as the essence in TCM.

V. History of TCM

With over 2000 years of development, TCM has its own sophisticated medical philosophy which originated from careful observation and critical thinking. With a long period of empirical clinical experience, TCM has been continuously developed to a high level, especially after the modern principles of the scientific methods were introduced.

Shennong Bencao Jing (Shennong Emperor's Classic of Materia Medica, 1st century C.E. Han dynasty), the first Chinese manual on pharmacology lists 365 medicines among which more than 15 including morinda root, caulis cistanchis, Chinese magnoliavine fruit, common cnidium fruit, epimedium and dendrobium nobile. have been widely used in treating sexual dysfunction by practitioners.

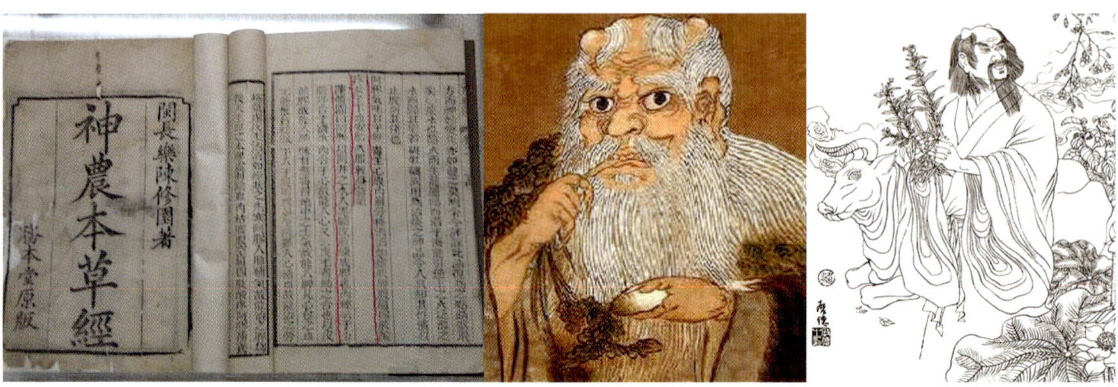

Figure 2. Shennong' s literature and author' s portrait of TCM

In the Sui Dynasty (581-618) , Chao yuan-fang mentioned that "kidney deficiency" played an important role in sexual dysfunction in his academic work (Zhu Bing Yuan Hou Lun). In his opinion, a combination of "kidney Yang and kidney Yin deficiency" was an important cause of sexual dysfunction and loss of libido. He was the earliest medical expert that proposed the etiology of sexual dysfunciton to be kidney deficiency. In the Tang Dynasty (618-907), the famous medical expert-Sun Si Miao attached great importance to kidney Yang in sexual life. Therefore, supplementing kidney yang was the major therapy. He listed 30 formulas such as Wu Bu Wan, Shen Qi Wan, Tian Xiong Wan and Shi Liu Huang San in the treatment of sexual dysfunction.

In the Ming Dynasty (1368-1644), supplementing kidney yang was the main therapy strategy in the treatment of sexual dysfunction. Zhang Jing-Yue was one of the representative medical experts of that period. He introduced more details on the etiology, mechanism and treatment of sexual dysfunction in his academic work (Jing Yue Quan Shu). Zuo Gui Wan and You Gui Wan were the typical formulas for supplementing kidney Yin and Yang deficiency respectively. Meanwhile, other practitioners put forward the etiology and therapy of ED from different angles. Wang Lun (author of the academic work Ming Yi Za Zhu of the Ming Dynasty) proposed that liver damp heat be the etiology and the solution was to clear the damp heat from the genitals with Long Dan Xie Gan Wan. Zhou Shen Zhai (author of the academic work Shen Zhai Yi Shu of the Ming Dynasty) put forward that Xiao Yao San combined with Bai Jili Wan was a mixed formula in the treatment of sexual dysfunction caused by liver qi stagnation.

Throughout the history of TCM the society has been dominated by men. This reality has lead to a focus on medical knowledge of Chinese medi`cine treatment of men's health and longevity. From a Chinese medicine point of view, the ability to obtain and maintain an erection is primarily the responsibility of the kidneys and liver. The deficiency control on "Yang Qi" results in erectile dysfunction, while the liver-channel transmits through the external sexual organs. Weaknesses reduce the kidney's physiological 'fire desire', while the liver-qi stagnation reduces physical fitness. If the liver qi stagnates for long enough, the blood will do as well.

VI. Current Prevalence of Sexual Dysfunction and Chinese Herbs for Sexual Medicine in China

Since 1990, many surveys have been conducted to investigate the prevalence of sexual dysfunction in different areas and different age groups in China. Of the four types of sexual dysfunction (lack of interest, erectile dysfunction, premature ejaculation (PE) and inability to reach orgasm), ED and PE have been the two most thoroughly studied.

1. Erectile dysfunction

Bai Q and his associates[2] conducted a cross-sectional, population-based survey in three cities (Beijing, Guangzhou and Chongqing) of China. Structured questionnaires were administered to 2 226 men, aged 20-86 years, by trained interviewers. The results showed that the age-adjusted prevalence of ED was 28.3% (mild 15.99%, moderate 7.14% and severe 5.21%). In men above 40 years, the prevalence was 40.2%. The prevalence of ED increased with age and age was positively correlated with ED. The prevalence of ED decreased with the increase in the education level. The prevalence of ED was 63.59%, 30.48%, 24.72% and 21.85% in men with elementary school or lower, middle school, high school, and college or higher degrees, respectively. In the sociodemographic variables, spouse companionship and living conditions were positively correlated with ED. IIn the sociodemographic variables, spouse companionship and living conditions were positively correlated with ED. In the medical variables, histories of cardiovascular diseases, diabetes and hyperlipidaemia were positively correlated with ED. Of the lifestyle factors, smoking was not correlated with ED, while the duration of smoking and the cigarette consumption were positively correlated with ED. The prevalence of ED elevated with the increase in cigarette consumption and duration. The risk of ED was higher in subjects having smoked for more than 10 years and in heavy smokers (daily cigarette consumption >20) than that in others. Alcohol drinking is negatively correlated with ED. The prevalence of ED was lower in drinkers than in nondrinkers. The duration of drinking was positively correlated with ED. The prevalence was significantly higher in subjects having drunk for more than 20 years than that in others. Weekly alcohol consumption was not correlated with ED. Zhang ZC et al[3] investigated the prevalence of ED in the Beijing urban area. The prevalence rate of ED among married men in Beijing was 39.1%, and the prevalence rate of ED over 40 years was 54.5%. ED was strongly correlated with age. The prevalence of ED was 7.3%, 9.4%, 32.0%, 51.1%, 66.8%, and 79.8% in the <30 years group, 30-39 years group, 40-49 years group, 50-59 years group, 60-69 years group and >70 years group respectively. The prevalence rate of complete ED in 60-69 years group was nearly 5 times as in 50-59 years group. The prevalence rate of ED in diabetes and vascular disease cases were 52.6% and 46.9% respectively. Smoking and education level were not correlated with ED. Jiang H[3] conducted an Asian Men' s Attitudes to Life Events and Sexuality (Asian MALES)-China study. A total of 2,055 men aged 20-75 years were included using a standardized questionnaire. The results indicated that the overall rate of ED in the Asian MALES-China was 5.9%. The rate of self-reported ED increased with age. The prevalence of ED was 2%, 2%, 4%, 8%, and 11% in men in the 20-29 years group, 30-39 years group, 40-49 years group, 50-59 years group, >60 years group respectively. A higher rate of ED was reported in men with comorbid medical conditions and risk factors, including cardiovascular disease, hypertension, dyslipidaemia, benign prostatic hyperplasia and depression, and so were the rates of these comorbid conditions in ED patients.

2. Premature ejaculation

Lau JT and his colleagues[5] investigated the prevalence and factors associated with sexual dysfunction among younger married men living in rural China. An anonymous questionnaire was self-administered by the husbands of 298 randomly selected married women aged 20 to 39 years. The results showed that the prevalence of premature ejaculation was 19.5%.

Liang CZ[6] conducted a survey to investigate the prevalence and risk factors of sexual dysfunction in Chinese men with chronic prostatitis. The prevalence of premature ejaculation and erectile dysfunction accounted for 26% and 15%, respectively; 7.7% had both premature ejaculation and erectile dysfunction. There was a negative correlation between prevalence and age, and with the duration of chronic prostatitis.

So far, a lot of traditional Chinese medicine compound formulas single monomer have been used to treat sexual dysfunction. The effectiveness and the mechanism for these formulas have been explored.

3. Chinese compound formulas

The Shugan Yiyang (SGYY) capsule is a Chinese traditional patent medicine which was based on the theory of "Impotence could be treated by regulating Gan (liver)". The regulation of Gan means soothing Gan to disperse depression, promoting blood circulation to remove obstruction from collaterals and meridians, and to get rid of impotence.

Qi Wang and his colleagues studied the pharmacological effect of the Shugan Yiyang (SGYY) capsule on erectile function. In the animal experiment, they found the SGYY capsule could remarkably reduce the incubation period of erection, ejaculation and innovate the sexual desire, erection, and ejaculation on both rats and rhesus monkeys. The weight of the prostate, seminal vesicles, and testes in rat along with the serum testosterone level of rats increased while the weight of thymus decreased. It can also diminish the luminar of vein and reduce the venous outflow while the transmission of the peripheral nervous system remained stable. It indicated that the SGYY capsule can remarkably improve erectile activity, sexual desire and ejaculatory activity. The mechanism of the SGYY capsule may be related to the increase of androgen and adrenocortical hormone levels as well as the reduction of penile venous outflow[7].

4. Single chinese herbs

1) *Szechwan lovage rhizome*

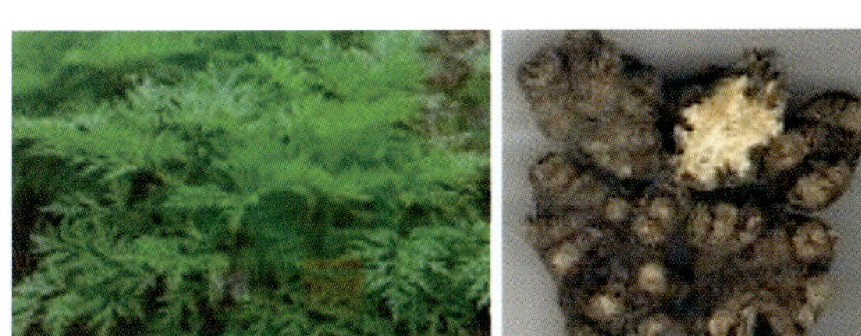

Figure 3. *Szechwan lovage rhizome*

Szechwan lovage rhizome is the dried root of ligusticum chuanxiong hort, which is planted in SiChuan, JiangXi, HuBei, YunNan, GuiZhou, and other areas. It is warm-natured with a pungent flavor, and can be used to promote blood flow, eliminate wind and alleviate pain in traditional Chinese medicine.

Xiao H and his associates investigated the role of ligustrazine on relaxation of the isolated rabbit corpus cavernosum tissue in vitro. The effects were observed by using an experimental method of smooth muscle strips. The results showed that ligustrazine could significantly relax the cavernosal muscle contraction induced by PE in vitro. The results suggested that ligustrazine inhibited calcium ion influx[8]. Chuanxiongzine was also effective in relaxing cavernosal muscle precontracted by PE in vitro. Its relaxing effect may be enhanced by increasing cGMP and cAMP levels in the corpus cavernosum[9].

2) *Angelica sinensis*

Angelica sinensis is the dried root of angelica. Angelica sinensis is warm, sweet and acrid in property and flavor, and its function in Chinese traditional medicine is to increase the blood flow, regulate menstruation and alleviate pain.

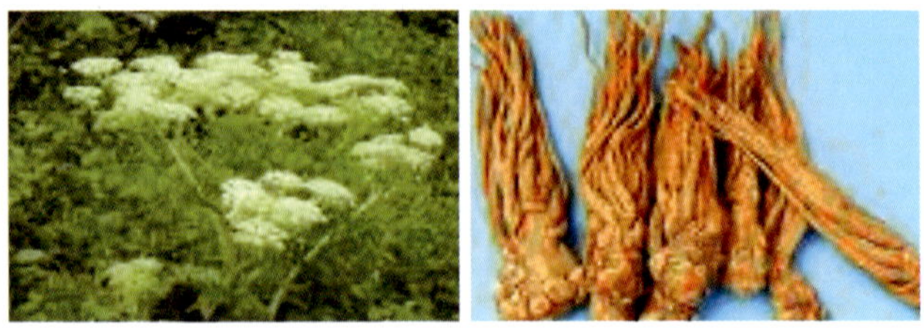

Figure 4. *Angelica sinensis*

Hu WL and his associates explored the change of nitric oxide synthase (NOS) activity in penile tissues after a crushing injury to the cavernous nerves (CN) and the effect of local injection with an Angelica Sinensis (AS) solution. The results indicated that the mean value of NOS activity of AS group was (1.360 ± 0.139)U/mg · prot, which was 77.4% of the normal group and significantly higher than that of the control group[(0.945 ± 0.098) U/mg · prot, which was only 53.8% of the normal group. The author concluded that crushing injury to CN could make NOS activity decrease in penile tissue and local injection with AS solution could avoid its decreasing to some extent[10].

3) *Ginseng*

Ginseng is the root of the Araliaceae plant, grown in Jilin, Liaoning and other provinces. Ginseng contains 5.22% ginsenosides, comprising more than 20 kinds of ginsenosides, among which, contents of ginsenoside Rb, Rc and Rg are the highest. Choi et al[11] found that ginsenoside could relax the corpus cavernosum in a concentration dependent manner, and also enhance the loose effect of corpus cavernosum induced by acetylcholine. LNNA

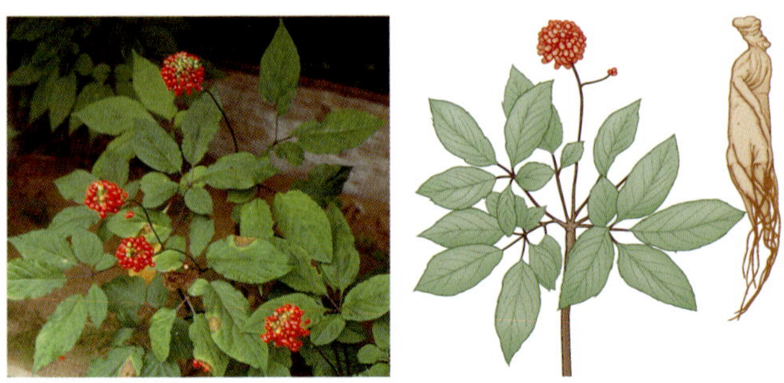

Figure 5. *Ginseng*

and oxyhaemoglobin could weaken such effect, while SOD could strengthen the effect, which showed ginsenoside could promote the endothelial cells to release NO so as to induce corpus cavernosum relaxation.

4) *Notoginseng*

Also named Panax, Notoginseng is mainly grown in Yunnan and Guangxi Provinces. Its main active ingredient is Notoginseng Triterpenes. Yang JL et al[12] observed the effect of Notoginseng Triterpenes on corpus cavernosum of humans, monkeys and dogs, then discussed its mechanism. The result showed that PNS had no effect on the affinity index and maximal effect of accumulated NE concentration and effect curve on dog's penile blood vessel, but it could inhibit the contraction effect of NE on corpus cavernosum, which meant that PNS was not a competitive antagonist of NE receptor. PNS induced the corpus smooth muscle to relax in a concentration dependent manner. LNNA could completely inhibit the dilation of the corpus smooth muscle by PNS, but this kind of inhibitive effect could be inversed by L-arginine, which meant PNS activated NOS and then caused the endothelial cells to release NO to relax the corpus cavernosum.

5) *Folium ginkgo*

Also named Folium ginkgo bilobae, it is a kind of leaf of the Ginkgoaceae plant which grows all over the country. Its main components are flavonoid and terpene lactones. Paick et al[13] researched the influence and mechanism of GBE on the corpus cavernosum of ED patients and rabbits by invitro perfusion and electrical stimulation.

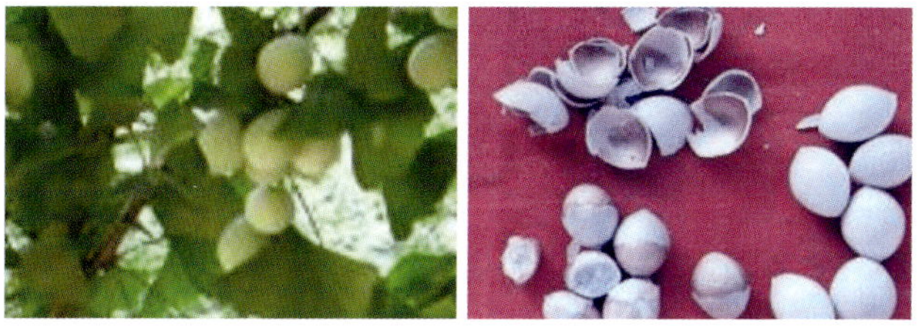

Figure 6. *Folium ginkgo*

6) *Common cnidium fruit*

It is the fruit of Umbelliferae cnidium monnieri, which grows in most of China. Its main physiological components are coumarin and also naphtha and flavonoids. Chen et al[13] observed the loose effect of Osthole on the corpus cavernosum of rabbits, and found that Osthole could relax the corpus cavernosum induced by PE in a dose dependent manner, which suggested that Osthole loosened the corpus cavernosum by increasing NO release from endothelial cells and inhibition of PDE.

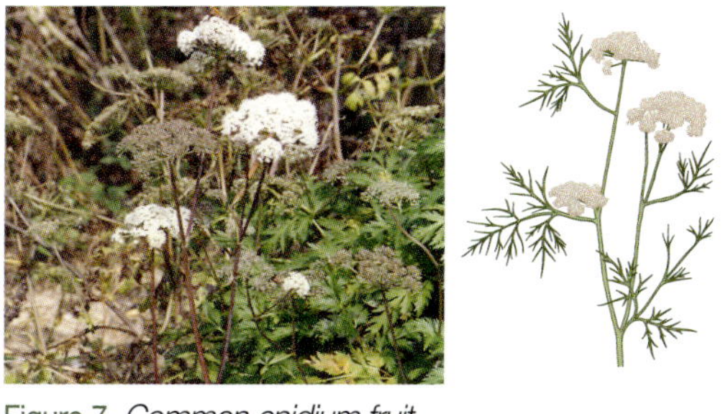

Figure 7. *Common cnidium fruit*

7) *Evodia rutaecarpa*

Also named Fructus evodiae, it is a kind of Rutaceae plant which mainly grows in Guizhou, Guangxi, Yunnan, Sichuan, Hunan and Shanxi provinces. It contains alkaloids, limonin, and naphtha. Chiou et al[14] found Evodia rutaecarpa could relax the contraction of the corpus cavernosum induced by PE in a concentration dependent manner. Furthermore, Evodia rutaecarpa could increase the loose effect of the corpus cavernosum and concentration of cyclic nucleotide induced by sodium nitroprusside and electrical stimulation. This kind of effect could be inhibited by Zaprinast.

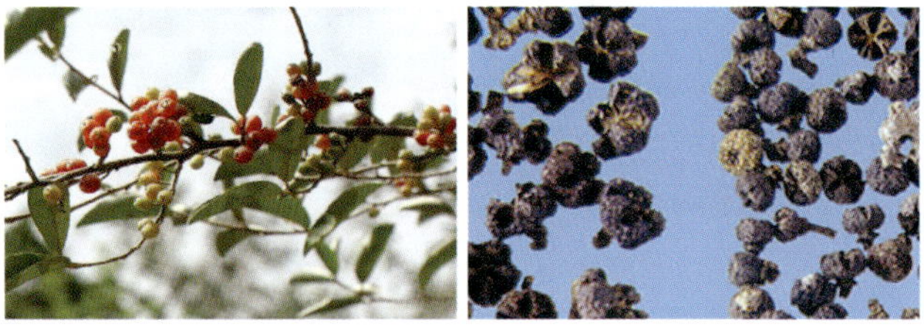

Figure 8. *Evodia rutaecarpa*

8) *Epimedium*

Epimedium (alias Herba Epimedii), is a perennial herb with 30 to 40 cm height. It grows in Heilongjiang, Jilin, Liaoning, Shandong, Jiangsu, Jiangxi, Hunan, Guangxi, Sichuan, Guizhou, Shanxi and Gansu provinces of China. From the aerial parts of Northeast Epimedium (Epimedium koreanum Nakai), four compounds were isolated and identified as hyperin, icarisid II, icarisid I and icariin according to physical and chemical data and spectral analysis. Icariin (ICA) is one active component of Epimedium. Recently the studies demonstrated that ICA may have neurotrophic effects and phosphodiesterase type 5 inhibiting effects[16]. In Traditional Chinese Medicine, Epimedium could invigorate the kidney yang, strengthen bones and tendons, and eliminate rheumatism. It could be used for patients with Kidney impotence, nocturnal emission, premature ejaculation, waist and knee flaccidity soft, cold limbs and chills.

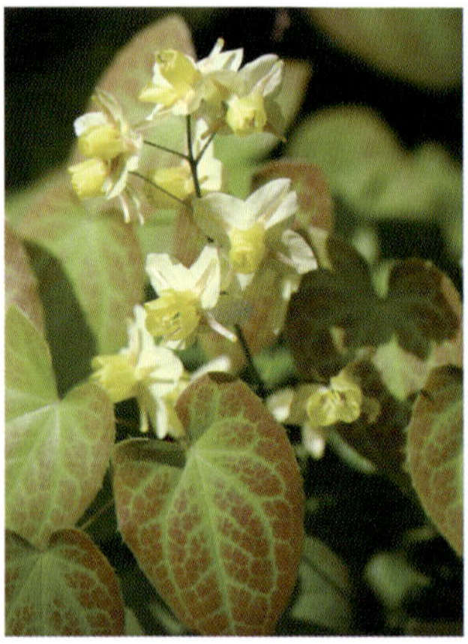

Figure 9. *Epimedium*

9) *Berberin*

It is a compound extracted from the rootstalk of Rhizoma coptidis. People found that other Chinese medicine like phellodendron, arcangelisia loureiri and radix berberidis also contained berberin. Chiou et al[17] observed the effect of berberin on the excised corpus

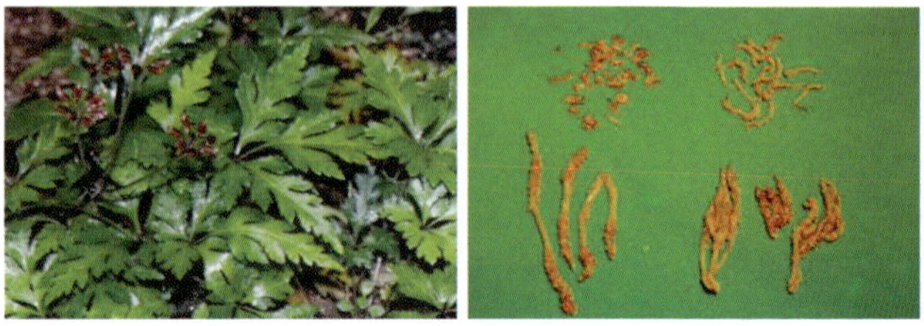

Figure 10. *Berberin*

cavernosum of rabbits and the ICP change in the corpus cavernosum after the injection of berberin into the corpus cavernosum. They found that berberin could relax the tissue of the corpus cavernosum. Its mechanism was not through nerve tract, adrenoreceptor or muscarine type cholinergic receptor, but through NO release from endothelial cells and regulation of the activity in the sensitive potassium channel which caused relaxation of the corpus cavernosum.

10) *Morinda officinalis how*

Morinda officinalis How (Rubiaceae) is the dry root of morindae officinalis which is widely used for medicinal purposes in China. It is used to nourish "Kidney-Yang" and strengthen the bone and muscle indicated for impotence, emission, enuresis, infertility, and to treat cold and dampness syndromes such as rheumatism, pain and fatigue[18].

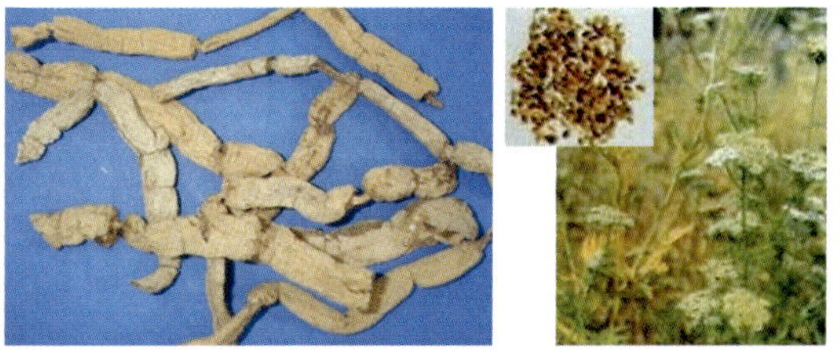

Figure 11. *Morinda officinalis how*

Recently, studies on Morinda officinalis How including chemical ingredients and relevant pharmacological properties have been performed. Iridoids isolated from M. officinalis have displayed obvious antinociceptive and anti-inflammatory effects[19]. Three polysaccharides MP-1, MP-2, and MP-3 were isolated from hot water extract of Chinese medicine Morinda officinalis through 95% ethanol precipitation and gel-filtration chromatography (DEAE-Sepharose CL-6B column and Sephadex G-75 or G-100 column). MP-1 was identified as an insulin-type fructan with simple linear (2→1)-linked structure. Both MP-2 and MP-3 were acidic polysaccharides which consisted predominantly of galacturonic acid, arabinose and galactose. Partial structure characterization of MP-3 was carried out by partial acid hydrolysis and periodate oxidation. The total polysaccharides of the herb were tested in a mice weight-loaded swimming model and were found to have anti-fatigue activity[20]. Xiao Fengxia and Lin Li studied the pharmacological action of the oligosaccharides which were extracted from Morinda officinalis How which could invigorate the kidney and strengthen Yang in TCM. The experiments were conducted to study how the oligosaccharides affect the hatching rate and sexual vitality of Drosophila melanogaster. They found that the oligosaccharides could significantly increase the hatching rate and sexual vitality. So they concluded that the oligosaccharides extracted from Morinda officinalis How can invigorate the kidney and strengthen Yang[21].

In addition, Morinda officinalis How has the function of warning Yang therefore, if the patients have such symptoms as thirst or yellowish or reddish urine, it is inadvisable to take Morinda officinalis How according to TCM.

11) *Herba cistanche*

Herba Cistanche is the dry stem of Cistanche deserticola Y.C.Ma., which is widely distributed in North Africa, Arabia, and Asian countries. It has been traditionally used as a promoting agent of blood circulation and treatment of impotence, sterility, lumbago, body weakness, and as a tonic. From the extract, new phenylethanoid oligoglycoside constituents, kankanosides F and G, and an acylated oligosugar, kankanose, were isolated together with 14 known compounds. The structures of these new compounds were determined on the basis of their chemical and physicochemical evidence. In addition the principal constituents kankanoside F, kankanose, echinacoside, acteoside, and cistanoside F, showed vasorelaxant activity, and several structural requirements for the activity were clarified[22].

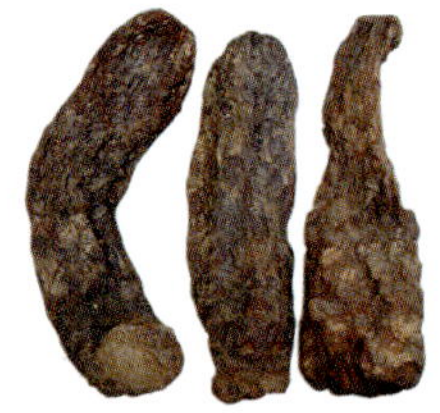
Figure 12. *Herba cistanche*

Through investigation, Wu B and Fu YM assumed that Glycosides of cistanche can adjust the oxidant / antioxidant balance of body function in aging mice, which suggested that glycosides of cistanche play a role in the antioxidant and anti-aging process[23]. Yang HX and his colleagues[24] studied the effect of cistanche deserticola on lacmte dehydrogenase (LDI-I) isoenzyme glycogen and nitric oxide synthase 3(NOS3)of liver in the mice burden swimming and explored relevant molecular mechanisms of anti-sports fatigue. They found Cistanche deserticola could decrease LDH5, protect the liver of the mice burden swimming and accelerate glycogen accumulation by increasing expression of NOS3 to protect liver and improve physical capacity recovery. Gong MJ et al[25] investigated the antifatigue effect of caulis cistanchis on mice with yang asthenia and they found the decoction of caulls cistanchis can improve anti-fatigue effect on the mice with yang asthenia.

According to TCM, patients with asthenic yin causing excessive pyrexia and diarrhea are forbidden to take this medicine.

12) *Semen cuscutae*

Semen cuscutae is a well known Chinese medicine first recorded in the famous book "Shen Nong' s Herbal" as an upper grade drug. It has been used in China to treat impotence and seminal emission as a tonic for thousands of years. Modern pharmacological experiments suggest that it has many biological properties, such as improving sexual function, regulating the body's endocrine and immune system, and antioxidation[24]. The Pharmacopoeia of the People's Republic of China (Version 2005) specifies Semen cuscutae as the dried ripe seeds of Cuscuta chinensis lam. Semen cuscutae is widely used as a tonic, as an aphrodisiac, to nourish the liver and kidneys and treat impotence and seminal emission[27, 28].

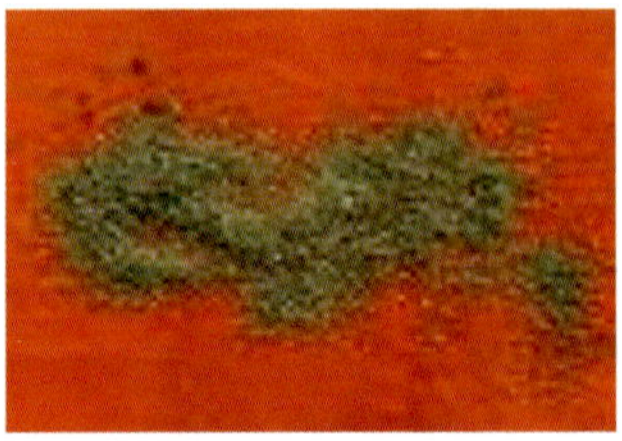
Figure 13. *Semen cuscutae*

Yang JX and his colleagues[29] investigated the effect of the total flavones from Semen cuscutae (TFSC) on the kidney-yang deficient in the male mouse, especially on hormone levels and the androgen receptor (AR) mRNA and protein level in the kidney and testicle. ICR male mice were separated into six groups, and except for the normal group, hydrocortisone was injected intraperitoneally to create the kidney-yang deficiency. The groups were then treated with TFSC, methyltestosterone and Jinkui ShenqiWan except for the normal group and control group. 14 days after administering, testosterone levels in the total serum were analyzed by radioimmunoassay, AR mRNA levels measured by real time RT-PCR and protein levels by immunohistochemistry. From the results, the control group had the lowest testosterone level, AR mRNA level and protein level, and the TFSC can reverse the reduction of testosterone level, AR mRNA level and protein level induced by the hydrocortisone. According to the study, they assumed that TFSC treatment might reverse kidney-yang deficiency symptoms by restoring the levels of testosterone and AR mRNA and protein expression in the kidney and testicle.

13) *Lycium barbarum l.*

The fruit of Lycium barbarum (in the family Solanaceae), also called Fructus Lycii, has been used for thousands of years in traditional Chinese medicine and is one of the dietetic Chinese medicines that have been officially recognized as being both food and a Chinese medicine. The pharmacological activities associated with L. barbarum include hypoglycemic, immunomodulation, anti-hypertension, lipotropic, protecting hepatic function, anti-aging, anti-fatigue, antioxidant and so on[30].

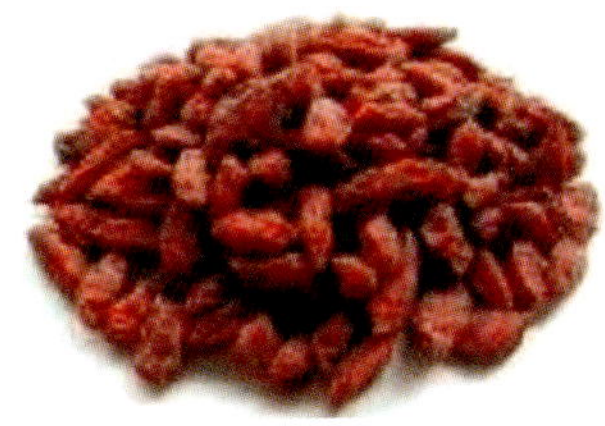

Figure 14. *Lycium barbarum l.*

Its red fruit contain 18 kinds of amino acids (six times higher than bee pollen), all 8 essential amino acids (such as isoleucine and tryptophan) and 21 trace minerals (the main ones being zinc, iron, copper, calcium, germanium, selenium, and phosphorus)[31]. The red fruit is the richest source of carotenoids, including beta-carotene (more beta-carotene than carrots), of all known foods or plants on earth. It contains 500 times the amount of vitamin C by weight than oranges, making them second only to camu camu berries as the richest vitamin C source on earth. It also contains vitamins B1, B2, B6, and vitamin E[32].

Lycium barbarum polysaccharides(LBP) has been identified as one of the active ingredients responsible for its biological activities. In both in vitro and in vivo studies, the results showed that LBP was an effective anticancer compound. In vivo, LBP could dose-dependently decrease tumor weight and increase the amount of splenocytes, proliferation of activated T cells, NK activity and TNF-a levels in S180-bearing mice[33]. In vitro, 20-1,000 mg/L LBP could inhibit the growth of human leukemia HL-60 cells in a dose-dependent manner and decrease the membrane fluidity[34]. LBP can also fortify the immune system and has been found to be a powerful secretagogue (a substance that stimulates the secretion of rejuvenative human growth hormone by the pituitary gland)[35, 36].

Li XM[37] isolated polysaccharides from dried Lycium barbarum fruit by boiling water extraction, then used the polysaccharides on the diabetic rats by intraperitoneal injection. At the end of the experiment, oxidative indices in blood, liver and kidney of all groups were examined. The results showed that administration of LBP could restore abnormal oxidative indices to near normal levels. Therefore he assumed that LBP was effective in the protection of liver and kidney tissue from damage in STZ-induced diabetic rats and that LBP may be of use as an antihyperglycaemic agent.

Lycium barbarum polysaccharides, the main active components of Fructus lycii, have been proven to enhance the response of SAMP aged mouse T splenic cells to SRBC, in which concentration-dependent increase in free calcium ion was detected in splenic cells and celiac macrophages[38]. Lycium barbarum glycopeptide 3 (LBGP3), one of the polysaccharides, plays a critical role in the above-mentioned response. It was reported that LBGP3 enhances the proliferation of splenic cells in aged mice and activates the function of monocytes by increasing the expressions of IL-2 and TNF-αmRNA and protein levels in a dose-dependent manner[39]. However, little is known about the effect of LBGP3 on aged T cells from the viewpoint of apoptosis. In the present research, the effect of LBGP3 on apoptosis of T cells in aged mice was examined and the expression of certain apoptosis-related proteins was detected. The results show that LBGP3 could efficiently reverse apoptotic resistance of T cells in aged mice and is thus a promising drug to modulate the aging process.

The fatty acid in Lycium barbarum was separated by saponification. The result shows the unsaturated fatty acids are comparatively abundant in the Lycium barbarum and account for 45.59% of the total. Among them, the content of linoleic acid is up to 30.92%, which is mainly unsaturated. In addition a small amount of linolenic acid has been detected. It is also necessary for the human body. It can debase blood pressure and hyperlipidaemia accommodation and strengthen the pancreatic function. Lycium Barbarum is good for health protection[40].

5. Chinese medicine monomer

1) *Icariin*

Icariin (2-(4'-methoxylphenyl)-3-rhamnosido-5-hydroxyl-7-glucosido-8-(3'-methyl-2-butylenyl)-4-chromanone) ($C_{33}H_{40}O_{15}$; Mw=676.65Da)

Epimedium (known as Yinyanghuo in China) is used in traditional Chinese medicine as a potent enhancer of erectile function. Present studies indicate that icariin is a flavonoid with a rhamnose as a ligand, which is one of the major active components in epimedium and has many biological effects, such as improving cardiovascular function, hormone regulation, immunological function modulation, and anti-tumor activity[41].

To clarify the effective site of icariin in the therapeutic action on erectile dysfunction (ED), Xin ZC and his colleagues isolated PDE5 from human platelet and PDE4 from rat liver tissue. The potencies of selectivity of icariin and papaverine on PDE5 (PDE4/PDE5 of IC(50)) were 167.67 times and 4.54 times, respectively. It indicated that icariin is a cGMP-specific PDE5 inhibitor that may be developed into an oral effective agent for the treatment of ED[42].

Furthermore, Ning H, Xin ZC and their colleagues isolated PDE5 isoforms (PDE5A1, A2, and A3) and insect the cDNA of PDE5 isoforms to cells with baculoviruses as vector. As a result, they found that icariin was inhibitory to all three PDE5 isoforms with similar IC50 values, which were approximately three times greater than those for zaprinast[43].

Many researchers found that icariin could improve erectile function but the mechanism was not clear until now. Most of the researchers focus on the NO-cGMP-PDE5 pathway. Some of the investigations were introduced as follows:

To investigate the effect of icariin on erectile function and the expression of nitric oxide synthase (NOS) isoforms in castrated rats, Liu WJ, Xin ZC and their colleagues found that oral treatment with icariin (98.6% purity) for 4 weeks potentially improves erectile function. This effect is correlated with an increase in percent of smooth muscle and the expression of certain NOS in the corpus cavernosum of castrated rats. These results suggest that icariin may have a therapeutic effect on erectile dysfunction by NOS[44].

Chronic oral treatment with icariin increases the intracavernosal pressure and restores the eNOS expression in the corpus cavernosum of arteriogenic erectile dysfunction rats. So icariin may have a long-term therapeutic effect on ischemia/hypoxia induced ED[45]. Tian L, Xin ZC and their colleagues found that icariin can increase intracavernous pressure (ICP) without influence on mean systematic arterial blood press (MBp) and this effect is inhibited by N (omega)-nitro-L-arginine (LNNA) and H-[1,2,4] oxadiazolo [4,3,-a] quinoxalin-1-one (ODQ) significantly. It indicated that icariin regulated the activity of NO-cGMP signal pathway on the corpora cavernosa (CC) to enhance erectile function by oral therapy[46]. In addition , Tian L, Xin ZC and their colleagues found that icariin may have a long-term therapeutic effect on ischemia/hypoxia induced ED through the NO-cGMP signal pathway[45]. Xu HB and his colleagues also found that icariin could enhance the production of bioactive NO in the short-term (after a 5 min incubation, Pb0.05). In concert with other effects, the protective effects of icariin on endothelial cells may contribute to the cardiovascular protective effects[47]. Ning H, Xin ZC and their colleagues also found that icariin was able to enhance cGMP levels in the cavernous smooth muscle cells treated with sodium nitroprusside[43]. It was further evidence for icariin that the regulation of the NO-cGMP signal pathway plays an important role in the enhancement of erectile function. Chung Byunghee and his colleagues found that icariin could stimulate angiogenesis by activating the MEK/ERK- and PI3K/Akt/eNOS -dependent signal pathways and may be a useful drug for angiogenic therapy[48]. Icariin could also enhance the blood and oxygen supply to the penis by angiogenesis, especially in arteriogenic erectile dysfunction.

As we know, oxidative damage is one of the harmful factors to cavernous smooth muscle cells which have a direct relationship with erectile dysfunction of the penis. Icariin is the major component in epimedium which was widely used for the treatment of atherosclerosis, neuropathy and erectile dysfunction in Chinese traditional medicine. Recently, Zhao F and his colleagues determined the antioxidative effect of icariin against oxidative DNA damage induced by 2,2'-azobis (2-amidinopropane) dihydrochloride (AAPH), and thought that icariin is a concentration-dependent chemopreventor in protecting DNA against radical-induced damage[49]. In the present investigation, icariin against oxidative injuries may be achieved via decreasing of caspase expression[50]. So the cavernous smooth muscle cells can be protected by icariin from being oxidated.

Chronic mild stress (CMS) is suggested to produce abnormalities in the hypothalamic-pituitary-adrenal (HPA) axis and hypothalamus-Pituitary-thyroid (HPT) axis. Stress may play an important role in the mechanism of erectile dysfunction. Recent research suggested that icariin possessed potent antidepressant-like activities which were at least in part mediated by improving the abnormalities in the HPA axis functions[51].

Zhang ZB and his colleagues found that icariin has testosterone mimetic properties and has therapeutic potential in the management of hypoandrogenism[52].

2) Neferine

Neferine ($C_{38}H_{44}N_2O_6$;Mw=624.77Da)

Lian zi xin, which is the embryo of the lotus seeds has been used in Chinese traditional medicine as a sedative, antipyretic and hemostat agent, indicating that it may possess many effects. Neferine is one of the major active components extracted from this plant. Recently it has been proven to be effective in the treatment of ED, but the mechanisms are not well known yet.

Chen J, Liu JH, and their colleagues studied the relaxant effect of six extractions from Chinese Herbs (neferine, tetrandrine, kakonein, scutellarin, ginsenoside Rg1 and ginsenoside Rb1) on the corpus cavernosum tissue of rabbit in vitro and found that neferine had greater functions than the other five extracts.[53] To further investigate the relaxation mechanism of neferine (Nef), a bis-benzylisoquinoline alkaloid extracted (isolated) from the green seed embryo of Nelumbo nucifera Gaertn in China, on rabbit corpus cavernosum tissue in vitro, the effects of Nef on the concentrations of cyclic adenosine monophosphate (cAMP) and cyclic guanosine monophosphate (cGMP) in isolated and incubated rabbit corpus cavernosum tissue were recorded using ^{125}I radioimmunoassay. As a result, Nef did not affect this concentration of cGMP, either in the presence or in the absence of a guanyl cyclase inhibitor. Also, sodium nitroprusside (SNP, a stimulator of cGMP production)-induced cGMP production was not enhanced by Nef. It was concluded that Nef can enhance the concentration of cAMP in rabbit corpus cavernosum tissue, probably by inhibiting phosphodiesterase activity[54].

Chen J and his colleagues carried out research on the relaxation mechanisms of neferine (Nef) on rabbit corpus cavernosum tissue in vitro. Strips of rabbit corpus cavernosum were mounted in organ chambers for the study and the effects of Nef were examined on isolated muscle strips. The results suggested that Nef possessed a relaxant effect on rabbit corpus cavernosum tissues which was attributable to the inhibition of extracellular Ca2+ influx and the inhibition of release of intracellular stored Ca(2+), but not mediated by the release of nitric oxide, prostaglandins or by the activation of potassium channels[55].

3) Tetrandrine (Tet)

Tetrandrine ($C_{38}H_{42}N_2O_6$;Mw=622.76Da)

Tetrandrine (Tet) is a bioactive component of the Chinese herb Han-Fang-Chi. It is a bis-benzylisoquinoline alkaloid which has been used to treat patients with silicosis, autoimmune disorders and hypertension for decades. Recently, it has been found to have the function of treating ED.

In recent studies, the relaxation mechanisms of tetrandrine (Tet) on the corpus cavernosum smooth muscle have been investigated. Liu JH, Chen J and their colleagues isolated the corpus cavernosum smooth muscle cells from New Zealand white rabbits and cultured them in vitro for research. As a result, Tet inhibited the Ca (2+) influx from the extracellular site via voltage-activated Ca (2+) channel and alpha (2)-adrenoceptor-operated Ca (2+) channel. At a high concentration, Tet might inhibit the cytosolic calcium pool release in cultured corpus cavernosum smooth muscle cells. This inhibitory action on [Ca(2+)](i) might be one of the relaxation mechanisms of Tet on the corpus cavernosum smooth muscle[56].

4) Tetramethylpyrazine

Chen Z and his colleagues found that tetramethylpyrazine (TMP) can inhibit rabbit PCSMC [Ca2+]i significantly by suppressing the voltage-dependent calcium channel and cytosolic calcium pool release. The effect, similar to Ver, signifies the important mechanism of erectile dysfunction (ED) therapy[57].

VII. Summary

After years of development, clinical and basic research of Chinese herbal medicine has improved greatly and yielded many clinical research findings. To further evaluate the effects and clinical applications of herbal formulations in male sexual dysfunction, well-designed prospective randomized controlled trials are needed. A consensus regarding TCM diagnoses, indication and contraindication of herbal formulations would be helpful.

In basic research, the progress of modern biotechnology will lead to a better understanding of this mechanism and bioavailability of the medicine. At the same time, the discovery of new active ingredients is an ongoing challenge.

REFERENCES

1. Andrew S. Crimmel, Chad S. Conner, Manoj Monga. Withered Yang: A review of Traditional Chinese Medical treatment of male infertility and erectile dysfunction. Journal of Andrology 2001;22:173-182.
2. Bai Q, Xu QQ, Jiang H, Zhang WL, Wang XH, Zhu JC. Prevalence and risk factors of erectile dysfunction in three cities of China: a community-based study. Asian J Androl 2004;6:343-348.
3. Zhang ZC, Sun B, Liu YS, Chen Q, Xin ZC, Guo YL. The prevalence of erectile dysfunction in 1247 married men in Beijing urban area. Chin J Urol 2003;24:855-857.
4. Jiang H, Zhu JC. Chinese Men' s Attitudes to Life Events and Sexuality: Prevalence of Erectile Dysfunction and Related Health Concern s Among Chinese Men in Asian MALES Study. National Journal of Andrology 2006;12:1048-1052.
5. Lau JT, Wang Q, Cheng Y, Yang X. Prevalence and risk factors of sexual dysfunction among younger married men in a rural area in China. Urology 2005;66:616-622.
6. Liang CZ, Zhang XJ, Hao ZY, Shi HQ, Wang KX. Prevalence of sexual dysfunction in Chinese men with chronic prostatitis. BJU Int 2004;93:568-570.
7. Wang Q, Ni P, Wu WP, Xia ZY. Study of Shugan Yiyang capsule on erectile dysfunction. Zhongguo Zhong Yao Za Zhi 2005;30:58-63.
8. Xiao H, Liu J, Yin C, Wang T, Chen J, Fan L,et al.Effects of ligustrazine on the contraction of isolated rabbit corpus cavernosum strips. J Huazhong Univ Sci Technolog Med Sci 2005;25:565-567.
9. Xiao H, Liu J, Yin C, Wang T, Chen J, Fan L, et al. Effect of chuanxiongzine on the relaxation of isolated rabbit corpus cavernosum tissues. Zhonghua Nan Ke Xue 2004;10:636-639.
10. HU WL, Hu LQ, Cheng B, Hong WX. Effect of Angelica Sinensis on NOS Activity in Penile Tissues of Rats after Crushing Injury to Cavernous Nerves. Zhonghua Nan Ke Xue 2001;7:11-13.
11. Choi YD, Rha KH, Choi HK. In vivo and in vitro experimental effect of Korean red ginseng on erection[J]. J Urol 1999; 162:1508-1511.
12. Yuan J, Guo W, Yang B. 116 cases of coronary angina pectoris treated with powder composed of radix ginseng, radix notoginseng and succinum. J Tradit Chin Med 1997; 17:14-7.
13. Paick JS, Lee JH. An experimental study of the effect of ginkgo biloba extract on the human and rabbit corpus cavernosum tissue. J Urol 1996;156:1876-80.
14. Chen J, Chiou WF, Chen CC, Chen CF. Effect of the plant-extract osthole on the relaxation of rabbit corpus cavernosum tissue in vitro. J Urol 2000;163:1975-80.
15. Chiou WF, Huang YL, Chen CF, Chen CC. Vasorelaxing effect of coumarins from Cnidium monnieri on rabbit corpus cavernosum. Planta Med 2001;67:282-4.
16. Shindel AW, Xin ZC, Lin G, et al. Erectogenic and neurotrophic effects of icariin, a purified extract of horny goat weed (Epimedium spp.) in vitro and in vivo. J Sex Med. 2010;7:1518-28.
17. Chiou WF, Chen J, Chen CF. Relaxation of corpus cavernosum and raised intracavernous pressure by berberine in rabbit. Br J Pharmacol 1998;125:1677-84.
18. Xiao PG. Modern Chinese Materia Medica, Chemical Industry Press, Beijing, 2002.
19. Choi J, Lee KT, Choi MY, Nam JH, Jung HJ, Park SK, et al. Antinociceptive anti-inflammatory effect of Monotropein isolated from the root of Morinda officinalis. Biol Pharm 32 Bull 2005;28:1915-18.
20. Zhang HL, Li J, Li G, Wang DM, Zhu LP, Yang DP. Structural characterization and anti-fatigue activity of polysaccharides from the roots of Morinda officinalis. Int J Biol Macromol 2009;44:257-61.
21. Xiao FX, Lin L. A preliminary study on the effect of Morinda officinalis How on invigorating the kidney and strengthening yang. Food and Drug 2006;8:45-6.

22. Yoshikawa M, Matsuda H, Morikawa T, Xie H, Nakamura S, Muraoka O. Phenylethanoid oligoglycosides and acylated oligosugars with vasorelaxant activity from Cistanche tubulosa. Bioorg Med Chem 2006; 14:7468-75.
23. Wu Bo, Fu YM. Study on Anti-lipid peroxide Effect of the Glycoside of Cistanche in the subacute aging mice. Chinese Pharmacological Bulletin. 2005;21:639.
24. Yang HX, Yang Y, Yan XH. Experimental study of anti-sports fatigue effect mechanisms of Cistanche Deserticola. Chinese Journa1 of Information on TCM 2008;15:24-6.
25. Gong MJ, Liu XM, Wang LW. Study on antifatigue effect of Caulis Cistanchis on the mice with yang asthenia. Guiding Journal of TCM 2007;13:8-10.
26. Ye M, Li Y, Yan Y, Liu H, Ji X. Determination of flavonoids in Semen Cuscutae by RP-HPLC. J Pharm Biomed Anal 2002;28:621-8.
27. Du XM, Kohinata TK, Guo YT. Components of the ether-insoluble resin glycoside-like fraction from Cuscuta chinensis. Phytochemistry 1998,48:843-50.
28. Pan HJ, Sun HX, Pan YJ. Adjuvant effect of ethanol extract of Semen Cuscutae on the immune responses to ovalbumin in mice. J Ethnopharmacol 2005;99:99-103.
29. Yang J, Wang Y, Bao Y, Guo J.The total flavones from Semen cuscutae reverse the reduction of testosterone level and the expression of androgen receptor gene in kidney-yang deficient mice. J Ethnopharmacol 2008;119:166-71.
30. Yu MS, Ho YS, So KF, Yuen WH, Chang RCC. Cytoprotective effects of Lycium barbarum against reducing stress on endoplasmic reticulum. Int J Mol Med 2006;17:1157-61.
31. Cui KR, Xing GS, Liu XM, et al. Effect of hydrogen peroxide on somatic embryogenesis of Lycium barbarum L. Plant Science 1996;146:9-16.
32. Tan AM, Huang YQ, Qu SS. Determination of the respiratory burst of polymorphonuclear leukocytes by microcalorimetry. J Biochem Biophys Methods 1998;37:91-4.
33. Liu JL, Zhang LH, Qian YK. Immune tumor-inhibition of Lycium barbarum polysaccharide on S180-bearing mice. Chinese Journal of Immunology 1996;12:115-7.
34. Gan L, Hua ZS, Liang YX, Bi XH. Immunomodulation and antitumor activity by a polysaccharide-protein complex from Lycium barbarum. Int Immunopharmacol 2004;4:563-9.
35. Luo Q, Li ZN, Huang XL, Yan J, Zhang SH, Cai YZ. Lycium barbarum polysaccharides: Protective effects against heat-induced damage of rat testes and H2O2-induced DNA damage in mouse testicular cells and beneficial effect on sexual behavior and reproductive function of hemicastrated rats. Life Sciences 2006;79: 613-21.
36. Zhang M, Chen HX, Huang J, Li Z, Zhu CP, Zhang SH. Effect of Lycium barbarum polysaccharide on human hepatoma QGY7703 cells: Inhibition of proliferation and induction of apoptosis. Life Sciences 2005;76:2115-24.
37. Li XM. Protective effect of Lycium barbarum polysaccharides on streptozotocin-induced oxidative stress in rats. International Journal of Biological Macromolecules 2007;40:461-5.
38. Lu G, Zhang S H, Xu H B, et al. A polysaccharide-protein complex from Lycium barbarum 33 upregulates cytokine expression in human peripheral blood mononuclear cells. Eur J Pharmacol 2003;471:217-22.
39. Deng HB, Cui DP, Jiang JM, Feng YC, Cai NS, Li DD.Inhibiting effects of Achyranthes bidentata polysaccharide and Lycium barbarum polysaccharide on nonenzyme glycation in D-galactose induced mouse aging model. Biomed Environ Sci 2003;16:267-75.
40. Fang X, Meng QX, Sun MZ, et al. Analysis of Fatty Acid of NingXia-Lycium by GC-MS. Journal of Gansu Sciences 2009;21:37-9.
41. Chen XJ, Guo BL, Li SP, Zhang QW, Tu PF, Wang YT.Simultaneous determination of 15 flavonoids in Epimedium using pressurized liquid extraction and high-performance liquid chromatography. J Chromatogr A

2007;1163:96-104.

42. Xin ZC, Kim EK, Lin CS, Liu WJ, Tian L, Yuan YM, et al. Effects of icariin on cGMP-specific PDE5 and cAMP-specific PDE4 activities. Asian J Androl 2003;5:15-8.
43. Ning H, Xin ZC, Lin G, Banie L, Lue TF, Lin CS. Effects of icariin on phosphodiesterase-5 activity in vitro and cyclic guanosine monophosphate level in cavernous smooth muscle cells. Urology 2006;68:1350-4.
44. Liu WJ, Xin ZC, Xin H, Yuan YM, Tian L, Guo YL.Effects of icariin on erectile function and expression of nitric oxide synthase isoforms in castrated rats. Asian J Androl 2005;7:381-8.
45. Tian L, Xin ZC, Liu WJ, Yuan YM, Liu G, Chen L, et al. Effects of icariin on the erectile function and expression of nitrogen oxide synthase isoforms in corpus cavernosum of arteriogenic erectile dysfunction rat model. Natl Med J China 2004,84:954-7.
46. Tian L, Xin ZC, Yuan YM, Fu J, Liu WJ, Wang LL.Effects of icariin on intracavernosal pressure and systematic arterial blood pressure of rat. Natl Med J China 2004;84:142-5.
47. Xu HB, Huang ZQ. Icariin enhances endothelial nitric-oxide synthase expression on human endothelial cells in vitro. Vascular Pharmacology 2007;47:18-24.
48. Chung BH, Kim JD, Kim CK, et al. Icariin stimulates angiogenesis by activating the MEK/ERK and PI3K/Akt/eNOS-dependent signal pathways in human endothelial cells.Biochem Biophys Res Commun 2008;376:404-8.
49. Zhao F, Tang YZ, Liu ZQ. Protective effect of icariin on DNA against radical-induced oxidative damage. J Pharm Pharmacol 2007;59:1729-32.
50. Wang YK, Huang ZQ. Protective effects of icariin on human umbilical vein endothelial cell injury induced by H2O2 in vitro. Pharmacol Res 2005;52:174-82.
51. Pan Y, Kong LD, Li YC, et al. Icariin from Epimedium brevicornum attenuates chronic mild stress-induced behavioral and neuroendocrinological alterations in male Wistar rats. Pharmacol Biochem Behav 2007;87:130-40.
52. Zhang ZB, Yang QT. The testosterone mimetic properties of icariin. Asian J Androl 2006;8:601-5.
53. Chen J, Liu JH, Wang T, et al. The relaxation effects of six extracts from Chinese herbs on the corpus cavernosum tissue of rabbit in vitro. Zhonghua Nan Ke Xue 2005;11:793-5.
54. Chen J, Liu JH, Wang T, et al. Effects of plant extract neferine on cyclic adenosine monophosphate and cyclic guanosine monophosphate levels in rabbit corpus cavernosum in vitro. Asian J Androl 2008;10:307-12.
55. Chen J, Qi J, Chen F, et al. Relaxation mechanisms of neferine on the rabbit corpus cavernosum tissue in vitro. Asian J Androl 2007;9:795-800.
56. Liu JH, Chen J, Wang T, et al. Effects of tetrandrine on cytosolic free calcium concentration in 34 corpus cavernosum smooth muscle cells of rabbits. Asian J Androl 2006;8:405-9.
57. Chen Z, Liu JH, Yin CP, Chen J, Xiao HJ. Effects of tetramethylpyrazine on cytosolic free calcium concentration in penis corpus cavernsum smooth muscle cells in rabbits. Zhonghua Nan Ke Xue 2003;9:331-4.

Editorial Comment

Traditional Chinese medicine (TCM) is a holistic modality derives from ancient oriental philosophy, whose concept believes that human body have an intimate interaction with the outer environment and have a set of inner homeostatic interconnected system maintained by yin-yang balance and wu-xing harmony. In this system, the zhang-fu organs in the body are connected by meridians and nourished by several elements, including jing (vital essence) , qi (vital energy), shen (vital spirit) and blood. According to TCM philosophical theories, disease can result from the imbalance in yin-yang which is disturbed over a period of time. Briefly, the diagnosis of TCM would look for and classify the "pattern of disharmony", and the treatment would attempt to restore the balance in yin and yang and subsequently bring the physical, emotional and spiritual aspects of the individual into harmony.

As a form of primary healthcare, TCM has been employed in China and its neighboring countries for thousands years. However, even though the Chinese herbal remedies and acupuncture have been widely used in western public for decades as well, TCM has until very recently been considered as part of complementary and alternative medicine (CAM) by health authorities in western countries. Whereas the theory of TCM is complicated and not easily explained by modern science, it is very important to explore the TCM with modern scientific perspectives and verify its safety and efficacy by rigorous clinical studies. As an excellent expert in andrology, Prof. Xin, along with his colleagues, has made significant contributions to modernize the TCM and apply it in sexual dysfunction clinic.

Here, in this chapter, Prof. Xin introduced the general principles of TCM, explained the diagnosis and treatment features of sexual dysfunction using the TCM theories and detailedly represented the Chinese experienced formulas, single herbs and TCM monomers with respect to sexual dysfunction using plenty of illustrations. Over thousands of years of development, practitioners of TCM have established a comprehensive framework for diagnosing and treating sexual dysfunction. Empirically, lots of TCM compound formulas and herbs have been identified with significant benefits to sexual function. Thus, TCM herbal medicine is considered to be promising sources of new drugs development and increasing studies have emerged to determine and understand the active ingredients. In this field, Prof. Xin has devoted considerable efforts in exploration of icariin, which is a major active compound in epimedium, to improve erectile function. In our group, ongoing studies evaluating neferine and tetrandrine, which have potential effects to relax the corpus cavernosum, have been conducted.

Taken together, TCM originated in ancient period and rooted in traditional oriental cultures, it still seems to hold promise in the novel drugs development for sexual dysfunction in this new era. However, the lack of evidence-based scientific data has limited TCM application and further efforts should be made to validate the numerous TCM compound formulas and herbs.

Jihong Liu, M.D., Ph.D.
Wuhan, China

Chapter 3

Indian Perspective

Ayurvedic Sexual Medicine in India

K Swayam Prakash, Sudhakar Krishnamurti

I. Introduction

Ayurveda is the oldest medical science. It is still in practice in India. Erectile dysfunction, premature ejaculation and infertility in both male and female are described in Ayurveda. Ayurveda literally means knowledge of life (Ayu = life, Veda = knowledge).

There is no exact date for the earliest Ayurvedic teachings. The first named teachers are Agnivesa and Susruta, who are said to have lived as early as 1500 B.C. Though the exact century is disputed (Ray and Gupta, 1965), at some time between 600 B.C. and 100 A.D. the traditional Indian knowledge was edited and systematized in two texts, Agnivesa in the Caraka (or Charaka) Samhita and Susruta in Susruta Samhita (Samhita = collection). The former deals mainly with medicine and the latter mainly with surgery. These two collections became the basis for the Ayurvedic texts that are still used today. The oldest surviving written text (Hoernle, 1987) dates from between the second and fourth centuries A.D. It is found in what is known as the Bower manuscript, and consists of quotations from the Caraka in a Buddhist medical compilation, the Navanitaka. Bower discovered the manuscript in 1890 in Kuchar, in far western China, north of Kashmir.

Sudhakar Krishnamurti, M.D.
Andrologist, Microsurgeon & Director Andromeda Andrology Center, First Floor, Topaz: Greenlands Rd. P.O. Box 1563, Somajiguda, Hyderabad 500 082 AP, India, E-mail: sudhakar1957@gmail.com

II. Erectile Dysfunction in Caraka Samhita

An erection problem, which is different from a desire problem, is clearly explained in the Caraka Samhita as: Even though a man is constantly desirous of sexual intercourse with a partner who is cooperative, he, because of the looseness (absence of erection) of the phallus becomes incapable of performing the sexual act. Even if he only rarely attempts the sexual act, he gets afflicted with dyspnoea as well as perspiration in the body, and gets frustrated in his determined efforts. His phallus becomes loose (because of the lack of erection), and he does not ejaculate any semen. These are the general signs and symptoms of erectile dysfunction. (Caraka Samhita; Cikitsasthana: chapter XXX, verse 1551$\frac{1}{2}$-157.) Various aphrodisiac herbs and drugs are mentioned in the *Caraka Samhita*.

Caraka recognized that inadequacy of arousal in some cases may be the responsibility not of the female partner, but of the male' s dependency or fixation on a specific stimulus of the type that today might be characterized as paraphilic. He mentioned in particular irshyaka and samskaravahi. Irshyaka (irshya = envy, jealousy) signifies that a male' s arousal, erection and orgasm with his own partner is dependent upon the stimulus of watching the copulation of another couple. Samskaravahi (samskara = to improve; vahi = practice) signifies that arousal may improve with the help of various auxiliary practices. The practices themselves were not specified by Caraka; however, they are mentioned by name in the Susruta Samhita (the collection of Susruta) as follows:

Sougandhika (su = good; ghandha = smell) signifies that a male' s arousal and erection is dependent on the stimulus of smelling the vagina of his partner.

Asekya (swallow) signifies that a man' s arousal, erection, and orgasm with his own female partner is dependent on the stimulus of first being able to suck another man' s penis so as to taste and swallow his semen.

Kumbhika (catamite; anal penetration) signifies that a man' s arousal, erection, and orgasm with his own female partner is dependent on the stimulus of his first being able to have another male penetrate him in anal intercourse.

For erectile dysfunction and infertility in the male, vajikarana treatment is advised. There are eight branches of Ayureveda. One branch is vajikarana (vaji = stallion, karana = to make), which translates as making a man stallion-like in performing sexually. The factors which make a man capable of entering into sexual intercourse with stallion-like vigour and which make him capable of performing excessive sexual intercourse are called "vajikarana". To achieve the goal of maintaining an erection and postponing ejaculation, vajikarana recommended various psychological and pharmacologic aphrodisiacs. Vajikarana promotes fertility also. Many of the prescriptions mentioned in vajikarana are successfully tried in male infertility. Ayurvedic drugs improve sperm counts, and the motility and percentage of normal forms also. Vajikarana facilitates recreative and procreative aspects of male health. An exhilarating woman is recommended as the best aphrodisiac. In the Caraka Samhita it is stated that:

"The sense objects even singly are exceedingly pleasant. What is to be said of the female physique, stationed collectively? And in that sense, objects located in woman are more pleasure giving, because there is special pleasure in woman. The progeny too, is dependent on woman."

The aphrodisiacs mentioned in Caraka Samhita can be classified into three groups - food recipes, pharmacologic prescriptions, and psychological stimuli. All these aphrodisiacs are said to increase sukra, the vital fluid. In addition to being responsible for life and health, sukra is responsible also for libido, sexual attraction and fertility. In the male, sukra is depleted chiefly by excessive loss of semen. To replenish a deficiency of sukra, aphrodisiacs are advised to be taken regularly. In this way, a man can unfailingly perform the sexual act. Replenishment of sukra is said to be through the essence of the food eaten.

On the aspects of food recipes, Milk is said to increase sukra instantaneously. Similarly, black lentil powder also increases sukra. These two foods are commonly used by some Indians, especially by newlywed couples, who keep them at the bedside. Among other food recipes, soups made from the flesh of various animals and birds have been given prime importance. A few such recipes read as follows.

'If one takes milk eating sparrow meat up to saturation, he does not get his organ slackened nor is there loss of sukra in night.'

'Pounded fish meat flavored with asafoetida gum, rock salt and coriander leaves should be mixed with flour and cooked in ghee (clarified butter) to make pupalika cakes. These cakes are bulkpromoting, strengthening, and exhilarating. They increase charm, ensure progeny, and promote semen profusely.'

1. Mucuna pruriens

One drug, which is extensively mentioned as an aphrodisiac, is Mucuna pruriens, the cow hage plant. Seeds of this plant are considered to increase sukra. Today, this drug is also used by Ayurvedic physicians for the treatment of Parkinsonism.

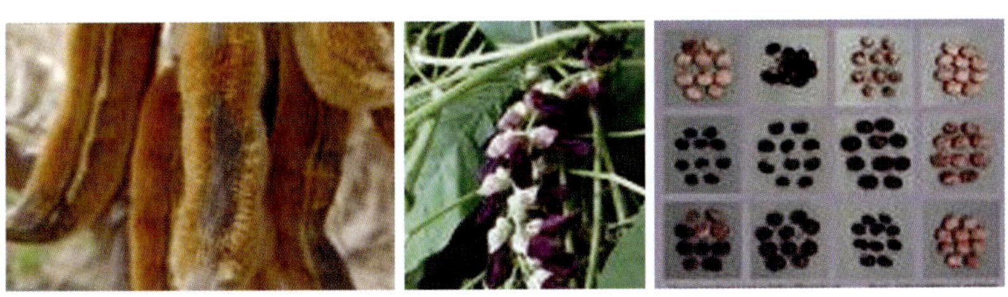

Figure 1. *Mucuna pruriens*

M. pruriens possesses significantly higher antiparkinson activity than l-dopa in the 6-hydroxydopamine (6-OHDA) lesioned rat model of Parkinson' s disease.

M. pruriens cotyledon powder treatment significantly restores the endogenous levo-dopa, dopamine, norepinephrine and serotonin content in the substantia nigra. Nicotine adenine dinucleotide (NADH) and coenzyme Q-10, that are shown to have a therapeutic benefit in

Parkinson' s disease, were present in the M. pruriens cotyledon powder. The seed powder of a leguminous plant, and a natural source of levo-dopa, this may have advantages in the long-term management of Parkinson' s disease (PD),

The seed powder of the leguminous plant, Mucuna pruriens has long been used in traditional Ayurvedic Indian medicine for diseases including parkinsonism, Levo-dopa (L-dopa) was first isolated from the seeds of M pruriens in 1937 and when the value of L-dopa for the treatment of PD became known, scientific interest in plants rich in L-dopa was revived.

Various findings suggest that M. pruriens formulations may actually have a higher bioavailability than standard L-dopa preparations.

Mucuna pruriens is considered to be an important vajikarana drug, capable of promoting the semen and sexual vigour. It is mentioned in the texts that the ascetics are reluctant even to utter its name on account of its powerful aphrodisiac properties!

In addition to its aphrodisiac property, atmagupta has been found to exert an antidepressant effect in patients suffering from depression neurosis (Singh and Tripathy, 1982). Modern science recognizes that depression and neuroses can be etiologic or aggravating factors in sexual dysfunction in both genders.

2. Withania somnifera

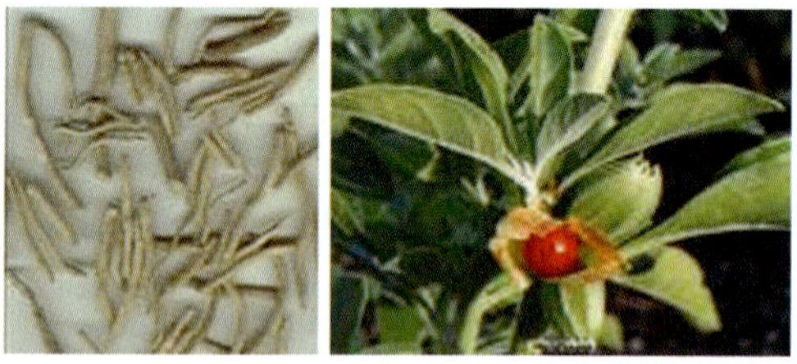

Figure 2. *Withania somnifera*

Known in India for centuries as Aswagandha, this plant is considered the Indian Ginseng, and has been used for centuries in Ayurvedic medicine to increase longevity and vitality. Therapeutically, it is mainly used for joint pains, sleeplessness, and tuberculosis. Various research supports its versatile pharmacological potential, confirming antioxidant, anti-inflammatory, immune-modulating, and anti-stress properties, both in the whole plant extract as well as in its separate constituents.

Ashwagandha is rated highly by Ayuvedists as a rejuvenating drug which is capable of imparting long life, youthful vigour and good intellectual powers. The root is its officinal part. This is bitter in taste, 'hot' in action, germicidal, aphrodisiac, and diuretic. It is used in ulcers, fever, cough, dyspnoea, consumption dropsy, impotence, rheumatism, toxicosis and leucoderma. The drug is a good tonic. It improves physical strength and is prescribed in all cases of general debility. Ashwagandharistam, Cyavanaprasam, Valiya Narayana thailam etc. are some of the important preparations using the drug.

Singh and Malaviya (1978) and Singh and Tripathy (1982) have demonstrated the psychotropic efficacy of the drug and found that the drug is very effective in the treatment of anxiety neurosis. The drug has also been found to possess significant anti-tumour activity (Singh et al., 1986).

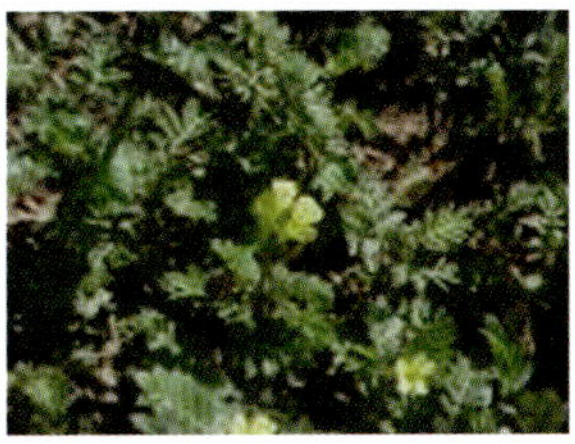

Figure 3. *Tribulus terrestris*

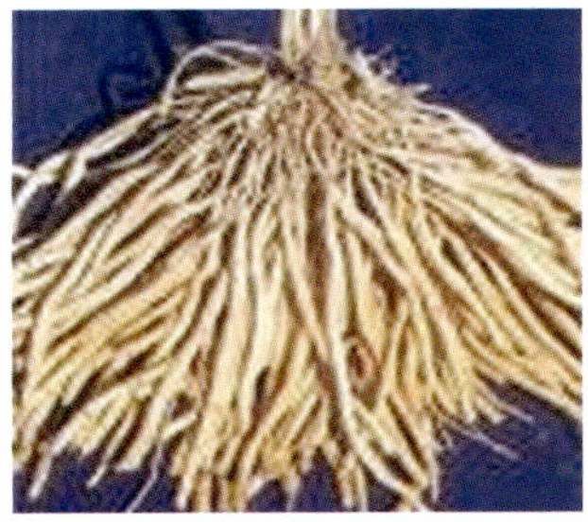

Figure 4. *Asparagus racemosus*

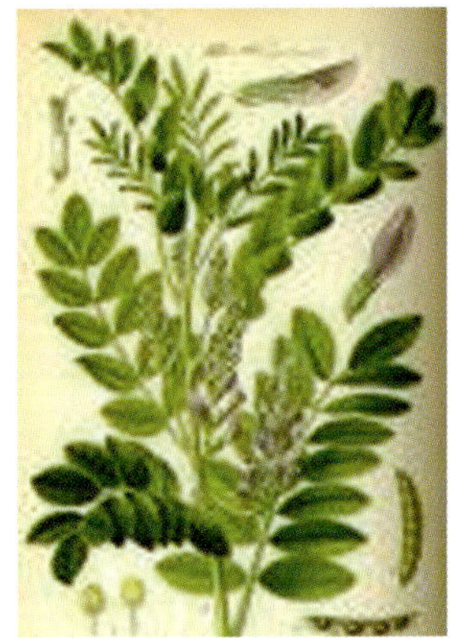

Figure 5. *Glycyrrihizza glabra*

3. Tribulus terrestris

Tribulus terrestris is a nutritional supplement, the physiological and actual effects of which are debatable. The main claimed effect is an increase of testosterone anabolic and androgenic action through the activation of endogenous testosterone production. Even if this biological pathway is not entirely proven, T terrestris is regularly used by athletes.

Methanolic and aqueous extracts of Tribulus terrestris possess significant antihypertensive activity in spontaneously hypertensive rats. The antihypertensive effects appeared to result from a direct arterial smooth muscle relaxation, possibly involving nitric oxide release and membrane hyperpolarization.

This is one of the ten drugs that constitute the group dasamula (ten roots). Due to the diuretic action of the fruits, Tribulus terrestris is found to be highly beneficial in renal calculus, difficult micturition, chronic cystitis and other genito-urinary disorders. It is also cooling, demulcent, tonic and aphrodisiac, promotes strength and digestive power, and is useful in cough, difficult breathing, diabetes, piles, rheumatism, dropsy, burning sensation, impotence and diseases of the heart (Nadkarni, 1954:1230; Kolammal, 1978. 2:57). Fruit, which is the officinal part, enters into the composition of preparations like Dasamularistam, Brhatyadi kasayam, Himasagaratailam, Vastyamayantakaghrtam, etc.

The pharmacognosy of the roots of T terrestris has been studied by Ansari and Prasad (1970).

4. Asparagus racemosus and Glycyrrihizza glabra (licorice)

Of these, the Samhitas say, 'One who uses ten grams of licorice powder mixed with ghee and honey, along with milk becomes continuously impelled with sex urge' .

5. Hygrophilia spinosa

Known as Kokilaksa, this plant is considered a reputed remedy for arthritis. It is a sweet, sour, bitter, cold, aphrodisiac that promotes strength and appetite. Its seeds are sweet and astringent. They promote sexual vigour and strength, and arrest abortion.

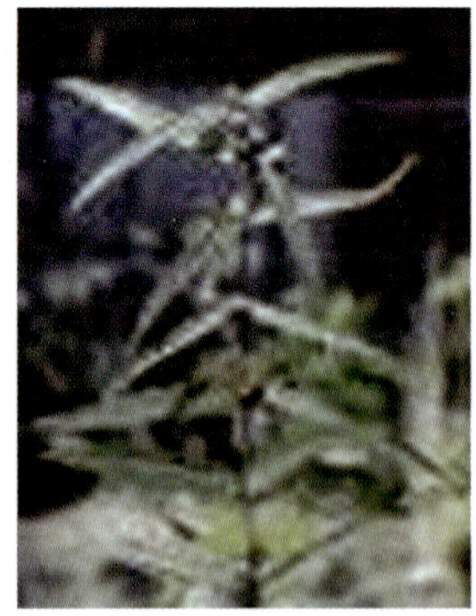
Figure 6. *Hygrophilia spinosa*

6. Curculigo orchioides

Known in India as musali, this is a reputed rasayana (rejuvenative) drug and a good aphrodisiac. It is sweet, bitter, viriligenic, roborant, easily digestible, diuretic and tonic. It improves the complexion and is useful in general debility, impotence, jaundice, urinary diseases, leucorrhoea and menorrhagia (Mooss, 1978 : 83, Sharma, 1983:561).

7. Pueraria tuberosa

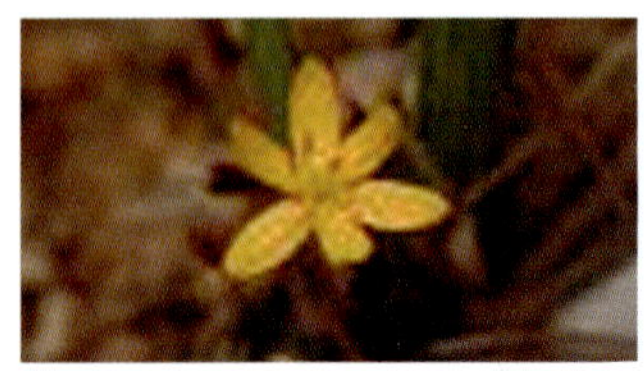
Figure 7. *Curculigo orchioides*

Vadari, as P tuberosa is known to Indians, is an important constituent of many Ayurvedic formulations and, according to the texts, the drug source is the subterranean tubers (varahikanda, vidarikanda) of a woody climber (vrksavalli) which have the shape of the tusk of a boar (varahi, grsti) or conical and curved like a pitcher (carmakaraluko) with abundant milky juice (ksiravalli, ksirakanda, payasvini). The drug is sweet (svadukanda), cooling, promotes strength and complexion, improves voice, enhances breast milk and semen production, overcomes vitiated pitta and vata and cures burning sensation. The drug is recommended in all cases of general debility and rheumatism (Aiyer and Kolammal, 1962. 5: 34-35). The important preparations using the drug are Vidaryadi ghrtam, Dasamularistam, Cyavanaprasam, etc.

8. Psychological stimuli

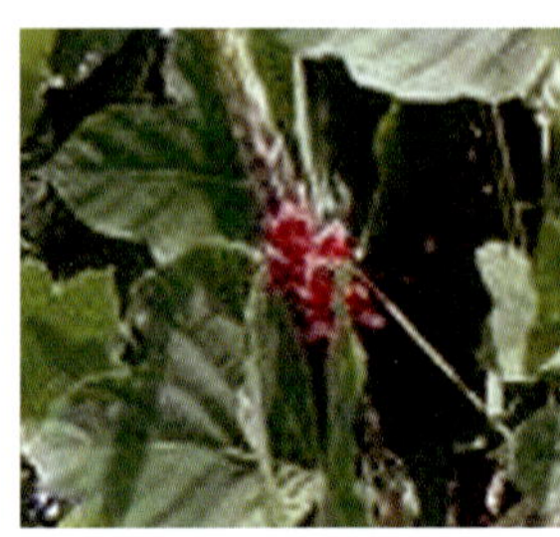
Figure 8. *Pueraria tuberosa*

Various psychological stimuli can influence sexual function. The following are said to decrease interest in the sexual act:

'old age, anxiety, diseases, fasting and excessive sexual indulgence: Even a saturated man does not get potency for the sexual act due to wasting, fear, lack of confidence, grief, finding fault with women, ignorance of enjoyment with women, lack of determination and interest, etc..'

Other psychological stimuli are said to augment sexual power:

'The youthful person who is free from fear and disorders; who takes diet with ghee and milk, cohabits frequently, and has strong determination, performs sexually with woman like a bull. This person also performs the sexual act like a bull, if he confides with his close friends and colleagues who are successful in endeavors, companionable, equally expert in psychic condition, similar in age and endowed with excellence of family, and who are also noble, kind, moral, joyful, free of pain and anxiety, similar in ideals, sincere, dear and sweet-spoken. He gets stimulated by massage, anointing, bathing and by receiving perfumes, garlands and adorations, by having a comfortable house, bed and chairs, and untorn favorite clothes. In addition, the chirping of favorite birds, tinkling of ornaments of women, and stimulation by gentle pressing of his body by his favorite women, turn him on.'

'A person who indulges in the sex act regularly does not get any obstruction in the seminal channels. Therefore, he gets more of sexual power. Persons who have accomplished their objectives have a natural inclination for sex acts. A person, whose mind is afflicted with grief, is not capable of sexual intercourse. By massage etc. the semen gets accumulated because of excitement, and thereafter,its ejaculation is the natural consequence. Because of this the virility of a person increases.'

These are the ways of the Caraka Samhaita with respect to aphrodisiacs: dietary recipes dominated by protein substances, herbal drugs like seeds of Mucuna prurience and licorice powder, and psychological factors like a comfortable house, fragrance, pleasant atmosphere, dear friends, massage, women, and an anxiety free and disease free state. These will increase sukra, the vital fluid and sexual power. Caraka advised also to take aphrodisiacs regularly so that the power to perform the sexual act can be retained till seventy years of age and beyond.

9. Aphrodisiacs in Later Ayurvedic Texts

In Ayurvedic texts written after the 12th century A.D., new aphrodisiacs make their first appearance. Sodhala, who is said to have lived in the 12th century A.D., in his Gadanigraha mentioned for the first time the medicinal uses of a plant, originally grown for its fibers, and is today known as Indian hemp or Cannabis sativa. In Sanskrit, this medicinal plant is bhanga.

In today' s Indian vernacular its drug is bhang or ganja. In Spanish it is marijuana, and in Arabic hashish. In medieval Ayurvedic texts, bhanga was said to increase libido. In the female, it was said to contract the vagina. For this purpose, powdered India hemp, three parts, nutmeg, opium and wild turmeric (Berberis aristrata) one part each should be mixed together and kept in the vagina.

In the 12th century A.D., Sodhala mentioned opium for the first time in Ayurvedic literature. It is considered to increase sexual capacity by postponing ejaculation. In Ayurvedic terminology, it is known as sukra stambana (stambana means to stop, or to sustain).

Sarangadhara Samhita, another Ayurvedic book which is said to have been written in the 13th century A.D., mentioned various preparations which can postpone ejaculation and prolong the sexual act. One such preparation reads as follows.

'Powders of Anacyclus pyrethrem (pellitory), dry ginger, long pepper, saffron, nutmeg, clove, sandalwood, ten grams each, and opium forty grams, are all mixed together. One gram of this powder taken with honey, daily, by either male or female desirous of coitus, gives them endurance. It prolongs the sexual act by postponing ejaculation.'

III. Summary

In the ancient classical Ayurvedic teachings, conservation of sukra, the life force, equated with semen, was given utmost importance. Conversely, voluntary stopping of ejaculation was also prohibited, as it was said to result in impotence. To maintain the balance of vital fluids in the body, regular use of sukra-augmenting foods and drugs, was advised. From the 12th century onwards, the Ayurvedic pharmacopoeia included herbal aphrodisiacs, namely, ganja, opium and nutmeg, which are today known as the sources of psychoactive substances. But prolonged use of these substances results in sukra kshaya and ultimately leads to impotence and damage to testicles. Herbal aphrodisiacs mentioned in ayurveda are purportedly giving encouraging results in erectile dysfunction and premature ejaculation. They are also useful in the treatment of anxiety and depression. Atmagupta showed encouraging results in the treatment of Parkinsonism. In Gujarat, India, Ayurvedic University ayurvedic aphrodisiacs were tried as growth promoters in children.

REFERENCES

1. Caraka Samhita Editorial Board. (1949). The Caraka Samhita (Vol.3). Jamnagar, India; Jamnagar Shree, Gulabkunverba Ayurvedic Society.
2. Hoernle, A.F.R. (Ed.) (1987). The Bower manuscript: Facsimile leaves, Nagari transcript, Romanised transliteration and English translation with notes (3 vols., facsimile of 1893 ed.). New Delhi: Aditya Prakashan.
3. Kim, Young Chan and Tan Hui Meng, (1993) APSIR Book on Erectile Dysfunction, The Asia Pacific Society for Impotence Research.
4. Kunjilal Bhishasratna (2002), (Eng. Trans.), Susruta Samhita, Varanasi, Chowkhambh Sanskrit Series Office.
5. Money J and Musaph H (1988 ed.) Hand book of sexology, vol. 6. Amsterdam, Elsevier.
6. Money. J, Joshi V.N. and Prakasam K.S. (1992). The Present and Future Prevention, Newbury Park, Sage publications.
7. Ray, P., and Gupta, H. (1965). Charaka Samhita: A scientific synopsis. New Delhi: National Institute of Sciences of India.
8. Sharma, P.V. (1983). Caraka Samhita: Agnivesa' s treatise refined and annotated by Caraka and redacted by Drdhabla. Varanasi: Chowkhambha Orientalia.
9. Sharma R.K., Dash Bhagawan (Eng. Translators) Caraka Samhita. Vol. V. (2005), Varanasi, Chowkambha Sanskrit Series Office.
10. Sivarajan,VV, Indira B. Ayurvedic drugs and their plant sources, (1998), New Delhi, Oxford and IBH Publishing Co. Pvt. Ltd.

Chapter 4

Indonesian Perspective

Increasing Need for Herbal as Sexual Performance Enhancer

FX Arif Adimoelja, Johannes Soedjono

I. Introduction

Currently, increasing the need for herb at an medicine in academic level has unconsciously governed the scientific modern medicine with more and more people are trending to use these healing herbs. Even physicians are often unaware that the drugs they prescribe are of herbal origin daily. The lay people as well as academics and physicians assume that synthetic phyto-pharmaceutical compounds are free from unwanted side effects or that they may exert only weak adverse reactions compared to modern chemical pharmaceuticals. Regretfully, green pharmaceuticals are often only used when modern medicine with her chemical pharmaceuticals fail to cure diseases. In other words, the green pharmaceuticals will only be applied as an alternative, "last resort" choice in medicine.

II. Phyto-pharmaceuticals in Asia, Indonesia and the Modern World

In Indonesia phyto-pharmaceuticals are sold as dietary food supplements and can be easily

---

FX Arif Adimoelja, M.D., Ph.D.
Andrology Sub Department, "Dr. Ramelan" Naval Teaching Hospital Reproductive Health Unit, School of Medicine, Hang Tuah University, Jl. Gadung No.1, Surabaya 60244, Indonesia, Tel: +62-31-594.4218, Fax: +62-31-593.0792, E-mail: ariclin@indo.net.id

bought over the counter. Unlike modern medicine, phyto-pharmaceuticals are not subjected to evaluation by the *Food and Drug Administration* (FDA) Control of the Republic of Indonesia (Badan POM).

Any drugs of herbal origin, regardless of whether a traditional products (home industrial product), modern processed and/or scientifically extracted (the phyto-chemical ingredients analyzed and standardized) and clinically tested products are allowed to be marketed over the counter. All are categorized as "*jamu*" (a local form of herbal medication).

However there has been numerous instances where many herbal medications, traditional or modern and processed "*jamu*" are reported to be contaminated with heavy metals and/or mixed with synthetic chemical drugs. This lack of regulation and standardization which may lead to a multitude of problems can be considered as the pitfalls of today' s phyto-pharmaceuticals.

An exclusive survey performed in the USA on ten "Herbal Sex Pills" reported that 9 out of 10 such pills did not contain the right compositions as stated in their brochures. The conclusion reached was that the sexual thrill experienced by the users were the results of mere fantasy, rather than the effect of the herbal pill itself (L.D. Sharlip, 2002). In fact, most herbal medications and phyto-pharmaceutical drugs are invariably composed of more than one herbal-extract and this method of using different components in a 'concoction' is thought to potentiate their herbal strength / power. Unfortunately, sometimes these different phyto-chemical components may interact with each other and give rise to undesirable side effects. The efficacy and safety of any herbal product (whole dry extract) is so far only attributed to a single plant product (e.g. Gingko biloba extract). When more (than one) herbal product is being combined, the interaction of all these phytochemical components with each other may influence the efficacy and safety of the combined phyto-pharmaceutical product. The evaluation of such combined herbal mixture requires a large number of basic as well as evidence-based studies that may be costly and time consuming.

III. Aphrodisiac, Performance Enhancer, Health Food Supplements and Elixir for Youth

All over the world and in particular Asia and Indonesia, herbs products are commonly used as aphrodisiacs, performance enhancers and "anti-aging" drugs. Their popularity leads to more intense research on herbs products. The extraction procedure of different herbs are becoming better analyzed and standardized. It has undergone a significant progress over the years, making it well positioned in the modern world and medicine. Phyto-pharmaceuticals were often marketed as health food supplements and "elixir for youth". They may be used to prevent and treat diseases because it was claimed that their phyto-pharmaceutical ingredients contain a diversity of vitamins and minerals that may stimulate the production of nitric oxide (NO) and NO-synthase to promote vascular and microvascular dilatations, to reduce oxidative stress and promote cerebral flow (Gingko biloba extracts). Many of them are also purported as sexual performance enhancers to help improve penile rigidity and maintain erection during intercourse and in this way help to enhance sex life.

IV. Clinical Trial Sample of a Multi-Combination Herbal Product

Vi™, a multi-combination phyto-pharmaceutical product is claimed to 'improve men' s performance' (manufactured by Pharmaceutical Labs in Asia). VI™ has been sent to our Centre for the Study and Services for "Men' s Health, Reprcduction, Sexual Health and Aging" where we conducted a small seeding trial to test its efficacy in treating male patients with erectile dysfunction (ED).

Vi™ contains 27 ingredients, comprising of 25 different kinds of herbal extracts (phyto-pharmaceuticals) - each of which contributes to enhance sexual performance as has been known throughout history - and 2 chemo-pharmaceuticals namely Niacinamide (vitamin) and L-Arginine (known to be an important chemical product for sexual performance). The 25 different kinds phyto-pharmaceuticals are: Panax ginseng, Notoginseng, Tribulus, Cordyceps, Polygonum, Epimedium, Cistanche, Gastrodia, Pinellia, Limonium, Gingko, Astragalus, Psoralea, Angelica Sinensis, Wild Yam, Marinda, Rehmania, Carthamus, Ginger, Ganoderma, Eucommia, Cuscuta, Maca, Eurycoma Longifolia and Guarana.

1. Method

12 (twelve) male subjects with mild to moderate ED were evaluated and the results of a continuous treatment with Vi™ two capsules daily were assessed with the International Index of Erectile Function-5 (IIEF-5), Sexual Encounter Profile (SEP), and post-treatment global assessment questionnaires. All subjects had to follow all study requirements and procedures. They were also advised not to take other medications or ED treatments during the clinical trial period. All subjects had to complete and sign a consent form before enrolling in the study.

2. Study design

The study was conducted at our Centre for the Study and Services for "Men' s Health, Reproduction, Sexual Health and Aging" / Andrology Clinic at the Naval Hospital Dr. Ramelan, Surabaya, Indonesia.

A pre-post test study design was applied. Twelve male subjects with mild to moderate ED completed the study. Baseline data (from past medical and sexual function history, IIEF questions and their history after their last sexual activity) were obtained after a "wash-out period" (from a treatment-free run-in period) of one month. After the "wash-out period" all subjects were given Vi™ two caps daily for 4 weeks. All subjects were instructed to have intercourse twice a week. All subjects had to complete IIEF-5 forms and a set of global assessment questionnaires at the end of the study. Subjects were also asked to complete their written past history and SEP questionnaires after each sexual intercourse activity. Any adverse events and side effects were instructed to be reported and the IIEF-5 questionnaire had to be completed at the end of each week.

3. Inclusion criteria

All male married subjects at the age of 47-71 years old suffering from ED for at least six months (defined as having difficulty in achieving or maintaining erection for successful intercourse) were eligible. All subjects had to be of good mental health and have stable sex partners.

4. Treatment regimen

Subjects were instructed to take 2 capsules daily in the morning on an empty stomach for four weeks. They were instructed to make at least two attempts at sexual intercourse per week and report any attempt responses in their diary.

5. Results

After 4 week of treatment, a significant improvement of their sexual function measurements were observed. At baseline the mean EF domain score was 13.83, consistent with mild to moderate ED. After finishing the 4-week-long trial, a significant increase of their mean EF domain score to 17.00 ($P<0.012$) was observed. None of the subjects regained normal sexual function (defined as EF = 26). The successful penetration rate increased significantly from 25.70% at baseline to 76.60%. The intercourse completion rate increased significantly from 35.00% at baseline to 81.90% (as assessed by the two SEP questions).

6. Conclusions

Vi™ indeed was shown to be effective in increasing sexual performances in terms of improving and maintaining penile rigidity. A longer period of trials involving a larger number of subjects should be performed in the future to get better insights into the dynamic pharmaceutical interactions between the different phyto-pharmaceutical substances involved. Last but not least, the purity of this pharmaceutical product can be determined.

REFERENCES

1. Adeniyi AA, Brindley GS, Pryor JP, et al. Yohimbine in the treatment of orgasmic dysfunction. Asian J Androl. 2007 May;9(3):403-7.
2. Adimoelja A. Pharmacodynamic interaction of Medicinal Plant-extract. EDACT Meeting, JW Marriott, Jakarta, Indonesia, May 10-11, 2003.
3. Adimoelja A and Sartono. S. Chemical and Phyto-pharmaceuticals to us or not to use in Sexual Medicine. Seminar on Sexual Medicine, NUH, Singapore, July, 8-9, 2006.
4. Bone, K., *Clinical Applications of Ayurvedic and Chinese Herbs - Monographs for the Western HerbalPractitioner*. Phytotherapy Press, Warwick, Australia, 1996. (KEB)
5. Brown GA, Vukovich MD, Martini ER, et al. Effects of androstenedione-herbal supplementation on serum sex hormone concentrations in 30- to 59- year-old men. Int J Vitam Nutr Res. 2001; 71:293-301.
6. Carey MP, Johnson BT. Effectiveness of yohimbine in the treatment of erectile disorder: four meta-analytic integrations. Arch Sex Behav. 1996;25(4):341-360.
7. Carlson JJ, Farquhar JW, DiNucci E, et al. Safety and efficacy of a ginkgo biloba-containing dietary supplement on cognitive function, quality of life, and platelet function in healthy, cognitively intact older adults. J Am Diet Assoc. 2007 Mar;107(3):422-32.
8. Cicero AF, Derosa G, Brillante R, et al. Effects of Siberian ginseng (Eleutherococcus senticosus maxim) on elderly quality of life: a randomized clinical trial. Arch Geronto Geriatr Suppl. 2004; 69-73.
9. Coleman CI, Hebert JH, Reddy P. The effects of . Panax ginseng on quality of life. J Clin Pharm Ther. 2003; 28:5-15.
10. Ebadi M. Pharmacodynamic Basis of Herbal Medicine. 2nd Ed. CRC Press, Taylor and Francis Group, Boca Raton, 2007.
11. Gauthaman K, Adaikan PG, Prasad RN. Aphrodisiac properties of Tribulus Terrestris extract (Protodioscin) in normal and castrated rats. Life Sci 8-9-2002; 71: 1385-96.
12. Gruenwald J (Ed). PDR for Herbal Medicines, 4th Ed. Medical Economics Company, Inc.. Montvale. 2000.
13. Ramawat K.G. (Ed.).Herbal Drugs: Ethnomedicine to Modern Medicine. Springer-Verlag, Berlin-Heidelberg, 2009.
14. Sharlip I.D. Herbal sex thrive on fantasy, more than fact. Newark Star Ledger, January 30, 2002.
15. Ulbricht C, Basch E, Ulbricht C, et al. Wild yam (Dioscoreaceae). J Herb Pharmacother. 2003;3(4):77-91.
16. Vogler BK, Pittler MH, Ernst E. The efficacy of ginseng. A systematic review of randomized clinical trials. Eur J Clin Pharmacol. 1999; 55:567-75.

Chapter 5

Japanese Perspective

The Japanese Experience of Phytotherapy in Sexual Medicine

Yasushi Miyagawa, Akihiko Okuyama

I. Background

1. Introduction

Nowadays, phytotherapy in the forms of herbal remedies and health foods are widely used throughout Japan. These plant materials have been characterized and classified as either medicine or food by the Ministry of Health and Welfare of the Japanese Government. Among these plant materials, Kampo (which literally means the "Han Method" of the Chinese herbal system that developed during the Han Dynasty) is utilized as pharmaceutical products such as extract granule and formulation. Kampo medicines have been accepted by the National Health Insurance and have been fully integrated into the modern health care system in Japan since 1971. Current sales of Kampo medicines are approximately 100 billion yen or 1.2% of the total pharmaceutical sales. Of these, approximately 80% of the sales are from Kampo formulation for prescription which are covered by the health insurance, and the remaining 20% are from over-the-counter (OTC) Kampo formulation which are not covered by the health insurance.[1]

Kampo medicine and Western medicine differ fundamentally in methodology and philosophy. Western medicine addresses the disease itself and works directly on the cause, and treats the disease by removing the cause. On the other hand, Kampo medicine takes a holistic approach by emphasizing the body' s overall balance and works to build the individual' s natural resistance and

Yasushi Miyagawa, M.D., Ph.D.
Department of Urology, Osaka University Graduate School of Medicine, 2-2, Yamadaoka, Suita, Osaka, 565-0871, Japan. Tel: +81-6-6879-3531, Fax: +81-6-6879-3539, E-mail: miyagawa@uro.med.osaka-u.ac.jp

healing capacity and thereby indirectly treats diseases. In Kampo medicine, the mind and the body are inseparable and the goal to treat the person on all levels by accounting for the individual' s constitution and characteristics, and by harmonizing the entire body to heal from within. This difference appears to come from different ways of thinking that are rooted in each culture. Western medicine is based on natural science and aims to understand nature theoretically through analysis and verification. On the other hand, Kampo medicine is based on natural philosophy and pursues ways in humans can coexist with nature through harmony and adaptation, empirically and comprehensively[1].

This chapter summarizes Kampo medicine and sexual medicine in Japan and has been into four sections: 1. History of Kampo in Japan; 2. Current status of Kampo medicine in sexual medicine and its efficacy and side effect; 3. Future trend of Kampo medicine in sexual medicine and the stance to research work for the new drugs from plant gene resources in Japan; 4. Prevalence of sexual medicine in Japan.

2. History[2]

Although there are no accurate historical records, it is probable that there were several folklore medicines in ancient Japan. Some Chinese medical works were introduced to Japan as early as the 4th or 5th Century, coming first by way of Korea, which had adopted Chinese medicine by that time. Historical records indicate that the Chinese written language was adopted in Japan during this period so that the people could learn from China about Buddhism, Confucianism, governmental organization, and the divination arts, opening the way for study of Chinese medicine.

The basic texts of Chinese medicine and Materia Medica was brought to Japan during the 7th through 9th centuries. This led to the publication of the most important historical text on Chinese medical theory and practice in Japan called the Ishimpo (The Essence of Medicine and Therapeutic Methods). This oldest surviving Japanese medical treatise, with 30 individually titled scrolls, was written by Yasuyori Tamba in 984 and is now a national treasure of Japan. The Ishimpo is a compilation of medical knowledge and theories from more than 100 Chinese texts that were prevalent during the Sui Dynasty (589-618) and Tang Dynasty (618-907). The herbal formulas that were included in the Ishimpo were mostly comprised of plant materials with low toxicity. These were supplemented by relatively safe minerals or mineralized compounds such as oyster shell, dragon bone, gypsum, and talc. For example, these calcium-based materials are used in the following formulas: Minor Bupleurum Combination (Xiao Chaihu Tang), Cinnamon and Hoelen Formula (Guizhi Fuling San), Hoelen Five Formula (Wuling San), Pueraria Combination (Gegen Tang), and Tang-kuei and Peony Formula (Danggui Shaoyao San). The Ishimpo is also notable for preserving some of the Taoist sexual manuals from the Han Dynasty (206BC-220) to the Tang Dynasty (618-907). The principal formulas, the accompanying medical theories and practices of the Ishimpo dominated Kampo medicine until the end of the 15th century.

Soon after the publication of the Ishimpo, Japan underwent a period of cultural and economic isolation from the end of the 9th century until the end of the 14th century. However, a few Japanese scholars still managed to travel privately to China despite the limited amount of interaction that was exchanged. These scholars developed distinctive schools of medical thought as epitomized by the Goseiha school of Sanki Tashiro (1465-1537) whose work was based on Li Dongyuan (1180-1251) and Zhu Danxi (1281-1358), which focused on the center-tonifying and yin-tonifying principles respectively, as well as on the Five Element theory. Later, the Kohoha school was developed by Todo Yoshimasu (1702-1773), which claimed that most disease was caused by an invasion of pathogenic toxin, not unlike the other two schools of the Jin Yuan period (Fire-purging and Wind-clearing) and the later treatise of the Wenbing Hiuichun (1587) describing the so-called four levels of disease, written by Gong Tingxian (1522-1619). Thus, Kampo medicine attained its strength and independent status in Japan with contribution of the several Japanese physicians and their Schools of Kampo at the end of 16th century.

During the 17th century, modern Western medicine was introduced to Japan from Holland and became known as "Rampo" (Dutch medicine) to distinguish itself Kampo which competed with it at that time. After the Meiji Restoration in 1868, the Japanese government rapidly westernized all fields; from the 1880s, traditional medical practices were officially prohibited and mandated all physicians to train in and graduate from Western medical schools. However, the people's support for traditional medicine as a cultural heritage prevented complete extinction of Kampo. Kampo revived during the first half of the 20th century by prescriptions that survived the test of times and by enthusiastic Western-trained doctors who were interested in returning to their classical roots in medicine. The government granted approval for the invention of several proprietary drugs containing Kampo medicines? which in turn gained much support from the people as primary health care remedies. A Committee of clinicians and pharmacists that formed under the Central Pharmaceutical Affairs Council organized, evaluated and selected traditional prescriptions to be tested in clinical trials and observed for their efficacy and safety. Based on these findings, the Committee developed a standard recommendation for each formulation regarding the quantity of the components, directions for use, dosage, and indications for administration. Diseases that required modern medical treatment were excluded from the sphere of indications of the prescriptions. In 1976, the Japanese government officially approved 82 Kampo prescriptions for coverage by the National Health Insurance and as over-the-counter (OTC) remedies. In addition, the Department of Pharmaceutical Affairs of the Ministry of Health and Welfare approved 210 herbal formulas (including the 82 already mentioned) for use in medical facilities. They were available as OTC remedies but not all of them were approved for coverage by national health insurance. The use of herbal drug products in hospitals and clinics were promoted as prescription drugs. Reflecting the growing interest in herbal medicine, the total expenditure on the production of Kampo formulations reached $80 million in 1977.

3. Today

At present, the Japanese health ministry officially recognizes over 220 Kampo formulas and more than 150 of these are covered by the national health insurance. It is currently estimated that as many as 50% of all doctors in Japan use some form of Kampo medicine and that there are in excess of 10,000 pharmacies dispensing Kampo formulations. Kampo medicine is taught in traditional academic and clinical setting to medical doctors and pharmacists who wish to specialize in herbal medicine. These are the only two professions licensed to practice and prescribe herbal medicine in Japan today. However, there is a large number of Kampo specialist doctors who have studied in the formal tradition of apprenticeship and those generally practice under the license of a collaborative physician. These individuals often have far superior knowledge and training in the medicine and are sought out by patients all over Japan. It is common for patients to seek for OTC or prescription herbal medicine from their local pharmacy or physician. It is also common for hospital inpatients to receive Kampo medicines concomitantly with their orthodox medication regime. Currently, 148 Kampo formulations are recognized by the Ministry of Health, Labor and Welfare and covered by the health insurance.

OTC Kampo formulations have a production value of approximately 1/4 to 1/5 of Kampo prescriptions, and they compromise 2.9% of the entire OTC sales. Along with the prescriptions, the OTC production value had reached its peak of 30 billion yen in 1992 and dropped thereafter. Sales have only recently recovered in part due to heightened awareness of lifestyle-related diseases and great hope in Bofutsushosan (Fang-Feng-Tong-Sheng-San) as an anti-obesity drug.

Surveys that have been conducted in Japan revealed that Kampo medicines are mainly used to treat the following symptoms and disorders: unidentified complaints, menopausal disorders, autonomic ataxia, infertility, sexual dysfunction, acute upper respiratory tract infection, constipation, chronic hepatitis, cough/phlegm, loss of appetite, malnutrition or nutritional abnormalities, muscle cramps, acute or chronic bronchitis, and allergic rhinitis. Of these conditions, approximately 35% of physicians use Kampo as the treatment of choice for unidentified complaints, menopausal disorders and autonomic ataxia. There is no data on the percentage of Kampo medicine use for sexual dysfunction. A recent publication of guideline for erectile dysfunction from the Japanese Society for Sexual Medicine (JSSM) did not even mention Kampo as a time-honored pharmacotherapy, even though Kampo is offiically approved by National Health Insurance system.

4. Future trends

As demands for Kampo increase in Japan, the adoption of Kampo medicine education at medical schools is also rapidly increasing. Kampo education, which was offered at only 24 medical schools as recently as 1997, was offered at all 80 medical schools in Japan by 2004. Moreover, in 2002 the Ministry of Education, Culture, Sports, Science and Technology issued a model core curriculum for medical education, in which general knowledge of Japanese Kampo medicine became a part of the basic requirement for graduation. Through the implementation of this model core curriculum, the importance of Kampo medicine knowledge for physician was officially acknowledged. Universities with pharmacology and pharmaceutical sciences have also incorporated Kampo medicine into their program, whose core curriculum includes the basic concepts of Kampo medicine, knowledge of Kampo formulations and crude drug constituents. Kampo medicine is expected to grow in Japan and worldwide with increasing public and professional interest and greater approval from the medical community. Several leading pharmaceutical companies are setting higher standards for quality assurance and conducting rigorous researches to establish scientific evidence.

In this social milieu, basic and clinical trials of Kampo medicines are rapidly progressing to identify the mechanisms of actions related to its efficacy through pharmacological tests using animal models and other methods. Appropriate methodologies for evaluating Kampo' s efficacy are also being investigated for future research purposes. Collectively., these endeavors are gathering scientific evidence of Kampo' s efficacy. For example, the results of placebo-controlled double-blind trials have shown that Shosaikoto improves liver function in patients with chronic hepatitis, Daiokanzoto improves constipation, and Shoseiryuto effectively improves allergic rhinitis. Further research and scientific evidence of Kampo are expected to promote the combination therapy of Kampo and Western medicine.

5. Prevalence of sexual medicine in Japan

The NIH Consensus Development Panel on Impotence has defined male erectile dysfunction (ED) as the inability to achieve and maintain an erection of the penis sufficiently to complete satisfactory sexual intercourse, a definition that gained worldwide acceptance. A recent review article[4] estimated that at present, 5-20% of all adult males worldwide experience moderate to complete ED. This proportion is expected to further increase with the aging population, doubling by the year 2025[5]. An epidemiological survey was conducted in Japan with a questionnaire using the same format as the Massachusetts Male Aging Study (MMAS)[6]. Subject selection was based on the basic resident registry, and the survey was conducted using a postal and visit format. This allowed an accurate statistical survey and an accurate estimation of the prevalence of this condition on a national scale. A total of 2000 subjects randomly selected from 100 locations around Japan were surveyed, with a 55.2% response rate. As with the MMAS, the prevalence of ED rose with age. From the prevalence found in the survey, 11,300,000 Japanese males aged 30-79 were estimated to have moderate to complete ED[7]. The rapidly aging population of Japan leads us to anticipate a further rise in ED patients in the future.

There are very few data available regarding female sexual dysfunction in Japan. A Japanese female cohort study,[8] including 2095 women aged 30 to 69 years (median 48), reported that the incidence of symptomatic orgasmic disorder, sexual desire disorder, arousal disorder, and lubrication disorder increased significantly and positively with age. The comparison of women in their 30s and 60s of the above mentioned disorders are as follows: 15.2% to 32.2%, 27.7% to 57.9%, 29.7% to 57.9%, and 12.5% to 51.2%, respectively. This rate of prevalence was comparable with women in the West, although this Japanese study failed to use validated FSD questionnaires.

II. The Phytotherapy Industry

1. The industry

About 2% of total drug expenditures in Japan are herbal medicines, the largest part of them provided by Tsumura and Co., with contributions from about 20 other manufacturers. They belong to two major industry organizations for medicinal plants in Japan, the Japan Kampo Medicine Manufacturers Association (http://www.nikkankyo.org/) and the Tokyo Crude Drugs Association (http://www.aa.alpha-net.ne.jp/shouyaku/index.htm).

2. Regulations

The Pharmaceutical Affairs Law regulates the import, distribution, and sale of natural medicines. In some cases, the products are also subject to provisions of the Plant Protection Law and the Domestic Animal Infectious Diseases Control Law. Materials imported for use in ordinary food, health food, and nutritionally enhanced foods are subject to provisions of the Food Sanitation Law and the Nutrition Improvement Law.

1) Plant protection law

This law is designed to prevent harmful plants, insect pests, and microorganisms from spreading to Japan. Items restricted under this law must be submitted for inspection to the plant protection station at the port of entry.

2) Pharmaceutical affairs law and pharmaceutical affairs regulations

In Japan, medicinal plants are classified into two groups based on the list of characteristics in the "Distinction between drugs and foodstuffs"; (1) Medicinal plants that are used exclusively as medicine (ie., cannot be used as food): 232 plant-based species, 21 animal-based species, 58 other species, e.g., Japanese Angelica (root), Astragalus (root), Phellodendron (bark), Coptis (rhizome, fibrous root), Rhubarb (rhizome), Aconite (tuberous root), etc, (2) Medicinal plants that are considered non-medicinal unless medicinal efficacy is clearly stated (ie., can be used as food as long as therapeutic claims are not made): 804 plant-based species, 65 animal-based species, 147 other species, e.g., Eleutherococcus senticosus (bark, root, root bark, leaf, flower, fruit), Bitter melon (fruit, root, leaf), Astragalus (stem, leaf), Phellodendron (leaf, berry), Coptis (leaf), Rhubarb (leaf), Ginseng (fruit, root, rhizome, leaf), etc.

The import and sales of natural medicines that fall under the category of pharmaceuticals according to the Pharmaceutical Affairs Law are subject to the provisions of this law. Products in this category include pharmaceutical ingredients and ingredients with claims of medicinal effects. When importing these products, it is necessary to obtain an import and sales license as well as a product-specific approval or license.

In 2007, the pharmaceutical affairs law was revised as part of the national attempt to promote self-medication. This allowed non-pharmacist, registered salesman to sell Kampo medicines. Due to these changes, the market was expected to show an upward trend in the years to follow. In 1975, 210 formulations were selected for OTC according to the internal regulations for "Guideline for OTC Kampo formulae". These formulae had the potential for approval in the recent years if their effects and indications matched the Guideline's effects and indications, and if sufficient data proving equivalence in quality as standard decoctions were presented. In 2008, the outdated internal regulations were rearranged, added and/or revised to update the effects and indications of the OTC formulations.

3) Food sanitation law

Whether a particular imported natural medicinal material is a food or a pharmaceutical product cannot be determined from its ingredients alone. Natural, medicinal substances may be imported for use as food provided that it is so stated and that no medicinal or health benefits are claimed. Materials that satisfy these conditions are subject to provisions of the Food Sanitation Law.

4) The Japanese pharmacopoeia (JP): standard of quality control

Crude drugs must meet The Japanese Pharmacopoeia (JP) criteria to qualify as medicine. In 2001, 121 crude drug species and their 52 powdered forms were listed in JP 14th edition (JP14). However, revisions and new advances from the non-JP crude drug standards (internal regulations for approval) after 2006 led to the addition of Supplement I in JP 15 in 2007 which expanded the list to 153 crude drugs and their 54 powdered forms. The following characteristics of crude drugs are standardized in the official monographs of JP: (1) Name, (2) Origin, (3) Medicinal part, (4) Preparation process, (5) Content of specific constituents (lower limit setting), (6) Description, (7) Identification, (8) Purity (includes heavy metals, arsenic, residual pesticides), (9) Loss of drying, (10) Total ash, (11) Acid-insoluble ash, (12) Extract content, (13) Assay. Some pharmaceutical companies devise their own in-house standards in addition to the legally minimal JP standards. Non-JP crude drug standards are used as a reference for drugs that are not listed in the JP, and each company must develop their own approval standards for drugs that are not listed in the former references.

5) Convention on international trade in endangered species of Wild Fauna and Flora (CITEC)

Natural medicines that fall under the provisions of CITEC are classified into three categories, each with its level of restrictions and import requirements. Prospective importers are advised to consult the Endangered Species of Wild Fauna and Flora Administration Section, Import Division, International Trade Administration Bureau, Ministry of International Trade and Industry. Prospective importers must also obtain an export certificate issued by a management authority of the exporting country.

3. Distribution channels

Kampo formulations are available from physicians as prescriptions and as OTC formulations from regular pharmacies. Kampo formulations for prescription have fixed national drug prices and are covered by the national health insurance which keep patient payments fractional.

Non-Kampo crude drug products may be used in OTC product but its detailed data of sales do not exist. Some of them may be delivered or mailed by practitioners via internet or retail shops. Health food can be bought through pharmacy, internet or retail shops in Japan.

III. The Products

1. Proprietary products (over-the-counter drugs)

Yombine is the only approved OTC drug for psychogenic erectile dysfunction and/or ejaculation disturbance which is manufactured in Japan. There are no known drugs that are manufactured in Japan for female sexual dysfunction. Several OTC drugs and or foods containing Maca are purported to have beneficial sexual effects for both men and women. However, data of their sales, efficacy and safety information have not been established yet.

2. Prescribed products

A total of four Kampo prescriptions are indicated for impotence and are manufactured in Japan and covered by the National Health Insurance. These are discussed in the section, "Clinical Experience" and introduced in Chapter Part II.

There are no known official and effective Kampo formulations for female sexual dysfunction.

IV. Clinical Experience

The characteristic of Kampo medicine practice in Japan today is that physicians are capable of prescribing both the Western drug and Kampo medicine. This is in contrast with the Chinese system where two separate physician licensures are required to practice Western medicine and Traditional Chinese Medicine. Application for approval for the manufacturing of Kampo formulations for prescription are based on the 1980 regulations, and no other formulations have been approved since then. This is because the current regulation mandates astringent data submission that is comparable to a new drug application with rigorous clinical trials. Unlike China, Japan does not have a separate approving system that is lenient toward empirical, traditional medicines.

The Kampo prescriptions which are applicable to impotence will be discussed successively.

1. Hachimijioganan

Hachimijiogan was developed by Zhang Zhong-Jing (150-219) in his Prescriptions of the Golden Chest at the end of the Eastern Han Dynasty. Hachimijiogan is composed of eight crude herbs: Rehmannia Root, Cornus Fruit, Dioscorea Rhizome, Alisma Rhizome, Poria Sclerotium, Moutan Bark, Cinnamon Bark and Powdered Processed Aconite Root. Although the pharmacological effects of Hachimijiogan have not proven yet, it is said that Rehmannia Root, Cornus Fruit and Dioscorea Rhizome have nutritious and tonic effect and that Moutan Bark has vasodilatatory effect. These may have some favorable effects on erectile function.

Ohyama et al.[9] reported a clinical study comparing the effect of Hachimijiogan on 26 patients with erectile dysfunction and 25 normal men. Judging by the questionnaires of both treated cohorts, efficacy rate in erectile function was 77% and 64%, respectively. In another study of Hachimijiogan, 32% of patients of the twenty-two Japanese patients diagnosed with psychogenic ED who participated in the study reported improvement of their erectile function[10].

2. Saikokaryukotsuboreito/ Keishikaryukotsuboreito

The original formula, Ryukotsuboreito, is frequently utilized for psychogenic ED patients to relieve of their anxiety, tension and depression. Saikokaryukotsuboreito is prepared by the addition of Saiko (Bupleurum Root) to Ryukotuboreito, while Keishikaryukotuboreito is made by the addition of Keihi (Cinnamon Bark) to Ryukotuboreito. Both prescriptions are differentially utilized according to "SHO". Sho is the set of patient' s symptoms at any given moment, and recognized in terms of Qi (well-being, energy, illness, vigour), Blood and Water (Body fluids); the eight categories (Yin-Yang, hypofunction and hyperfunction, heat and cold, superficies and interior); the five parenchymatous viscera; and the six stages of the disease (Taiyang, Shaoyang, Yangming, Taiyin, Shaoyin, Jueyin). Sho is broadly defined as Kampo diagnosis in the epistemic framework of Kampo' s perspective of illness, and provides the foundation for formulating treatment strategy.

Nagata et al. used Saikokaryukotsuboreito to treat aging men with psychogenic ED, and nine of 25 patients (36%) was reported curing of symptoms[11]. Tsujimura et al. also reported the effectiveness of Saikokaryukotsuboreito for eugonadal patients with late-onset hypogonadism-related symptoms whose sexual functions, as estimated by a self-reported questionnaire "Aging Male Symptom score", had significantly improved[12]. Tsujino et al. reported the combination therapy of Keisikaryukotuboreito with Cilostazol was more useful for patients with vascular ED patients than monotherapy of Cilostazol. It is probable that the vasodilatatory effect of Cinnamon Bark and Poeny Root play some role in improving ED[13]. However, all these reports fail to provide strong evidence of the usefulness of these Kampo prescription because of insufficient study design.

3. Goshajinkigan

Goshajinkigan is a traditional Chinese medicine formulation composed of ten herbs.14 One study compared the effect of limaprost, an oral prostaglandin E1 (PGE1) derivative, to the Goshajinkigan. The study investigated 50 patients with mild erectile dysfunction who showed a good erectile response to intracavernosal injection of 20 mg PGE1. Limaprost was administered to the first 25 patients (30 mg three times daily) and Goshajinkigan (7.5 g three times daily) to the next 25 patients for 8 consecutive weeks. Patients were evaluated according to their ability to achieve vaginal penetration and by a subjective assessment of erectile functions (i.e. penile rigidity and maintenance of erection) before and after the treatment, using a self-administered questionnaire. Objective measurements (e.g. nocturnal penile tumescence) were also evaluated. Four of the 24 patients taking Goshajinkigan succeeded in vaginal penetration. However, these positive responders did not experience a full erection[14].

4. Hochuekkito

Generally, Hochuekkito is indicated for patients with delicate constitution, reduced digestive functions, and severe fatigability of limbs presenting the following symptoms or conditions: summer emaciation, debility after illness, tuberculosis, anorexia, gastroptosis, cold, hemorrhoid, anal prolapse, uterine prolapse, impotence, hemiplegia, and hyperidrosis. Hochuekkito has been extensively used in Japan to treat male infertility and occasionally for erectile dysfunction. The proposed mechanisms of efficacy of Hochuekkito include the vasodilatory effects of Astragalus Root and Japanese Angelica Root, and the sedative or CNS-inhibitory effects of Citrus Unshiu Peel, Glycyrrhiza Root, Cimicifuga Rhizome and Ginger Rhizome. Nagao et al. treated psychogenic and organic ED with Hochuekkito and reported that 52% of the former and 19% of the latter was improved[15].

REFERENCES

1. Tsumura and Co. Kampo Fact Book. (http://www.tsumura.co.jp/english/kampo/fact/use/index.html)
2. Dharmanada S. KAMPO MEDICINE: The Practice of Chinese Herbal Medicine in Japan. (http://www.itmonline.org/arts/kampo.htm)
3. Kimoto Y, Nagao K, Sasaki H, Marumo K, Takahashi Y, Nishi S et al. JSSM Guidelines for erectile dysfunction. Int J Urol. 2008; 15: 564-76.
4. Kubin M, Wagner G, Fugl-Meyer AR. Epidemiology of erectile dysfunction. Int. J. Impot. Res. 2003; 15: 63-71.
5. AytaÇ IA, McKinlay JB, Krane RJ. The likely worldwide increase in erectile dysfunction between 1995 and 2025 and some possible policy consequences. BJU Int. 1999; 84: 50-6.
6. Feldman HA, Goldstein I, Hatzichristou DG, Krane RJ, McKinlay JB. Impotence and its medical and psychosocial correlates: results of the Massachusetts Male Aging Study. J. Urol. 1994; 151: 54-61.
7. Marui E. Epidemiology of erectile dysfunction and risk factors. Igaku-no-ayumi 2002; 201: 397-400 (in Japanese).
8. Hisasue S, Kumamoto Y, Sato Y, Masumori N, Horita H, Kato R et al. Prevalence of female sexual dysfunction symptoms and its relationship to quality of life: a Japanese female cohort study. Urology 2005; 65: 143-8.
9. Ohyama t, Maekawa M, Kashihara N. The effect of Hachimijiogan on impotence patients. Hinyokika Kiyo 1982; 28: 493-7 (in Japanese).
10. Nishizawa Y. The effect of Hachimijiogan on patients with impotence. Impotence 1986; 1: 81-9 (in Japanese).
11. Nagata H. The clinical efficacy f Saikokayrukotsuboreito and Rokumijiogan on patients with impotence. Impotence 1986; 28: 81-9 (in Japanese).
12. Tsujimura A, Takada S, Matsuoka Y, Nakayama J, Takao T, Miyagawa Y et al. Clinical trial of treatment with Saikokaryukotsuboreito for eugonadal patients with late-onset hypogonadism-related symptoms. Aging Male. 2008;11:9 5-9.
13. Tsujino T. Clinical experience of oral drugs for impotence patients: combination therapy of Keishikaryukotsuboreito and Vasodilator. The abstract book of the 11th annual meeting for Study of Urological Kampo. 1994; 1: 32-6 (in Japanese).
14. Sato, Y., H. Horita, H. Adachi, N. Suzuki, H. Tanda, Y. Kumamoto and T. Tsukamoto. Effect of oral administration of prostaglandin E1 on erectile dysfunction. Br. J. Urol. 1997; 80: 772-775.
15. Naao K. The present status of drug therapy for impotence. Sexual Science. 1994; 3: 66-9 (in Japanese).

Editorial Comment

In this chapter, Drs. Miyagawa and Okuyama present a comprehensive summary of Kampo medicine and sexual medicine in Japan. Although Kampo practice originated in China and was introduced into Japan as traditional Chinese medicine in the 6th century via Korea, Kampo medicine in Japan was modified to adapt to the environment and cultural practices of Japan in the 17th and 18th centuries (the Edo era). Kampo was temporarily eliminated from official medical education during the Meiji restoration when modern Western medicine was introduced to Japan mainly from Germany. However, many Japanese people support the use of traditional Oriental medicine, because Kampo medicine is based on natural philosophy and physiology in humans. At present, 147 Kampo products (as formulae) are available and about one billion US dollars are spent on Kampo products in Japan.

The authors divided this chapter into 4 sections: the History of Kampo in Japan, Current status of Kampo medicine in sexual medicine and its efficacy and side effects, Future trends of Kampo medicine in sexual medicine and the stance to research work for new drugs from plant gene resources in Japan, and Prevalence of sexual medicine in Japan. After presenting a comprehensive explanation in each section, they describe several representative drugs for sexual medicine. Yohinbin is the only approved OTC (over-the counter) drug for psychogenic erectile dysfunction. Although Hachimijiogan, which is composed of eight crude herbs, is approved for the treatment of benign prostate hyperplasia, this Kampo medicine may have some favorable effects on erectile function. Saikokaryukotsuboreito and Keishikaryukotsuboreito are both derivatives from Ryukotsuboreito, which is used for psychogenic erectile dysfunction, and used differentially according to the Kampo diagnosis "Sho." Goshajinkigan is a traditional Chinese medicine formulation composed of ten herbs. Hochuekkito is used not only for male infertility, but also for erectile dysfunction. The proposed mechanisms of action of Hochuekkito are its vasodilatory effects and sedative effects.

Japanese doctors recognize the Kampo diagnosis "Sho." and then choose the most suitable formula. Although the concept of "Sho" comes from the Zheng of traditional Chinese medicine, "Sho" is simplified according to Kampo theory. "Sho" is the patient' s symptoms at a given moment composed of Qi (well-being, energy, illness, vigor), Blood, and Water.

Kampo is now widely used in clinical practice in Japan and has been integrated into modern medicine, because Kampo medicine takes a holistic approach by maintaining the body' s overall balance and function. However, many components of the herbs contained in Kampo have complex pharmacological effects, which may induce toxic effects. Indeed, several adverse effects of Kampo have been reported. It is unclear how Kampo medicines are quoted and evaluated for efficacy and adverse effects. In the era of evidence-based medicine, Kampo medicine should also be evaluated according to clinical practice guidelines.

Mikio Namiki, M.D., Ph.D.
Kanazawa, Japan

Chapter 6

Korean Perspective I

Current Update of Phytotherapy for Sexual Dysfunction in Korea

Jong Kwan Park, Chen Zhao

I. Background

1. Introduction

Between 30-50% of the adult population in industrialized nations use some form of complementary and/or alternative medicine to prevent or treat a variety of health related problems[1, 2]. Sexual dysfunction is the most common disease in the aging male. Erectile dysfunction and premature ejaculation are two of the most frequent disorders in male sexual dysfunction. Erectile dysfunction is defined as the inability of the male to achieve an erect penis as part of the overall multifaceted process of male sexual function[3]. Aging is a complex process with multiple alterations to the physiological structure and functional responses of the penis. Premature ejaculation is the persistent or recurrent ejaculation with minimal stimulation before, on, or shortly after penetration and before the person wishes, which causes marked distress or interpersonal difficulty[4]. In a recent Korean epidemiological study, aging is an independent risk factor of erectile dysfunction and the study revealed that the prevalence of erectile dysfunction and premature ejaculation was 32.4% and 11% (intravaginal ejaculation latency time, IELT< 2 min), respectively[5].

2. Herbal medicine and functional food in Korea

Asia, especially Korea has been influenced by Chinese herbal medicine for many years with a

Jong Kwan Park, M.D., Ph.D.
Department of Urology, Medical School, Chonbuk National University, 634-18, Keumam-dong, Dukjin-gu, Jeonju, Jeonbuk 561-712, Korea. Tel: +82-63-250-1510, E-mail: rain@jbnu.ac.kr

long history of herbal/traditional and complementary medicine. The Asian region has a high usage to treat a variety of diseases. In Korea, the school of oriental medicine has a long history of 60 years (since 1948) and produced many herbal doctors and hospitals and also kept their own medical delivery system. Hospitals and clinics of oriental medicine have treated patients with complementary medicine. The prescription of herbal medicine (except functional foods) regulated by the Korean Foods and Drug administration (KFDA). Herbal medicines for a variety of diseases utilize a number of fruits and vegetables, acupuncture and moxibustion and the use of these materials in herbal medicine remains another important field of medical activity in Korea. In Korea herbal medicine has been delivered by oriental physicians.

Functional food has been supplied to the people followed by KFDA. The Korean government also regulates functional foods. Sales of Over the Counter (OTC) functional foods are thought to be approaching 770 million dollars[2]. There are two kinds of functional foods in the market, individual approval and notice forms. In notice form of functional food, 37 kinds have been registered. In individual approval form, 181 kinds have been registered. The individual approval form accounts for of 1% (27 million dollars) of the whole market for functional food.

3. Herbal medicine and functional food for erectile dysfunction

Men who suffer sexual dysfunction or women who have a husband with erectile dysfunction are particularly interested in the use of herbal or complementary medicine. They believe that herbal or complementary medicine is natural and, not only treats isolated symptoms but also maintains general well-being. It is often perceived that as a natural medicine, herbal medicine or functional food usually does not have significant side effects and is so much safer than western style medicine. The safety and efficacy of herbal medicine is most often based on anecdotal evidence, which was evaluated by informal longitudinal clinical studies performed by many ancestors. The mechanism of herbal medicine is unknown and not explained in the clinical study. The herbal medicine provides general health benefits beyond those related to erectile dysfunction. The Doctors of herbal medicine have treated patients with erectile dysfunction with herbal medicine such as Korean fresh ginseng, Korean white ginseng, Korean Red Ginseng, *Rubus Coreanus*, *Cornus officinalis*, Kugija, and mixtures. All kinds of herbal medicine have been referenced from 'Donguibogam' written by Heo Jun[6].

Western style medication gives a quick response, however herbal medicine on the contrary responds slower when used for treatment. Western style medicine is used as a single agent, however herbal medicine has been used with a mixture of many kinds of medicines, which has an additive or similar effect. People have thought that herbal medicine or functional food use different mechanisms to enhanced body function when it is in critical imbalance or deficiency in proper function. In erectile dysfunction, a cocktail method has been developed and used to treat the patient. The mixture targets different aspects of the mechanism of erection an libido.

4. Pharmacodynamic of phytochemicals

Herbal plants contain chemical compounds, vitamins, plant-hormones and minerals which are needed for a growing plant. These products protect the plant from noxious environments or harmful insects, which have to live together. Human bodies and animals need phytochemical compounds, hormones, vitamins and active elements to achieve a balanced metabolism for healthy living. The philosophy of using herbal medicine is to adopt and imitate the natural pharmacodynamic action that is already within the plant. Purifying phytochemicals to a single agent would imitate a synthetic chemical[7]. Western style medication may not look at the totality of the disease and instead focus on an instant erection. The herbal medicine acts by a dynamic interactive complicated process. Therefore, the purification of herbal medicine sometimes loses or weakens the effect compared to original phytochemicals or herbal medicine mixed.

II. Kinds of Herbal Medicine

1. Korean ginseng

Ginseng has been an essential herb in traditional Chinese medicine for many years. Ginseng cultivated in Korea is divided into three types, depending on how it is processed. Fresh ginseng (less than 4 years old), white ginseng (4-6 years old and dried after peeling) and red ginseng (harvested when 6 years old, steamed and dried)[8]. Traditionally ginseng has been used to restore and enhance the normal well-being of the body. Effects of ginseng reacts with the central nervous system, metabolism, immune function, and cardiovascular system. The principal active compounds in ginseng are ginsenosides, saponin glycosides. Over 20 different ginsenosides have been identified from extracts of the roots, leaves, and seeds of the ginseng plant.

Animal study: Ginsengs have been reported to enhance significantly copulatory behavior parameters in male rats and mice[9, 10]. Oral doses of powdered ginseng root sufficient to alter sexual behavior in male rats were as low as 10 mg/kg body weight and significant changes in libido were measured within one week of daily oral ginseng treatment[10]. Daily treatment of male mice with an extract of Korean ginseng (25-100 mg/kg, ip) or ginsenoside Rg1 (2.5-10 mg/kg, ip) produced a dose-dependent increase in the number of mice displaying copulatory behaviors (mounting, intromission, and penis licking). However, ginsenosides Rb1, Rb2, and Ro have no effect in sexual behavior. These data suggest that specific ginsenosides may be responsible for ginseng mediating actions on copulatory behavior[11].

2. Korean red ginseng (Panax ginseng)

Korean red ginseng belongs to Araliaceae and is grown in Korea and China. Korean red ginseng is one of the most commonly used ginseng products in Korea. There are many brand names of Korean red ginseng. Korean red ginseng contains numerous active compounds, the major active ingredients being triterpene glycosides known as ginsenosides[12].

The ginsenosides relax the penile smooth muscle though by nitric oxide cyclic GMP pathway, which may be related with improvement of erectile function and vascular endothelial function is improved by increasing the concentration of nitric oxide. Korean red ginseng increases nitric oxide (NO). The yields for water extract of Korean red ginseng extract from 100% ethanol extract of Korean red ginseng were 4.76%. The water extract of Korean red ginseng extract contains Ginsenoside-Re, -Rf, -Rg1, -Rg2, -Rg3 and other minor ginsenosides and components[13].

1) Animal study: In laboratory data, Korean red ginseng causes a dose-dependent relaxation by increasing of NO from corporal cavernosal tissue and vaginal smooth muscle of rabbit[14, 15].

2) Human study: In a clinical trial, approximately 60% of the patients taking ginseng had a therapeutic effect versus 30% for the placebo and drug groups. In randomized clinical studies, Korean red ginseng has beneficial effects in psychogenic erectile dysfunction[16]. The Korean red ginseng has the ability to increase NO levels or reduce fatigue, insomnia and depression[17, 18]. In another study, the dose of oral ginseng was 1,000 mg three times daily and the treatment for 8 weeks significantly improved IIEF scores compared to placebo (Ginseng; 16.4 ± 2.9 to 21.0 ± 6.3 versus control; 17.0 ± 3.1 to 17.7 ± 5.6). 66.6% reported improved erection, significant in the global efficacy question[19, 20]. Side effects of Korean red ginseng included headache, hypertension, tachycardia, insomnia, drowsiness and spontaneous regression during the first month were observed in 3.7% and delayed ejaculation was noticed in 7.4% during the second and third month of treatment[21].

3. Extract of tissue cultured Korean mountain ginseng

1) Human study: 1 g of extract of tissue cultured Korean mountain ginseng twice per day for 8 weeks significantly improved total IIEF from 29.78 ± 13.14 to 39.86 ± 15.29. Erectile function domain, orgasmic function domain, and sexual desire domain in tissue cultured Korean mountain ginseng extract group were significantly improved compared to the placebo group (11.89 ± 5.89 to 16.37 ± 7.08, 4.09 ± 2.49 to 5.32 ± 2.74, 4.32 ±1.59 to 5.85 ± 2.03, respectively). Minor headache was developed in 4.6% of the cultured Korean mountain ginseng group[22].

4. Ginko biloba

Ginkgo, like ginseng, is mentioned in the traditional Chinese pharmacopoeia. The main indications for ginkgo are peripheral vascular disease such as intermittent claudication and, more important, cerebral insufficiency. Ginko extract can improve vascular perfusion, and in German data, that improved chronic cerebrovascular insufficiency[23].

Ginkgo biloba extract contains flavonid glycosides, mainly composed of kaempferol, quercetin isorhamnetin with glucose or rhamnose and characteristic terpenes of ginkgolides, bilobalides[24]. These have acomplicated pharmacological action and improve not only damage to the vessel walls but also damage to the tension f blood vessels.

1) Animal study: In vivo study, ginkgo biloba extract relaxed corpus cavernosal tissue of human and rabbit in response to subfractions of nonginkgolide nonflavonoid fraction in a dose-dependent manner. However, ED 50 is too high and they suggested further fractionation should be needed[25].

2) Human study: In a clinical study, an extract of Ginko biloba, 60 mg for 12 to 18 months, blood perfusion improved after 6-8 weeks. 50% of the patients with erectile dysfunction regained erectile function after 6 months administration[26]. In a clinical study, sexual dysfunction caused by the use of elective serotonin reuptake inhibitor (SSRI) antidepressants improved in 76% in men when ginkgo extract, 209 mg/day was taken for approximately 1 month. Ginkgo also improves other sexual function, including enhanced desire, excitement, orgasm, and resolution[27]. Ginkgo can produce adverse events such as bleeding, nausea, headache, gastroenteric upset, diarrhea and anxiety

5. Rubus coreanus

Rubus coreanus, is used commonly in the treatment of several diseases in Korea. Rubus coreanus grows across the whole area of Korea. Rubus coreanus is a perennial shrub that is distributed in the southern part of Korea. The season also is very important for the efficacy. The most effective Rubus coreanus is reaped from the local area of Kochang. Fried unripe fruits of Rubus coreanus have been used for centuries as a herbal medicine, the safety has been proven in some degree. This crude Rubus coreanus is used for the management of impotence, spermatorrhea, enuresis, asthma, allergic diseases and it also has been used as a stomachic and tonic in Korea[28, 29].

1) Animal study: Extract of unripe Rubus coreanus relaxed the contracted rabbit penile corpus cavernosum smooth muscle by phenylephrine. The extract of 1, 3, 10, and 30 mg/mL unripe Rubus coreanus relaxed the penile smooth muscle by 8.3 ± 1.5%, 17.0 ± 4.4%, 69.7 ± 9.6% and 128.0 ± 13.9% in corporal tension respectively.

2) Human study: Controlled clinical study is going in the patients with erectile dysfunction in Korea.

6. Epimedium koreanum

Epimedium koreaum is used in traditional Korean herbal medicine as a potent enhancer of erectile function. Icariin is the main active component and has many biological effects, such as improving cardiovascular function, hormone regulation, immunological function modulation, and anti-tumor activity[30].

Animal study: In the study of sexual behavior in rat, the amounts of Epimedium koreanum are 300 mg/body weight per day and 600 mg/body weight per day for 10 days. In the results, the number of intromission increased to 23.3 ± 2.6 in 300 mg/kg body weight per day and to 20.1 ± 2.3 in 750 mg/kg body weight per day. The number of ejaculations increased from 2.6 ± 0.4 in E-01 group compared with 1.1 ± 0.3 in placebo group. Latent ejaculation period reduced 9.8 ± 1.5 min in E-01 group compared with 14.2 ± 1.8 min in placebo group[30].

7. Male silkworm extract (Nuegra™)

Nuegra is composed of male silkworm moth (Bombyx mori), Acantohpanax centicosus, Schizandra chinensis, Rubus Coreanum, L-glutamine, freeze-dried royal jelly, Lycium chinense Mill., tocopherol. Nuegra is a combined natural herbal product and enhances of masculinity without side effects. This is produced by prescription in Donguibogam and has been used for young and old men with reduced physical function, or strength, weak urinary function, or complaints off fatigue.

1) Animal study: In rats, Nuegra increased male hormone by 32.8% compared with 9.9% inthe sildenafil administered group. The nitric oxide content increased by 16.6% with Nuegra compared with 5.4% in the sildenafil administered group. Sperm count increased by 41% with Nuegra compared with 11.9% in the sildenafil administered group[31].

2) Human study: In a clinical study with 168 volunteers, they used 2 capsules 3 times per day for 4 weeks and they administered 3 capsules 3 times per day from 4 week for 2 weeks in the volunteer, who did not improve to 2 capsules 3 times per day. In 80 volunteers followed by per protocol, Nuegra increased testosterone from 4.4 nmol/L to 4.9 nmol/L. FSH increased from 7.7 mIU/mL to 8.0 mIU/mL without significance. There was a statistically significant improvement in the symptoms of fatigue, erectile dysfunction, impotence, weak urinary stream, muscular atrophy, and sleep disturbance from 2 weeks after administration. Nuegra produce mild adverse effects such as digestive difficulty, sputum production, temporary chest palpitation, drowsiness and increased stool frequency[32].

8. Garlic

Garlic has long been used as a spice and has been reported to possess medical and pharmacologic properties. Garlic has hypoglycemic, anticoagulative, antihypertensive and hypolipidemic properties. Garlic may enhance hormone regulated protein anabolism. There is no clinical data on improving erectile function, although garlic has been used for erectile dysfunction as a results of word of mouth.

Animal study: 0.8 g / 100 g body weight for 28 days increased testosterone content in the testis and decreased plasma corticosterone concentration.

9. Mixture of multiple plants

1) *Chonbo-204®*

Chonbo-204® is based on the Ojayounjonghwon described in 'Dong ui bo gam' and the oriental concepts of Yin and Yang[33, 34]. The major ingredients of the herbal formula are seeds obtained from five plants: *Cornus officinalis* Sieb. Et Zucc. (Cornaceae, 32%), *Rubus coreanus* Miq. (Rosaceae, 16%), *Cuscuta chinensis* Lam. (Convolvulaceae, 16%), *Lycium chinense* Mill (Solanaceae, 32%), and *Schizandra chinensis* Baill. (Schisandraceae, 4%) in different ratios (KH_2O_4: Korea Patent No.0364684). Mixture of the dried seeds of five plants is extracted with tap water (0.25 g/mL) for 3h by boiling. The extracts are filtered and concentrated in vacuum, and then lyophilized. This product was developed as a health supplement by Korea Medical Science Institute Co. Ltd., who is developing oriental herbal medicines. However it is not used anymore for human.

1) Animal study: In aged rats with diabetes mellitus, HF of 100 mg/kg body weight per day for 10 days restored the severely reduced peak intracavernous pressures. The penile expression levels of nNOS, eNOS and CaV-1, Ca^{2+}-dependent NOS activities and cGMP concentrations were increased significantly in the HF-treated rats. The extraction from 5 components was used with 100, 300 mg/kg body weight per day for 4 weeks in hypertensive rats. The intracavernous pressure/mean arterial pressure ratio was markedly increased in the treated group with KH-204 compared with placebo group. Endothelial and neuronal nitric oxide synthases were significantly increased in the treated group with KH-204 compared with the placebo group[35].

2) Human study: The commercial product (Chonbo-204®) is registered as a patent name of 'a herbal formula for improvement in penile erection and lasting effects' and is available as small tablets prepared with a water-extracted mixture.

Herbal formula of 30 g per day for 4 weeks significantly improved total IIEF from 42.45 ± 7.25 to 53.58 ± 11.87 compared with 41.90 ± 17.37 to 48.48 ± 17.22 in placebo group. Erectile function domain and overall satisfaction domain were significantly improved in herbal formula group compared with the placebo group. The level of side effect was 7.5% in both groups. The side effects were headache 2.5% and nausea 5%[34].

2) *SA1*

SA1 is a mixture of 9 Oriental herbs (Korean red ginseng, fermented soybean, Tribulus terrestris, Fructus Rubi, Fructus Lycii, Semen Cuscutae, Dioscorea Rhizome, Fructus Corni and Fructus Crataegi). These herbs are widely used as energizers and vitalizers in the indigenous system of medicine and have been alleged to improve sexual function in men. *In vitro*, SA1 significantly enhanced the relaxation responses to acetylcholine. SA1 significantly increased the ratio of intracavernous pressure to mean arterial pressure. The male rats used to examine the copulatory behavior were administered either the placebo or SA1 (30, 100, 300, 600 mg/kg) orally for 2 weeks. There was an overall increase in the copulatory behavior parameters in the SA1-treated rats[36].

10. SS Cream™

SS-cream is a topical agent derived from the extracts of nine natural products (Ginseng Radix Alba, Angelicae Gigantic Radix, Cistanchis Herba, Zanthoxylli Fructs, Torilidis Semen, Asiasari Radix, Caryophylli Flos, Cinnamoni Cortex, and Bufonis Veneum) for the treatment of premature ejaculation.

1) Animal study: SS-Cream prolonged mean latency of somatosensory evoked potential from 21.57 ± 1.86 msec to 23.09 ± 0.85 and 27.49 ± 2.4 in 30 and 60 minutes after application of SS-cream, respectively. SS-cream also decreased mean amplitude somatosensory evoked potential 1.83 ± 0.07 and 1.72 ± 0.05 uV in 30 and 60 minutes after application of SS-cream, respectively[37].

2) Human study: In a Phase III clinical study, the efficacy and safety of SS-cream was evaluated in 106 volunteers who had suffered from premature ejaculation. Mean ejaculatory latency time prolonged to 10.92 ± 0.92 minutes in the SS-cream group compared with 2.45 ± 0.29 in the placebo group. The percentage of patients who prolonged ejaculatory latency time over 2 minutes in the placebo and SS-cream groups was 15.09 and 79.81%, respectively. SS-cream had a sense of mild local burning and pain[38].

REFERENCES

1. Astin JA. Why patients use alternative medicine: results of a national study. JAMA 1998;279:1548-53.
2. KFDA. Analysis and prospect for the market of health functional foods and presentation of strategy for industry development in Korea. 2007 Report:82-4.
3. NIH Consensus Conference. Impotence. NIH consensus development panel on impotence. JAMA 1993;270:83-90.
4. American Psychiatric Associatin. Diagnostic And Statistical Manual of Mental Disoeders, DSM-IV, 4th Ed. Washington D.C., 1994, pp.509-11.
5. Ahn TY, Park JK, Lee SW, Hong JH, Park NC, Kim JJ, Park K, Park H, Hyun JS. Prevalence and risk factors for erectile dysfunction in Korean men: results of an epidemiological study. J Sex Med 2007;4:1269-76.
6. Huer, J., 1613. Ojayounjonghwon. Donguibogam (New edition, 1998), Namsandang, Korea, p. 603.
7. Adimoelja A. Phytochemicals and the breakthrough of traditional herbs in the management of sexual dysfunctions. Int J Androl 2000;23 (Suppl 2):82-4.
8. Yun TK. Panax ginseng--a non-organ-specific cancer preventive? Lancet Oncol 2001;2:49-55.
9. Kim C, Choi H, Kim CC, Kim JK, Kim MS. Influence of ginseng on mating behavior of male rats. Am J Chin Med 1976;4:163-8.
10. Murphy LL, Cadena RS, Ch ez D, Ferraro JS. Effect of American ginseng (Panax quinquefolium) on male copulatory behavior in the rat. Physiol Behav 1998;64:445-50.
11. Murphy LL, Lee TJ. Ginseng, sex behavior, and nitric oxide. Ann N Y Acad Sci 2002;962:372-7.
12. Kim YM, Namkoong S, Yun YG, Hong HD, Lee YC, Ha KS, Lee H, Kwon HJ, Kwon YG, Kim YM. Water extract of Korean red ginseng stimulates angiogenesis by activating the PI3K/Akt-dependent ERK1/2 and eNOS pathways in human umbilical vein endothelial cells. Biol Pharm Bull 2007;30:1674-9.
13. Kim JH, Hahm DH, Yang DC, Kim JH, Lee HJ, Shim I. Effect of crude saponin of Korean red ginseng on high-fat diet-induced obesity in the rat. J Pharmacol Sci 2005;97:124-31.
14. Choi YD, Xin ZC, Choi HK. Effect of Korean red ginseng on the rabbit corpus cavernosal smooth muscle. Int J Impot Res 1998;10:37-43.
15. Sun-Ouck Kim, Min Kyung Kim, Myeong Jeong Chae, Hwi Young Kim, Jong Kwan Park and Kwangsung Park. Effect of Koran red gingeng of the relaxation of clitoral corpus cavernosum in rabbit. Kor J Androl 2006;24:29-34.
16. Jang DJ, Lee MS, Shin BC, Lee YC, Ernst E. Red ginseng for treating erectile dysfunction: a systematic review. Br J Clin Pharmacol 2008;66:444-50.
17. Choi HK, Seong DH, Rha KH. Clinical efficacy of Korean red ginseng for erectile dysfunction. Int J Impot Res 1995;7:181-6.
18. Choi YD, Rha KH, Choi HK. In vitro and in vivo experimental effect of Korean red ginseng on erection. J Urol 1999;162:1508-11.
19. Hong B, Ji YH, Hong JH, Nam KY, Ahn TY.A double-blind crossover study evaluating the efficacy of Korean red ginseng in patients with erectile dysfunction: a preliminary report. J Urol 2002;168:2070-3.
20. de Andrade E, de Mesquita AA, Claro Jde A, de Andrade PM, Ortiz V, Paranhos M, Srougi M. Study of the efficacy of Korean red ginseng in the treatment of erectile dysfunction. Asian J Androl 2007;9:241-4.
21. Andrade EM, Messina LE, Alaron G, et al. Korean red ginseng in the treatment of erectile dysfunction: a prospective controlled double-blind clinical trial [abstract 1419]. J Urol 2003;169(Suppl 4):380.
22. Kim TH, Lee HL, Hahn EJ, Paek Kee-Yoeup, Park JK, Youn NY. The effects of tissue cultured mountain ginseng (Panax Ginseng C. A. Meyer) extract on male patients with erectile dysfunction. Asian J Androl 2009; in pressing

23. Moyad MA, Barada JH, Lue TF, Mulhall JP, Goldstein I, Fawzy A. Sexual Medicine Society Nutraceutical Committee. Prevention and treatment of erectile dysfunction using lifestyle changes and dietary supplements: what works and what is worthless, part II. Urol Clin North Am 2004;31:259-73.
24. Kleijnen J, Knipschild P. Ginkgo biloba. Lancet 1992;340:1136-9.
25. Siroka R, Sohn MH, Engelke B et al. Randomized placebo-controlled study on the effects of oral treatment with Ginkgo biloba extract in patients withd erectile dysfunction [abstract917]. J Urol 1998;159;240A.
26. Balon R. Ginkgo biloba for antidepressant-induced sexual dysfunction? J Sex Marital Ther 1999;25:1-2.
27. Paick JS, Lee JH. An experimental study of the effect of ginkgo biloba extract on the human and rabbit corpus cavernosum tissue. J Urol 1996;156:1876-80.
28. Lee SJ. 1996. Korean Folk Medicine. Publishing Center of Seoul National University: Seoul.
29. Moon GS. 1991. Constituents and Uses of Medicinal Herbs. Ilweolseogak: Seoul. 310-311.
30. Makarova MN, Pozharitskaya ON, Shikov AN, Tesakova SV, Makarov VG, Tikhonov VP. Effect of lipid-based suspension of Epimedium koreanum Nakai extract on sexual behavior in rats. J Ethnopharmacol 2007;114:412-6.
31. Ryu KS, Ahn MY, Lee HS, Kim I, Kim JW, Kim SH, Choi JH. The tonic effect of the extract from male silkworm (Bombyx mori L.) moth on rat. Intl J Indust Entomol 2002;5:123-6.
32. Kim DC, Kim YW, Park MS, Suh JK, Lee DS, Lee SH, Chun BH, Jun YK, Jeong BD, Ryu KS. Effects of the Nuegra from male silkworm extract on enhancement of the masculine function and activation of overall physical function. Intl J Indust Entomol 2002;5:109-22.
33. Park CS, Ryu SD, Hwang SY. Elevation of intracavernous pressure and NO-cGMP activity by a new herbal formula in penile tissues of aged and diabetic rats. J Ethnopharmacol 2004;94:85-92.
34. Kam SC, Choi SM, Jeh SU, Lee SH, Hwa JS, Jung KH, Kang CW, Hyun JS. Efficacy and safety of a herbal formula that mainly consists of Cornus Officinalis for erectile dysfunction: a double-blind, placebo-controlled study. Kor J Urol 2007; 48:741-7.
35. Sohn DW, Kim HY, Kim SD, Lee EJ, Kim HS, Kim JK, Hwang SY, Cho YH, Kim SW. Elevation of intracavernous pressure and NO-cGMP activity by a new herbal formula in penile tissues of spontaneous hypertensive male rats. J Ethnopharmacol 2008;120:176-80.
36. Park SW, Lee CH, Shin DH, Bang NS, Lee SM. Effect of SA1, a herbal formulation, on sexual behavior and penile erection. Biol Pharm Bull 2006;29:1383-6.
37. Xin ZC, Choi YD, Choi HK. Somatosensory evoked (SEP) and effect of SS-cream on rabbit. Kor J Urol 1996;37:867-71.
38. Choi HK, Jung GW, Moon KH, Xin ZC, Choi YD, Lee WH, Rha KH, Choi YJ, Kim DK. Clinical study of SS-cream in patients with lifelong premature ejaculation. Urology 2000;55:257-61.

Chapter 7

Korean Perspective II

Herbal Phytotherapy for Sexual Dysfunction in Korea

Jong Hee Park

I. Background

1. Introduction

From ancient times, human beings have resorted to various methods for the purpose of stimulating sexual desire and strengthen sexual function. To attain these goals, they have used not only aromatics, smoking, painting and music that can stimulate the nerve system, but also warm bath, sexual devices, etc. in physical terms, medicinal animals, plants and minerals in medical terms, and specific animals and plants, spices, alcoholic drinks, etc. in terms of food and drink.

If a human body is healthy, sex is also healthy, but a tired body and weakened health make it impossible to enjoy a satisfactory sex. Therefore, if we get rid of fatigue and improve our physical power, we will naturally feel sexual impulses that correspond to our ages and health extents. As a healthy stomach makes any food and drink digested and completely absorbed, so will a healthy sexual vitality gives greater satisfaction to a beautiful life.

A drug good for a vigorous sexual life must be helpful to physical health as well by boosting health, energy and rejuvenation, so a true energy booster is not a drug that simply stimulates the nerve system or a part of a human body. Consequently, s true energy booster refers to a medicine that can revitalize the functions of the whole body, promote health, stimulate seminal vesicle and thus strengthen sexual power. In Korea and China, studies have been made of energy boosters in

---

Jong Hee Park, Ph.D.
College of Pharmacy, Pusan national University, 30 Jangjeon-dong, Geumjeong-gu Busan 609-735, Korea. Tel: +82-51-510-2806 / 011-577-2806, Fax: +82-51-513-6754, E-mail: abpark@pusan.ac.kr

such terms since early times. Their results include all the invigorants seen in Korean and Chinese literatures on herbal medicine. We may refer to all the drugs for boosting health, energy, rejuvenation, perpetual youth and longevity as energy boosters. The natural drugs, including Korean herb medicines, have had their values recognized by numerous people that have tried them throughout a long period of about four thousand years.

This chapter is designed to selectively introduce the natusal drugs that have demonstrated their efficacies in boosting health, energy, rejuvenation and perpetual youth. Such natural drugs were originally developed China, but have been also in full bloom since they were introduced into Korea together with Buddhism. In terms of effect, they have been fully proven, thus establishing themselves as necessary medicines. Nevertheless, some drugs have not yet verified in terms of contemporary pharmaceutical chemistry. The following are herbal medicines that are mainly used to treat sexual dysfunction.

II. Korean Crude drugs in Sexual Medicine

1. Ginseng Radix

Ginseng is the most valued herb widely used in Korea, as well as in other Asian countries, especially China and Japan.

Origin: It is the dried root of *Panax ginseng* C. A. Meyer, Alariaceae. Wild ones are called wild moutain ginseng, while cultivated ones are called garden ginseng. Garden ginseng are two kinds. One is dried raw ginseng and another is steamed red ginseng. Wild mountain ginseng are mainly produced in Korean moutain and Jilin Province of China.

Distribution: Garden ginseng are mainly produced in Korea, China, and Japan.

Chemical constituents: Garden ginseng contains many valuable ingredients.

1. Essential oil; panacene, β-elemene
2. Monosaccaride; D-glucose, D-fructose, disaccaride; sucrose, maltose, trisaccharide-A, trisaccharide-B, trisacchsride-C
3. Saponins; ginsenoside R_0, a, b_1, b_2, c, d, e, f, g_1, g_2, oleanolic acid, 20-s-protopanaxidiol, 20-s-protopanaxatriol
4. Peptides
5. Antioxidants, fatty acids, alcohols, and vitamins.

Pharmacodynamic actions:

1. Sexual development

   For thousands of years, Korean folk medicine has used ginseng as a rejuvenating drug. Traditional Korean medical text claimed that ginseng is a drug which enriches the juice and

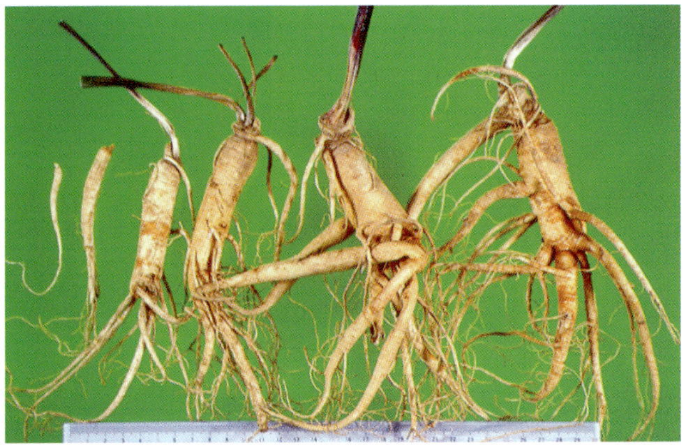

Figure 1. Ginseng from Korea

blood of the body.

2. Cardiovascular system

   Administration of ginseng to rats and rabbits with hypertension induced by partial renal artery constriction also produced a hypotensive effect.

3. Central nervous system

   Sakai reported several effects of ginseng extract, including a tranquilizing effect on the CNS.

4. Endocrine system

   Ginseng extract is the stimulating effect on the hypothalmopituitary suprarenal system.

5. Antidiuretic effect

   Ginseng extract is the stimulating effect on the anterior pituitary and increase secretion of ACTH, TSH, and gonadotropic hormones.

6. Metabolism

   Ginseng extract is the stimulating effect on carbohydrate, fat, and RNA and DNA metabolism.

7. Anticancer activity

   Ginseng extract can inhibit several types of cancer cell growth *in vitro*.

Indication:

1. The drug is used for the symptoms of shortness of breath, mental fatigue, faint and indistinct pulse.
2. The drug is prescribed for the symptoms of poor appetite, loose stool, dyspnea and spontaneous perspiration due to deficiency of the lung and kidney.
3. The drug is used for the treatment of insomnia, amnesia, palpitation.
4. The drug is used for the treatment of thirst due to impairment of body fluid and diabetes.

Administration and dosage:

5-10 g of ginseng are decocted solitary with slow fire. Decoctions of ginseng and other crude drugs are usually mixed together for internal use; 1-2g of powder are taken orally, 2-3 times each day.

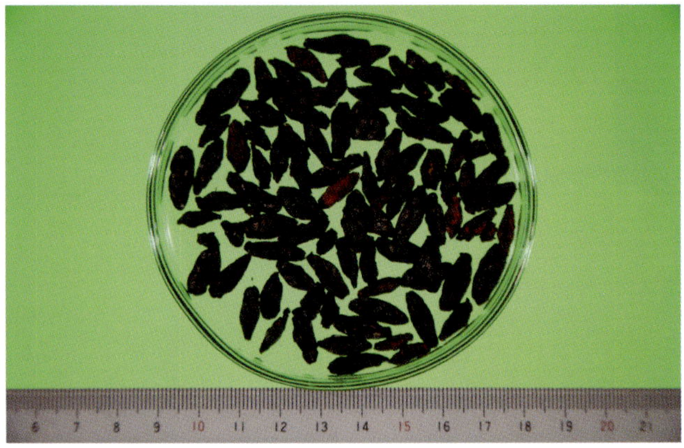

Figure 2. Wolfberry Fruit from Korea

2. Wolfberry fruit

Lycii Fructus

Origin: It is the ripe, dried the mature fruit of *Lycium chinensis* Mill., Solanaceae.

Distribution: It is mainly produced in Jin do, Shin An (Korea) and Quinghai, Gansu provinces (China).

Characteristics: Wolfberry fruit is spindle-shaped and slightly flat. Its surface is bright red or dark red in color. It is odorless, sweet and slightly sour in taste.

Chemical constituents: Wolfberry fruit contains betaine, vitamin A, B, B_2, C, zeaxanthin, physalein, carotene and polysaccharide.

Pharmacodynamic actions:

1. A water-based extract of Wolfberry fruit can lower blood pressure, blood sugar and stimulate the heart.
2. Wolfberry fruit include an increase in leukocyte count.

Indication:

1. It has the efficacies of nourishing the liver and kidney, and improving acuity of vision. It is usually prescribed for the patients with deficiency of the liver-yin(陰) and kidney-yin(陰).
2. It is effective in the treatment of hectic fever and cough due to yin(陰) deficiency.
3. Seminal emissions.

Administration and dosage:

6-12 g of the wolfberry fruit are decocted, take the decoction daily.

3. Angelica root

Angelicae Radix

Other name: Seung Geum Cho

Origin:

Korea: It is dried root of *Angelica gigas* Nakai, Umbelliferae.

China: It is dried root of *Angelica sinensis* (Oliv.) Diels.

Japan: It is dried root of *Angelica acutiloba* Kitagawa or *A. acutiloba* Kitagawa var. *sugiyamae* Hikino.

Distribution:

Angelica gigas Nakai is mainly prodeced in Gang Won Do of Korea.

Angelica sinensis (Oliv.) Diels is mainly prodeced in Gansu, Sichuan, Yunnan, Hubei provinces of China.

Angelica acutiloba Kitagawa is mainly prodeced in Japan.

Chemical constituents:

Angelica gigas Nakai contains a decursin, nodakenin, decursinol, nodakenetin, umbelliferone, imperatorun, and β-sitosterol.

Angelica acutiloba Kitagawa contains a ligustilide, n-butyllidenephthalide, n-butylphthalide, sedanoic acid lactone, senkyunolide E, F, H, I, angeloylsenkyunolide, bergapten, isopimpinellin, xanthotoxin, scopoletin, umbelliferone, and p-cymene.

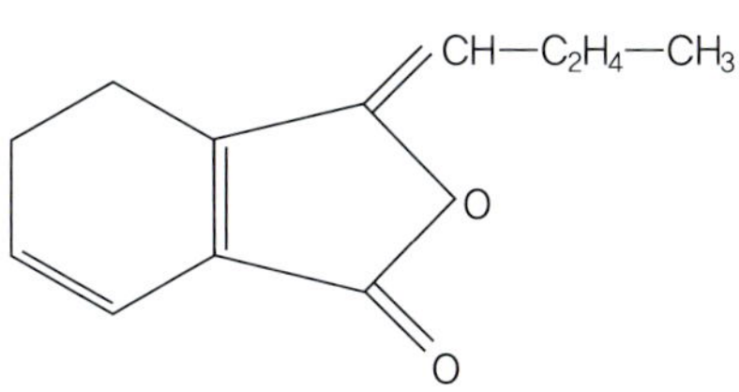

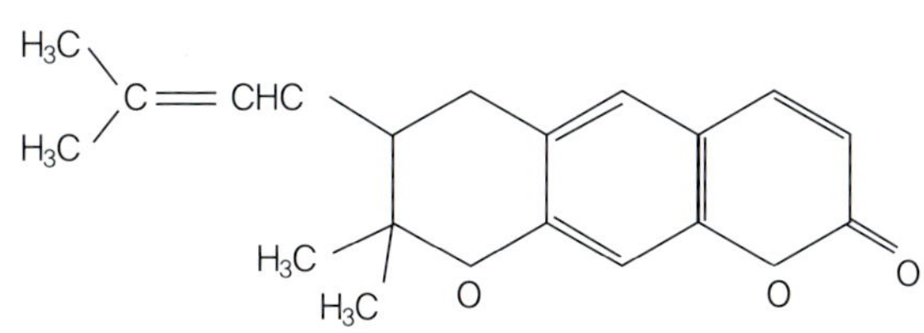

Pharmacodynamic action:

1. It has both stimulating and inhibiting actions on uterine muscles.
2. The volatile oil of Angelica Root inhibits brain activity, thus having the effect of sedation.
3. It promotes urine excretion.

Indication:

1. Irregular menstruation, amenorrhea and menorrhalgia.
2. Promoting blood circulation to stop pain.
3. Anemia
4. Headache, abdominal pain, chest pain, coronary heart disease.

Administration and dosage:

5-15 g, decocted in water for an oral dose.

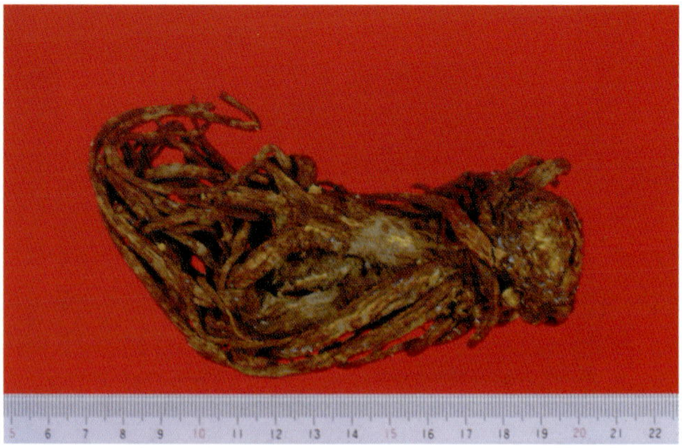

Figure 3. Angelica Root from Korea

4. Eucommia bark

Eucommiae Cortex

Origin: It is the dried the trunk bark of *Eucommia ulmoides* Oliv., Eucommiaceae.

Distribution: It is mainly produced in Guizhou, Hubei, Sichun and Yunnan of China, and Korea.

Characteristics: Eucommia Bark is crisp in texture and easy to break. The boken section is connected by silver-white, elastic, fine glue silks.

Chemical constituents:

Eucommia bark contains resin (7%), gutta-percha (2-6.5%), iridoid and lignan.

iridoid : ulmoside (=aucubigenin-1-β-isomaltose), aucubin, harpagide acetate, geniposide, geniposidic acid.

lignans : eucommin A, (+)-1-hydroxypinoresinol-4,4'-glucopyranoside, (+)-mediorecinol di-O-β-D-glucopyranoside, (-)-olivil-4', 4''-di-O-β-D-glucopyranoside.

Pharmacodynamic action:

1. The antihypertensive effect is mild, but long induration.
2. It has a diuretic and sedative effect.
3. It can decrease the absorption of cholesterol and also has an analgesic action.

Indication:

1. It effect nourishing the liver and kidney.
2. It strengthen the bones and muscles.
3. It prevent miscarriage.
4. It is efficacious in the treatment of dizziness and vertigo due to hyperactivity of liver-yang.

Administration and dosage:

5-10 g, decocted in water for an oral dose.

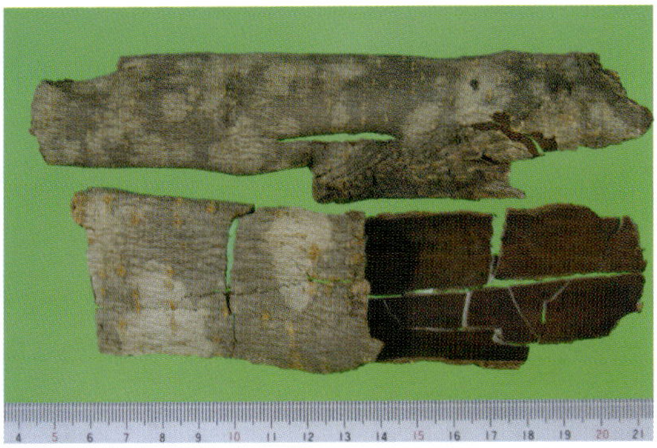

Figure 4. Eucommia Bark from Korean market

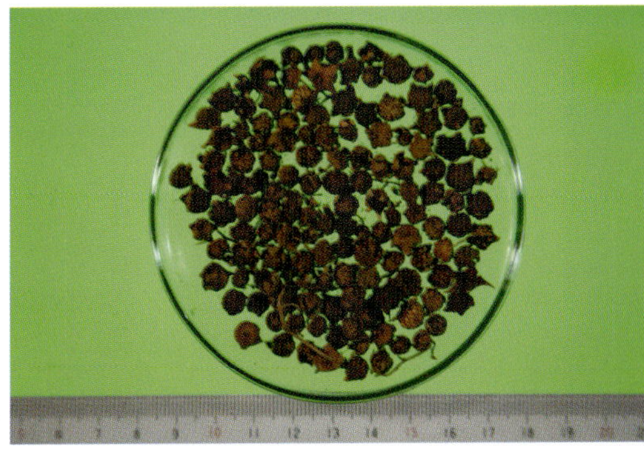

Figure 5. Raspberry from Korea

5. Raspberry

Rubi Fructus

Origin: It is the dried unripe fruit of *Rubus crataegifolius* Bunge or *Rubus coreanus* Miquel, Rosaceae.

Distribution:

It is mainly produced in Korea and in Zhejiang, Anhui, Hubei and Fujian provinces of China.

Chemical constituents:

It contains malic acid, citric acid, tartaric acid, and sugar.

Pharmacodynamic action:

1. It inhibits the growth of *Vibrio cholerae* in vitro.

Indication:

1. Nocturnal emission, impotence, enuresis, urinary frequency.
2. Blurring of vision.

Administration and dosage:

9-15 g daily for decoction.

6. Prepared lateral root of aconite

Aconiti Tuber

Other name: O Du, Cheon Ung

Origin : It is the lateral root of *Aconitum carmichaeli* Debx.,
Ranunculaceae. Usually Aconiti Tuber is cultivated to insure a more constant amount of aconitine.

Distribution:

It is mainly produced in Chinese provinces such as Sichuan and Shaanxi.

Chemical constituents:

It contains alkaloids(0.4-1.0%) such as aconitine, mesaconitine, jesaconitine, atisine, napelline, ignavine, higenamine (=dl- demethylcoclaurine), and coryneine chloride.

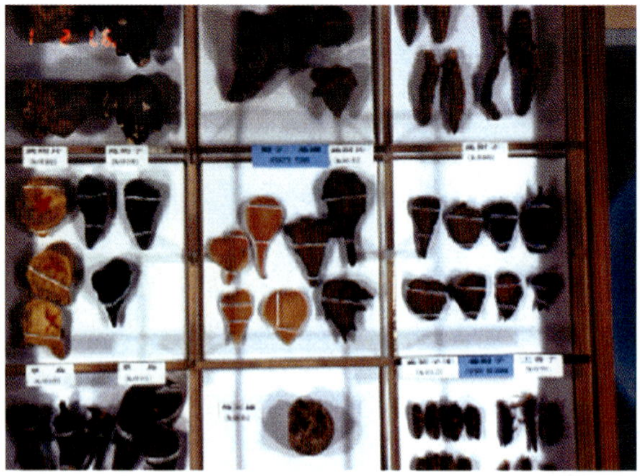

Figure 6. Prepared Lateral Root of Aconite from Korean market

Pharmacodynamic action:

1. Cardiotonic effect: The decoction has been proven to posses cardiotonic action, but the cardiotonic constituents are not aconitine-type alkaloids but rather hygenamine.
2. Analgesic effect: Aconitine possess definite analgesic actions.
3. Antiphlogistic effect.
4. Stimulation of the adrenalcortical system of the pituitary gland.
5. In low doses, aconitine slightly stimulates the central nervous system and peripheral motor nerves.
6. The unprocessed root is very toxic. Subcutaneous injection of aconitine at a dose of 0.4-0.5 mg/Kg cause such toxification phenomena as respiratory inhibition, hypersalivation, vomiting, motor paralysis.

Indication:

1. Impotence, emission
2. Shock
3. Urinary frequency, edema.
4. Diarrhea, conspitation
5. Arthralgia of shoulder joint.

Administration and dosage:

1.5-5 g daily for decoction.

7. Dogwood fruit

Corni Fructus

Origin : It is the pulp of the ripe fruit *Cornus officinalis* Sieb. et Zucc. of Cornaceae.

Distribution:

It is mainly produced in Zhejing, Henan, Anhui, Shaanxi of China and in Gu Rye, Nam Won of

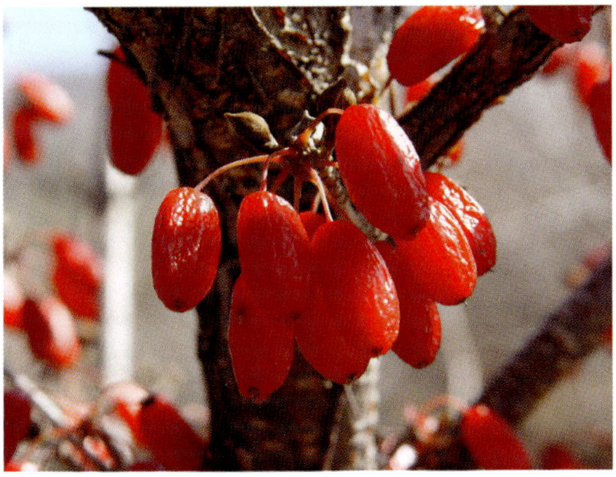

Figure 7. Dogwood Fruit

Korea.

Chemical constituents:

1. Triperpenoids; ursolic acid
2. Saponin; cornin
3. Organic acid; gallic acid, malic acid, tartaric acid.
4. Glycoside: loganin, sweroside, morroniside.

Pharmacodynamic action:

1. Diuretic effect: It promotes diuresis.
2. Antibacterial effect: It inhibits *Staphylococcus aureus*, *Shigella dysenteriae* and various dermatophytes.
3. Antihistamine actions.

Indication:

1. Weakness of the lower part of body and lower limb, emissions, impotence, urinary frequency.
2. General weakness, spontaneous sweating.
3. Dazziness, deafness.

Administration and dosage:

5-10 g, 30 g in large dosage, daily for decoction.

8. Chinese yam

Dioscoreae Rhizoma

Other name: San Uoo

Origin : It is the rhizome of *Dioscorea batatas* $D_{ECAISNE,}$ Dioscoreaceae.

Distribution:

It is produced in Xinxiang Prefecture of Henan Province is considered the best. It is also

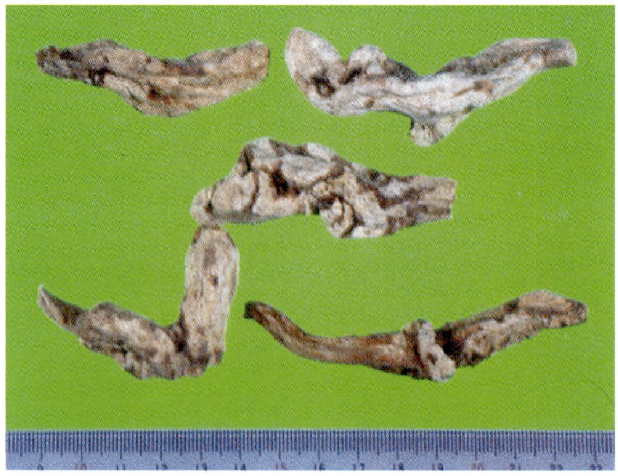

Figure 8. Chinese Yam from Korea

produced in Hebei, Shanxi of China, Japan and Korea.

Chemical constituents:

1. Starch 16% and protein
2. Sugar; glucose, fructose, sucrose
3. Amino acid; leucine, lysine, phenylalanine, valine
4. Phenol; batatasin I, III, IV, V
5. Glucosamine, choline, allantoin, etc.

Pharmacodynamic action:

Nutritive effect is probably due to its mucilage and nutrient content.

Indication:

1. Spermatorrhea due to deficiency of the kidney, or leucorrhagia, firequent urination, etc.
2. Deficiency of the spleen and stomach characterized by poor appetite, lassitude or loose stool and diarrhea.
3. Cough and dyspnea due to lung deficiency.
4. Diabetes or consumption of body fluid.

Administration and Dosage:

10-30 g, 60-250 g in large dosage, decocted in water for an oral dose.

9. Acanthopanax bark

Acanthopanacis Cortex

Origin: It is the dried bark of *Acanthopanax sessiliflorus* (Rupr. et Maxim.) Seem., Araliaceae.

Distribution:

It is produced in Hubei, Henan, Shaanxi, Anhui of China and Korea.

Chemical constituents:

It contains seagmin, savinin, acanthoside A, B, D, lignans, etc.

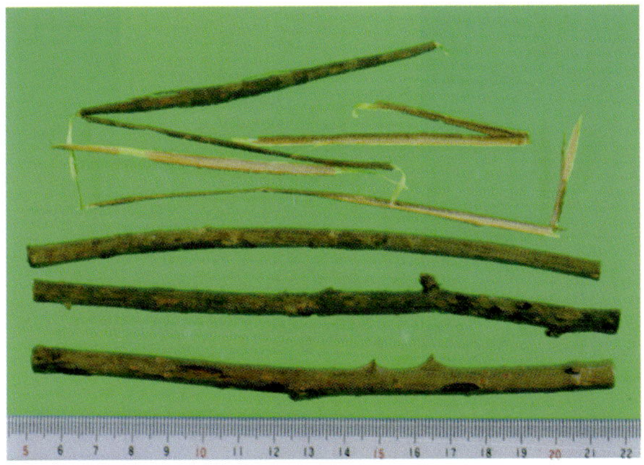

Figure 9. Acanthopanax Bark from Korea

Pharmacodynamic action:

1. Antiphlogistic effect.
2. Analgesic, antipyretic effect.
3. Effect on the cardiovascular system.
4. Adaptogenic effect.

Indication:

1. Strengthening the bone and muscle.
2. Chronic rheumatism with weakness of extremities, infantile paralysis.
3. Insomnia, excessive dreams.
4. Leukopenia.
5. Coronary heart disease.

Administration and dosage:

5-10 g, daily for decoction. It can also be taken in form of liquor infusion.

10. Desertliving cistanche

Cistanchis Herba

Origin: It is the pulpy stem with scales of *Cistanche deserticola* Y. S. Ma, Orobanchaceae.

Distribution:

It is mainly produced in Inner Mongolia, Gansu, Xinjing and Qinghai of China.

Chemical constituents:

It contains a boschnakoside, orobanin, boschniakinic acid and boschniakine, etc.

Pharmacodynamic action:

1. Tonifying and laxative effect.
2. Sialotic effect.
3. Hypotensive effect.

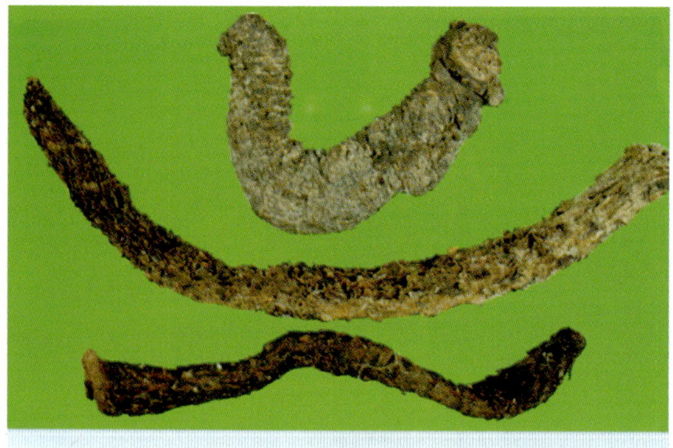

Figure 10. Desertliving Cistanche from Korean market

Indication:

1. Deficiency of the kidney characterized by impotency, cold pain in the loins and female sterility.

Administration and dosage:

10-20 g, daily for decoction.

11. Epimedium

Epimedii Herba, Epimedii Folium

Other name: Seon Ryung Bee, Bang Jang Cho.

Origin:

Korea; It is the whole ground part of *Epimedium koreanum* Nakai, Berberidaceae.

China; It is the whole ground part of *Epimedium sagittatum*, *E. grandiflorum* Morr.(=*E .macranthum Morr. et Decne)*, *E. brevicorum Maxim.*, and *E. cauminatum*, Berberidaceae.

Distribution:

It is produced in Shaanxi, Sichuan, Hubei, Shanxi of China and Korea.

Chemical constituents:

It contains a glycoside (epimidine), flavonoid (icariin=icaritin rhamnoside-glucoside), and olivil.

Pharmacodynamic action:

1. Aphrodisiac effect.
2. Hypotensive effect.
3. Antitussive, expectorant, and antiasthmatic effect.

Indication:

1. Impotence, lassitude of the loins and knees, frequent urination and female sterility due to deficiency of the kidney.

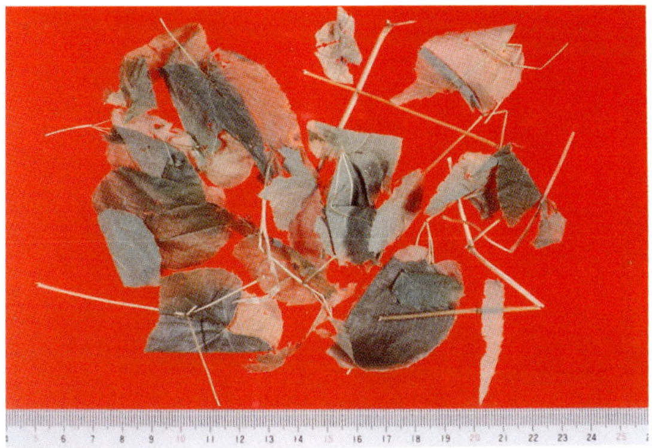

Figure 11. Epimedium from Korea

2. Arthralgia, muscular spasm, numb hands and feet due to wind-cold-dampness.

Administration and dosage:

5-10 g, daily for decoction.

12. Fleece-flower root

Polygoni Multiflori Radix

Origin: It is the dried root tuber of *Polygonum multiflorum* Thunb., Polygonaceae.

Distribution:

It is mainly produced in Hubei, Henan, Sichuan of China and Korea.

Chemical constituents:

It contains chrysophanol, emodin, 3, 5, 4' -tetrahydroxystilbene-2-0-β-D-glucoside, tannin, and fat, etc.

Pharmacodynamic action:

1. Purgative effect.
2. Cholesterol level-lowering effect.
3. Antiviral effect.
4. Cardiotonic effect.

Indication:

1. Fleece-flower root has the function of invigorating the liver and kidney.
2. Fleece-flower root is efficacious in the treatment of toxicosis, inflammation and constipation.

Administration and Dosage:

10-30 g, decocted in water for an oral dose.

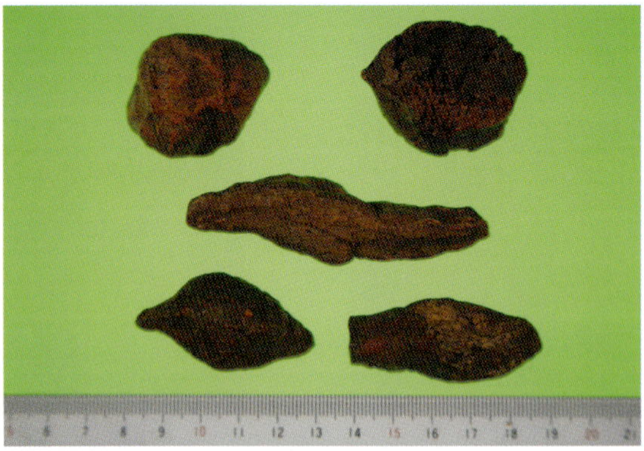

Figure 12. Fleece-flower Root from Korea

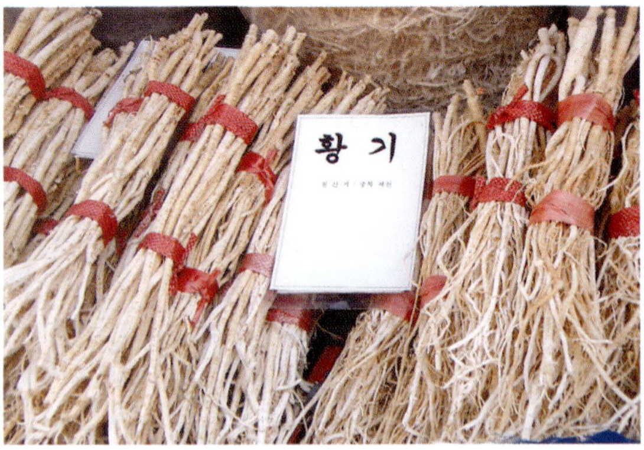

Figure 13. Astragalus Root from Korea

13. Astragalus root

Astragali Radix

Origin: It is the dried root of *Astragalus membranaceus* (Fisch.) Bunge, Leguminosae.

Distribution:

It is mainly produced in Shanxi, Heilongjiang of China and Korea.

Chemical constituents:

Flavonoid; 2, 4-dihydroxy-5, 6-dimethoxyisoflavone, formonetin, γ-aminobutylic acid.

Saponin; astragaloside I, II, III, IV, V, VI, VII, VIII, soyasaponin I.

Pharmacodynamic action:

1. Tonifying effect.
2. Diuretic effect.
3. Effect on nephritis
4. Cardiotonic effect.
5. Vasodilation effect.
6. Hypotensive effect.

Indication:

1. Invigorating the vital energy and elevating the spleen-yang.
2. Consolidating superficial resistance to stop sweating.
3. Promoting pus discharge and tissue regeneration.
4. It is used in the treatment of diabetes.
5. Promoting diuresis to reduce edema.

Administration and dosage:

10-30 g, decocted in water for an oral dose.

REFERENCES

1. Park, Jong Hee. The encyclopedia of Chinese crude drugs. Seoul: Shin il books; 2002. Book chapter.
2. Tsunneo Namba. The encyclopedia of Wakan-Yaku with Color Pictures. Osaka: Hoikusha Co.; 1993. Book chpater.
3. The Pharmacopia Commission of PRC. Pharmacopia of the people' s republic of China. Beijing: Chemical Industry Press; 1997. Book chpater.
4. W. Tang and G. Eisenbrand. Chinese Drugs of Plant Origin. Berlin: Springer-Verlag; 1992. Book chapter.
5. K. Takagi, M. Kimura, M. Harada, Y. Otsuka. Pharmacology of Medicinal Herbs in East Asia. Tokyo: Nanzando company; 1982. Book chpater.
6. Zhang Dianmin. English-Chinese Rare Chinese Materia Medica. Shanghai: Publishing house of Shanghai University of traditional Chinese medicine; 1989. Book chpater.
7. Zhao Zhongzhen. An Illustrated Chinese Materia Medica in Hong Kong. Hong Kong: Chung Hwa Book Co.; 2004. Book chpater.

Chapter 8

Korean Perspective III

Alternative Medicine in Female Sexual Dysfunction

Kwang Sung Park

I. Introduction

Female sexuality is an important women's health issue. It has been reported that 30% to 50% of women have some kind of sexual dysfunction.[1,2] Female sexual dysfunction is characterized by decreased sexual desire, decreased sexual arousal, difficulty in achieving orgasm, and painful sexual intercourse. There have been limited investigations of female sexual dysfunction, however, and few developments of medical therapies. Although several medications have been tried, such as estrogen, transdermal testosterone, yohimbine, apomorphine, and phosphodiesterase type 5 inhibitors,[3-9] no medications are currently approved for use in female sexual dysfunction. Alternative medicines have also been tried to ameliorate menopausal symptoms and to improve sexual function in women.

II. Herbal Medicine and Functional Foods in Female Sexual Dysfunction

Several herbal medicines have been tried for treating sexual dysfunction in women. One of the attractive alternative medicines for female sexual dysfunction is ginseng. Ginseng is a traditional

Kwang Sung Park, M.D., Ph.D.
Department of Urology, Chonnam National University Medical School, Sexual Medicine Reseach Center, Chonnam National University, 8, Hak-dong, Dong-gu, Gwangju, 501-757, Korea.
Tel: +82-62-220-6701, E-mail: uropark@gmail.com

Asian remedy for sexual dysfunction. Ginseng is a popular herb that has been used to ameliorate menopausal symptoms and to improve a woman's sense of wellbeing.[10] Recently, several reports have investigated the effect of Korean red ginseng (KRG) on female sexual function and dysfunction in both animal and human studies.[11-15] Another nutritional supplement or herbal medicine is ginkgo biloba. Ginkgo biloba is known to facilitate blood flow and to have a relaxant effect on smooth muscle tissue.[16]

1. Korean Red Ginseng Extract

1) Animal Study: In one study, KRG extract relaxed the rabbit vaginal strip in a dose-dependent manner up to 85% at a concentration of 20 mg/mL. The relaxing effect of KRG on the vaginal smooth muscle is in part mediated via K^+ channels, especially Ca^{2+}-activated K^+ channels.[11]

In a female castrated rat model study, vaginal blood flow tended to improve after pelvic nerve stimulation in the KRG treatment group. This finding was supported by the histologic finding that the vaginal epithelial layer and submucosal microvasculature showed improvement in the KRG treatment groups.[13]

2) Human Study: There have been 2 placebo-controlled, double-blind crossover clinical trials to evaluate the effects of KRG on female sexual function and dysfunction.[14,15] In healthy, married women aged 30-45 years (n=24), KRG improved sexual function and women's health-related quality of life without statistical significance. In this study, all the subjects exhibited trend for improvement in the sexual desire domain of the female sexual function index (FSFI), but no statistical difference was noted. There were no significant adverse events related to KRG.[14]

Another study investigated the effect of KRG on the sexual arousal response in menopausal women. In this study, 3 capsules of ginseng (1 g per capsule) or placebo daily were administered for 8 weeks. The KRG group had significantly improved scores on the sexual arousal domain of the FSFI from 3.10 ± 0.87 to 3.50 ± 0.72 ($p=0.006$). There were no severe adverse events after treatment with KRG extracts. However, two cases of vaginal bleeding were noted.[15]

There is also a report of a nutritional supplement, ArginMax®, which consists of extracts of ginseng, gingko, and damiana, L-arginine, multivitamins, and minerals. Of the 77 women over the age of 21 years who were interested in improving their sexual function, 34 received ArginMax and 43 received a placebo. After 4 weeks, 73.5% of the ArginMax group reported improved sexual satisfaction, compared with 37.2% of the placebo group ($p<0.01$).[17]

2. Ginkgo biloba

1) Animal Study: There have been no reports on the effect of ginkgo biloba on female sexual function or dysfunction in an animal model. However, there was an experimental study of the effects of ginkgo biloba extract on human and rabbit corpus cavernosal tissue.[16] Both human and

rabbit corpus cavernosal tissue showed a potent relaxation response to subfractions of the nonginkgolide nonflavonoid fraction of ginkgo biloba extract.[16]

2) Human Study: Women (n=99) aged 18-65 years who had sexual arousal disorder participated in a clinical study investigating the short- and long-term effects of ginkgo biloba extract (GBE) on sexual dysfunction. A single dose of 300 mg GBE had a small but significant facilitatory effect on physiological, but not subjective, sexual arousal compared to placebo. However, long-term GBE administration did not significantly enhance arousal responses beyond placebo. Therefore, it was suggested that a substantial placebo effect on sexual function exists in women with sexual concerns.[18]

III. Future Perspectives

Ginseng seems to be an attractive option for maintaining or improving sexual function in menopausal women. Further research is needed to establish the optimal treatment duration and dose of ginseng suitable for a specific category of female sexual dysfunction.

● REFERENCES

1. Laumann EO, Paik A, Rosen RC: Sexual dysfunction in the United States: prevalence and predictors. JAMA 1999, 281:537-44.
2. Lewis RW, Fugl-Meyer KS, Bosch R, et al.: Epidemiology/ risk factors of sexual dysfunction. J Sex Med 2004, 1:35-39.
3. Dennerstein L, Burrows GD,Wood C, Hyman G. Hormones and sexuality: Effect of estrogen and progestogen. Obstet Gynecol 1980;56:316-22.
4. Braunstein GD, Sundwall DA, Katz M, et al. Safety and efficacy of a testosterone patch for the treatment of hypoactive sexual desire disorder in surgically menopausal women: A randomized, placebo-controlled trial. Arch Intern Med 2005;165:1582-9.
5. Warnoock JK, Swanson SG, Borel RW, Zipfel LM, Brennan JJ, ESTRATEST Clinical Study Group. Combined esterified estrogens and methyltestosterone versus esterified estrogens alone in the treatment of loss of sexual interest in surgically menopausal women. Menopause 2005;12:374-84.
6. Arlt W, Callies F, van Vlijmen JC, Koehler I, et al. Dehydroepiandrosterone replacement in women with adrenal insufficiency. N Engl J Med 1999;341:1013-20.
7. Modell JG, May RS, Katholi CR. Effect of bupropion-SR on orgasmic dysfunction in nondepressed subjects: A pilot study. J Sex Marital Ther 2000;26:231-40.
8. Piletz JE, Segraves KB, Feng YZ, Maguire E, Dunger B, Halaris A. Plasma MHPG response to yohimbine treatment in women with hypoactive sexual desire. J Sex Marital Ther 1998;24:43-54.
9. Bechara A, Bertolino MV, Casabe A, Fredotovich N. A double-blind randomized placebo control study comparing the objective and subjective changes in female sexual response using sublingual apomorphine. J Sex Med 2004;1:209-14.
10. Amato P, Christophe S, Mellon PL. Estrogenic activity of herbs commonly used as remedies for menopausal symptoms. Menopause 2002;9:145-50.
11. Kim SO, Kim MK, Lee HS, Parj JK, Park K. The effect of Korean Red Ginseng extract on the relaxation response in isolated rabbit vaginal tissue and its mechanism. J Sex Med 2008;5:2079-84.
12. Kim SO, Kim MK, Chae MJ, Kim HY, Park JK, Park K. Effect of Korean Red Ginseng on the relaxation of clitoral corpus cavernosum in rabbit. Korean J Androl. 2006;24(01):29-34.
13. Kim So, Lee M, Xui Y, Ahn K, Hong HD, Kim SS, Park K. Effects of Korean Red Ginseng on the vaginal blood flow and structure in female castrated rats. Korean J Urol 2006;47(8):888-894.
14. Kim DI, Choi MS, Ahn HY. Efficacy and safety of Red Ginseng on women's health related quality of life and sexual function. J Ginseng Res 2009;33:115-26.
15. Oh KJ, Chae MJ, Lee HS, Hong HD, Park K. Effects of Korean Red Ginseng on sexual arousal in menopausal women: Placebo-Controlled, Double-Blind Cressover Clinical Study. J Sex Med 2010;7:1469-77.
16. Paick JS, Lee JH. An experimental study of the effect of ginkgo biloba extract on the human and rabbit corpus cavernosum tissue. J Urol 1996;156(5):1876-80.
17. Ito TY, Trant AS, Polan ML. A double-blind placebo-controlled study of ArginMax, a nutritional supplement for enhancement of female sexual function. J Sex Marital Ther. 2001;27(5):541-9.
18. Meston CM, Rellini AH, Telch MJ. Short- and long-term effects of Ginkgo biloba extract on sexual dysfunction in women. Arch Sex Behav. 2008;37(4):530-47.

Chapter 9

Singapore Perspective I

Evidence Based Phytotherapy in Sexual Medicine

P.Ganesan Adaikan, Balasubramanian Srilatha, Lang Chu Lau

I. Introduction

It was believed by practitioners of the homeopathic system of medicine that the method of treatment used by allopathic practitioners was an attempt against the process of disease. A well-known homeopathic proponent, Samuel Hahneman (1755-1843) introduced the term "allopathy" (Allo means against). The notion of countering the overreacting bodily function or an upheaval of endogenous transmitter or enzyme appears to be the mechanistic approach even in today's allopathic way of clinical management. For instance, the enzyme that converts angiotensin I to angiotensin II (leading to hypertension when in excess) can be curtailed by treating the patient with an inhibitor of angiotensin converting enzyme or an angiotensin receptor antagonist. This is a direct suppression of the end outcome of the bodily reaction (blood pressure) by inhibitor/antagonist without taking into consideration the cause of the aberration - hypertension, in this case. Some of the limitations to modern medicine are overcome by an array of biochemical diagnostic tools, disease markers, genomic and such other evidence-based pharmacotherapeutic principles. Similar contemporary advances have not taken place with other systems of medical sciences including homeopathic, ethnic traditional (Indian Ayuvedic or Chinese) and other alternative medicinal approaches using age-old herbal extracts (phytotherapeutics) or parts of animals.

P. Ganesan Adaikan, Ph.D., D.Sc.
Department of Obstetrics & Gynaecology, Yong Loo Lin School of Medicine, National University Hospital, National University of Singapore, NUHS Tower Block Level 12, 1E Kent Ridge Road, Singapore 119228. Tel: +65 6772 4128 / +65 9049 8636 E-mail: p_ganesan_adaikan@nuhs.edu.sg

Table 1. Hormonally sensitive phytochemicals

Puncture vine (Tribulus terrestris)
Red clover (Trifolium pretense)
Black cohosh (Cimicifuga racemosa)
Wild yam (dioscorea villosa)
Squaw vine (Mitchella repens)
False unicorn root (Helonius dioica, Chamaelirium luteum)
Gotu kola (Centella asiatica)
Chaste tree (vitex agnus castus)
Blue cohosh (Caulophyllum thalictroides)
Liquorice (Glycyrrhiza glabra)
Dong quai (Angelica sinensis)

Phytotherapy is probably the oldest form of medication known to mankind. Over the centuries, cultures around the world have intricately crafted the herbal pharmacopoeia through observations or trials and errors. Our oldest reference materials include the treatise on Chinese herbs written by the emperor Shen Nong in 2700BC, instructions on the use of medicinal preparations from the records of King Hammurabi of Babylon (1800BC) and some texts belonging to the ancient cultures of Mesopotamia, Egypt and India. Along these timelines, herbal medicines have evolved over the periods of Hippocrates (460-377BC), Galen (131-201AD), Johnson (1636-), Linnaeus (1761-) and Withering (1785-), to name a few. From the available records, we believe that in the medieval times, home-grown herbs were the only medications available for common ailments. Indeed, a number of the modern day medicines appear to have had their origins from plants either in the form of extracted active principles or synthetic mimics. Similarly, significant advancement in plant derived medicines in the last two centuries in such areas as central nervous system, anti-tumour and anti-inflammatory activities has led to the development and identification of active chemicals and understanding of their modes of action. As for man' s health related to sexuality, numerous age-old natural products have been historically claimed as 'aphrodisiacs' - a collective terminology, which describes improvement of arousal, libido and/or sexual energy and activity. Some known phyto-agents considered to be aphrodisiacs include tribulus terrestris, pausinystalia yohimbe, ptychopetalum olacoids, eurycoma longifolia, root of ginseng plant, ginkgo biloba and green oats extract; Several of these are also considered to be hormonal mimics (Table 1), however very few of them went through proper scientific methodology in the identification of the constituents and delineation of effectiveness and modes of action. We had the opportunity to explore and evaluate the pharmacological effects of TT (TT-with 48% of protodioscin extract as active ingredient) and Trifolium pretense (red clover) in our laboratory.

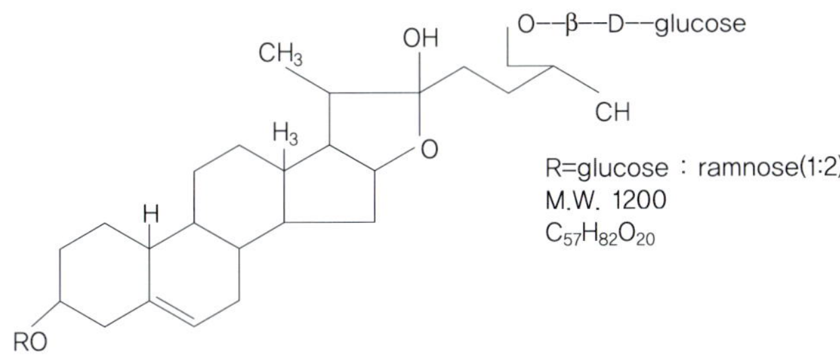

Figure 1. Chemical structure of protodioscin

II. TT Plant

TT, a perennial flowering plant, also known as puncture vine is distributed worldwide in Mediterranean, subtropical and desert climates. It is regarded as an aphrodisiac in the indigenous medicine of China, India, South Africa and Bulgaria and has other documented benefits such as in the treatment of urinary infections, cardiovascular and gastrointestinal diseases etc[1,2]. The steroidal saponins of furastanol type are considered to be the active principles mediating the biological effects of products derived from this plant. Apparently the activity of TT is dependent on the composition and concentration of these saponins which are not only distinctively influenced by the geographical origin of the plant material but also by the plant part and stage of development[3]. In a recent comparative investigation on phytochemicals, protodioscin (Figure 1) and prototribestin are identified as the main components in the aerial part of plant samples from Bulgaria, Turkey, Greece, Serbia, Macedonia, Georgia and Iran whereas the Vietnamese and Indian samples exhibit a totally different chemical profile[3]. The total content of saponins is highest in the leaves, followed by the stems and the fruits[3,4].

Many TT plant products are commercially marketed under various names such as Tribestan, Tribulus Maximus and Tribulus Terrestris. However, there are not many scientific studies on the actions/mechanisms to substantiate the various claims of TT as a liver tonic, nutritional supplement, vitalizer or aphrodisiac. While there is some evidence based on animal studies supporting the use of TT in sexual medicine, the outcome of human trials is inconclusive[5].

Protodioscin that constitutes 48% (dry weight) of TT extract (origin Bulgaria) had been reported to increase the serum levels of testosterone, luteinizing hormone[6] and dehydroepiandrosterone[7] in man. This observation was supported by our acute study on bolus intravenous administration of TT extract in primates that resulted in an increase in testosterone, dihydrotestosterone and dehydroepiandrosterone sulphate[8] - TT may thus increase testosterone level either by acting as a natural precursor to sex hormone or as a consequence of enhanced

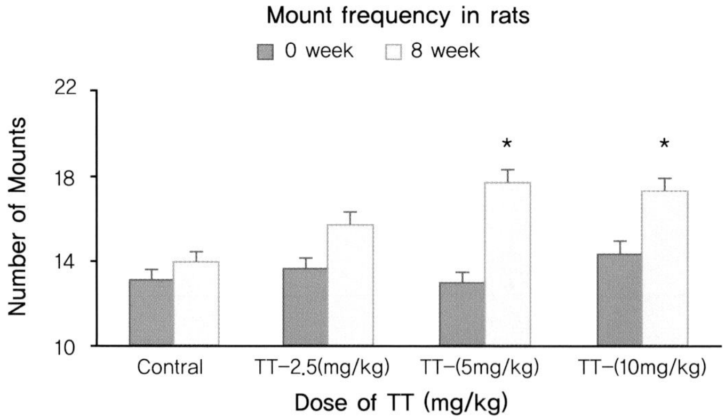

Figure 2. The number of mounts recorded in different groups of rats (n = 10). The results are compared between the control and the *Tribulus terrestris* (TT)-treated groups. The values are expressed as mean ± standard error of the mean. *Indicates significant differences ($p < 0.05$) from control [10].

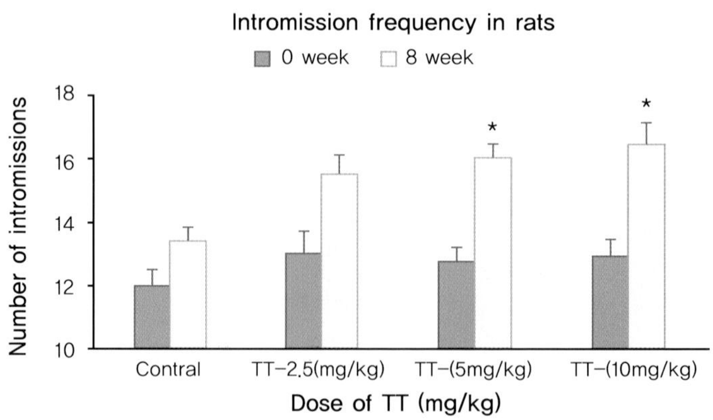

Figure 3. The number of intromissions recorded in different groups of rats (n = 10). The results are compared between the control and the *Tribulus terrestris* (TT)-treated groups. The values are expressed as mean ± standard error of the mean. *Indicates significant differences ($p < 0.05$) from control [10].

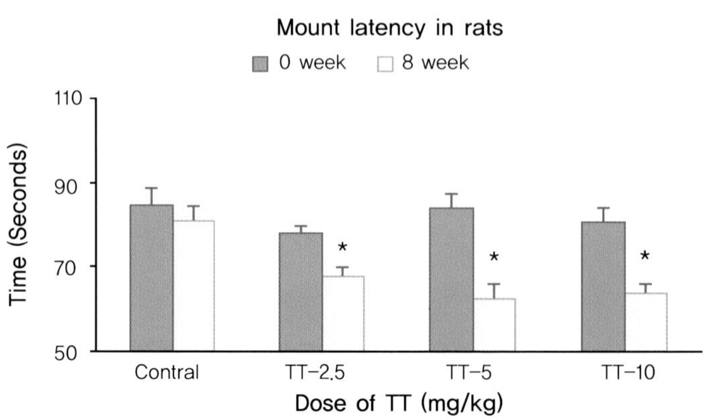

Figure 4. The mount latencies recorded in different groups of rats (n = 10). The results are compared between the control and the *Tribulus terrestris* (TT)-treated groups. The values are expressed as mean ± standard error of the mean. *Indicates significant differences ($p < 0.05$) from control [10].

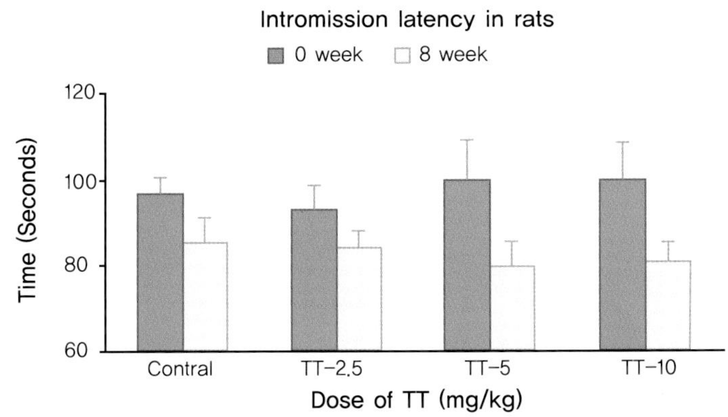

Figure 5. The intromission latencies recorded in different groups of rats (n = 10). The results are compared between the control and the *Tribulus terrestris* (TT)-treated groups. The values are expressed as mean ± standard error of the mean [10].

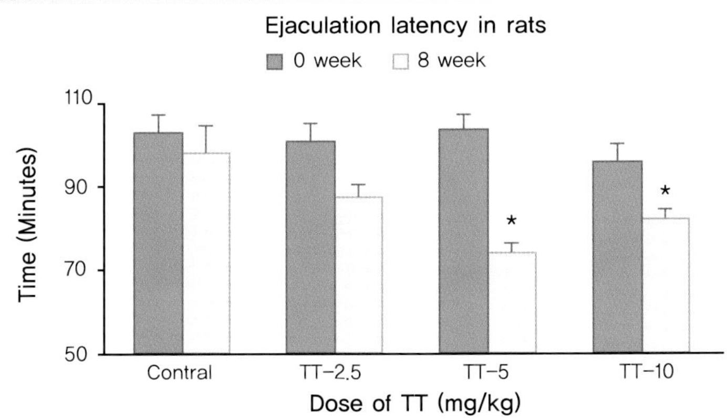

Figure 6. The ejaculatory latencies recorded in different groups of rats (n = 10). The results are compared between the control and the *Tribulus terrestris* (TT)-treated groups. The values are expressed as mean ± standard error of the mean. *Indicates significant differences ($p < 0.05$) from control [10].

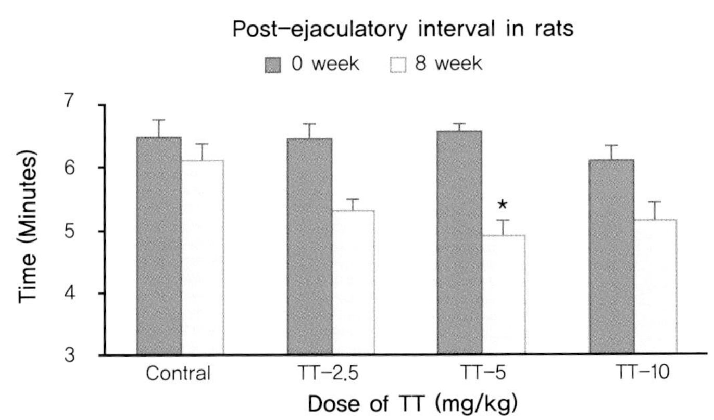

Figure 7. The postejaculatory interval recorded in different groups of rats (n = 10). The results are compared between the control and the *Tribulus terrestris* (TT)-treated groups. The values are expressed as mean ± standard error of the mean. *Indicates significant differences ($p < 0.05$) from control [10].

production of luteinizing hormone. The proandrogenic activity of TT suggests that it could contribute to improvement in sexual desire. However, a recent study on TT supplementation in young adult males failed to demonstrate either direct or indirect androgen increasing property[5].

The proerectile effect of TT has also been illustrated in several animal models of sexual function. Chronic treatment with TT extract marginally sensitizes the rabbit corpus cavernosum muscle to relaxation induced via cholinergic and nitrergic pathways[9]. In addition, improvement in libido, sexual activity (Figures 2-7) and intracavernous pressure response to cavernous nerve stimulation following oral administration of TT in rats were considered as positive markers of enhanced sexual performance[10]. The experimental evidences were based on a rat model of sexual behavior which was carried out in a room under dim red illumination. Each male rat was placed in a rectangular plexiglass chamber, 10 minutes before the introduction of a primed female, for the male rat to get acclimatized to the chamber conditions. The primed female rat was then introduced into the chamber and the following sexual behavior parameters were recorded:

1. Mount frequency - the number of mounts without intromission from the time of introduction of the female until ejaculation
2. Intromission frequency - the number of intromissions (characterized by pelvic thrusting and springing dismount) from the time of introduction of the female until ejaculation
3. Mount latency - the time interval between the introduction of the female and the first mount by the male
4. Intromission latency - the interval from the time of introduction of the female to the first intromission by the male
5. Ejaculation latency - the time interval between the first intromission and ejaculation (characterized by longer, deeper pelvic thrusting, a slow dismount followed by a period of inactivity)
6. Postejaculatory interval - the time interval between ejaculation and the first intromission of the following series.

The experiment was terminated when each male rat began to mount the female again after a brief period of inactivity (this period of refractoriness of the male rat to the female is usually observed after ejaculation) or following 30 minutes of sexual inactivity by the male rat from the time of introduction of the female into the testing chamber[10].

In castrated rats treated with TT, prostate weight, intracavernous pressure (Figure 8) and sexual behaviour parameters were significantly restored providing evidence that TT improved these characteristics possibly via its pro-androgenic property[11]. Furthermore, TT may exert a central mechanism of action since chronic treatment of rats with TT increased both nicotinamide adenine dinucleotide phosphate-diaphorase positive neurons (used to localize NOS neurons) and androgen receptor immunoreactivity in the paraventricular nucleus region, which is one of the important

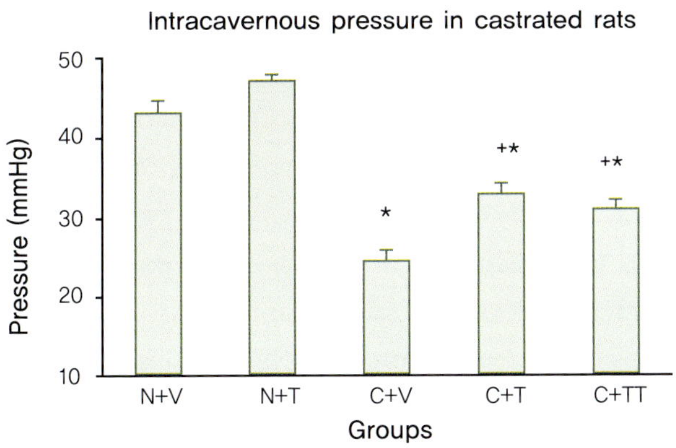

Figure 8. N = Normal rat; V = Vehicle; C = Castrated rat; T = Testosterone; TT = Tribulus terrestris extract. Intracavernous pressure recorded in the control and treated groups of rats (n = 8). The results are compared between a) the intact control and rest of the groups, b) the castrated control and rest of the castrated groups. The values are expressed as mean ± SEM. † and * indicates significant differences ($p < 0.05$) from control for a and b respectively [11].

areas of the brain involved in sexual function[12].

Besides steroidal saponins, a number of flavonoid glycosides have been isolated from TT. The existence of significant quantities of flavonoids in TT suggests that flavonoids should be evaluated for any pro-sexual activity as well. It is hoped that natural herbal preparations can be alternatives to synthetic anabolic hormones. They are selectively preferred as a form of testosterone replacement since some of them are shown to stimulate the body to produce natural testosterone and even dehydroepiandrosterone. In view of the fact that phytoandrogens are weaker than androgens, they may have lesser side effects. They are also claimed to have minimal feedback inhibition on testosterone biosynthesis in the body; however, this has to be proven.

III. Avena Sativa (Wild Oats, Green Oats, Oatstraw)

The active ingredients of Avena Sativa are saponins, flavonoids, minerals, alkaloids, Vitamins B1, B2, D, E, carotene and wheat protein, avenin.

Two different types of saponins have been isolated from oat kernels: the avenacoside-type pentacyclic triterpenoid saponins and the avenacin-type steroidal saponins. The structures of two avenacosides (avenacoside A and avenacoside B) and several of the avenacin-type saponins have been elucidated[13,14].

In alternative medicine, oats are becoming popular as herbal aphrodisiacs for enhancing sexual performance without serious side effects of natural hormones. Oats are noted to release testosterone that becomes bound to tissues for the biological effect[15]. It is also plausible that the steroidal saponins found in Avena Sativa probably act by displacing testosterone from its binding to SHBG. This purported action of oats can result in an increase in free, active bioavailable testosterone which is more effective at stimulating sex drive centers in the brain. The libido-enhancing mechanism of Avena Sativa is yet to be fully validated.

In the internet, Avena Sativa is claimed to be effective in treating impotence and premature ejaculation in men whereas it reportedly increased sexual desire in women. However, there is no evidence-based literature supporting the sexual properties of Avena Sativa in both male and female.

IV. Phytoestrogens

In addition to the phytoandrogens, other classes of environmental hormone substances have been identified; these include the functional mimics of oestrogens, antioestrogens, antiprogestins and antiandrogens[16]. Phytoestrogen, as the name implies, comprises oestrogen from the plant source with inherent ability both in vivo and in vitro to bind to the subtypes of oestrogen receptors (ER^{α} and ER^{β}) albeit with varying affinities[17]. Together with the increasing use of complementary or alternative medicines in the industrialized world, many perimenopausal women are turning to the natural substitutes, which have been purported to have fewer side effects, for relief of their vasomotor symptoms. Reports of the lesser prevalence of hot flushes in Asian women especially from Japan, compared to their occurrence in other parts of the world[18] may explain the therapeutic benefits of plant oestrogens. The potential health effects, which may also be related to improvement of atherosclerosis, cognitive or sexual functions and bone preservation, are being variously investigated by researchers worldwide with the pertinent intention of identifying tissue selective alternatives as the suitable form of non-hormonal therapy.

1. Understanding phytoestrogens

Chemically, the term phytoestrogen refers to the group of non-steroidal oestrogen mimetics which can be phenylpropanoids or simple phenols[19]. From a nutritional and health perspective, there are three major groups of such active plant agents. These include 1. isoflavones (present in legumes including peas, beans, lentils and soy (a common ingredient of the Asian diet), 2. lignans, found in nuts, cereals, berries, fruits, vegetables and also in high concentrations in flax seed (linseed) and 3. coumestans - found in alfalfa, bean sprouts and red clover[20,21]. Being structural analogues of endogenous oestradiol (E_2), the phytoestrogens share the phenolic ring which is also an important prerequisite for binding to target tissue oestrogen receptors[22]. Thus, they can act either as ER agonists or antagonists; their biological actions at the cellular and molecular levels are influenced by many factors including the level of exposure, bioavailability, receptoral status, endogenous E_2 level and the end organ or cell in question. Plant oestrogens are basically weak agonists (10^{-2} to 10^{-3}) when compared with circulating E_2 or oestrone. The preferential binding of these non-steroidal oestrogens to ER^{α} than ER^{β}[18] also indicates that they are capable of being more selective than the endogenous oestrogens, with the possibility of acting as natural selective oestrogen receptor modulators (SERMs)[21]. As in a classical reaction, the agonistic effect at the receptoral level may be mediated by activation of transcription whereas the antagonistic effect may be the result of mechanical occupation at the receptors and preventing of activation of DNA response elements. Additional antioestrogenic effects may be mediated by competing for the oestrogen biosynthesizing (aromatase) and metabolizing (17 beta-hydroxy steroid oxidoreductase type1) enzymes[23]. Furthermore, lignan and isoflavone phytoestrogens may also be antiandrogenic due to their effects in inhibiting conversion of testosterone to 5α-dihydrotestosterone[24] and increased synthesis of SHBG with further modulations in testosterone levels[25]. Due to their lesser affinity than E_2 for extracellular binding proteins such as SHBG and α fetoprotein, phytoestrogens may be available in higher free concentrations[16] for peripheral tissue effects. It has been shown that in spite of the lower oral bioavailability as demonstrated by time-resolved fluoroimmunoassay[26], the phytoestrogens can reach 3 to 5 folds higher target tissue levels[27].

Many commonly-consumed processed foods and soybean proteins contain significant amounts of isoflavones such as daidzein and genistein, either as the aglycone (unconjugated form) or the glycoside conjugates[28,29]. These compounds can be further activated by the microbial enzyme systems in the gastrointestinal tract to heterocyclic phenols with hormonal potentials[30]; however, the concentration of the active metabolites may vary widely between individuals consuming the same quantity of the plant hormones[20]. Nevertheless, both the precursors and metabolites retain adequate oestrogenic activity and pharmacokinetic studies indicate that they are handled by the body through similar endogenous pathways viz., transportation to the liver and elimination by kidneys[21]. Early interest in the possible oestrogen-like effects of soy was prompted by the discovery of extremely high levels of isoflavones in blood and urine of women after soy food consumption. A prototypical plant extract, red clover (Trifolium pretense L.) is a rich dietary source for the isoflavone subtypes formononetin (21.3%), biochanin A (18.2%) daidzein (0.6%), and genistein (0.4%).

2. Phytoestrogens for menopausal sexual dysfunction

The declining sexual functioning during the perimenopausal phase is attributed to reduced genital blood flow and vaginal dryness resulting from hypoestrogenism[31] as the symptoms of sexual dysfunction have been shown to improve with oestrogen replacement[32]. However, in the aftermath of the Women's Health Initiative report and the feared risks of heart disease, breast cancer and stroke with hormone therapy (HT)[33,34], there are well-justified consumer concerns regarding the side effects and long-term health impacts of conventional hormone replacement. Several other options have been widely considered as alternatives for alleviation of some of the menopausal symptoms [35,36]. Identifying suitable agents is particularly important since improvements in general health and quality of life have resulted in a rapid increase in a woman' s life expectancy where she spends nearly one-third of her life in the menopausal years. In our studies[37], we attempted to validate the therapeutic efficacy of phytoestrogen isoflavones for some of the menopausal sexual dysfunctional changes. The methods consisted of experimental trials on the efficacy of plant hormone preparations as compared to oestradiol (standard HT) on the parameters of bone mineral density, whole body and uterine weights, genital blood flow, clitoral cavernosal histology and serum levels of oestradiol and testosterone in ovariectomized and normal rabbits.

3. Scientific evaluation of phytoestrogen isoflavones

Thirty New Zealand White female rabbits were divided into five groups (n=6). One group served as the intact control group, while other groups underwent ovariectomy to serve as surgical menopausal models. Three of the ovariectomised experimental groups respectively were given 100 μg/kg oestradiol valerate (Progynova, Schering), 100 μg/kg daidzein (Sigma) and 6.68 mg/kg red clover extract (equivalent to 100 μg/kg of daidzein, which makes up 0.6% of the extract) daily as a suspension in water for 12 weeks. All the animals were weighed before and after treatment for effects on body weight. Following treatment, in-vivo vaginal blood flow response was measured in anaesthetized rabbits using laser Doppler flowmeter, before and after pelvic nerve stimulation. Vaginal lubrication was estimated by weighing cotton-tipped swab, prior to and following PNS. Blood was collected for serum hormone level quantification assays, uterine weights were taken and bone mineral density of the femur was measured using the Lunar DPX-L technique. The significant difference in results was compared with data from operated control rabbits.

In all groups, an increase in vaginal blood flow was observed after pelvic nerve stimulation. For instance, blood flow increased significantly in oestradiol (36%), daidzein (116%) and red clover isoflavone (59%) treated menopausal groups. No significant results were obtained in the measurement of body weight and vaginal lubrication changes. Treatment with E_2 increased average uterine weights significantly in the oestradiol treated rabbits (14.7 g) in comparison with ovariectomized control (2.6 g), red clover isoflavone (4.4 g) and daidzein (6.0 g) groups (Figures 9 (a-d) and 10). Bone mineral density was lowest in the ovariectomized control group (0.3467 g/cm^2) and highest in the red clover isoflavone-treated group (0.4012 g/cm^2). Preservation of bone mineral density was observed in other groups seen as 0.3785 g/cm^2 (control), 0.3798 g/cm^2 (oestradiol) and 0.3763 g/cm^2 (daidzein). Serum level of oestradiol was significantly increased in the oestrogen-treated group with minor changes in other groups.

Our studies provide the scientific basis that the use of isoflavones as non-hormonal replacement therapy may lead to significant increases in bone mineral density and vaginal blood flow for possible consideration as viable alternative to traditional regimens using synthetic

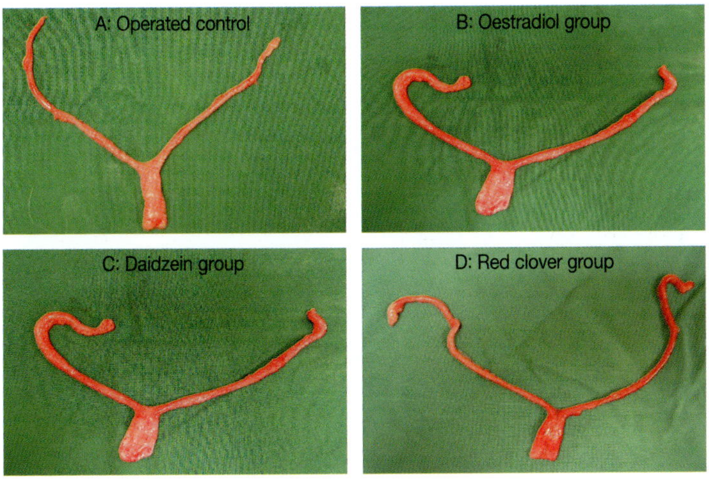

Figure 9. Gross appearance of rabbit uterus from different treatment groups. Note the significant proliferative change with oestradiol treatment (B).

oestrogens. Sexual arousal in women is a vasocongestive event resulting primarily from increased blood flow to the genital tract. Oestrogen plays a role in regulating vaginal vascularity through nitric oxide (NO) synthase[38] and menopause is associated with endothelial dysfunction due to absence of protective effect of endogenous oestrogens on vascular endothelium[39]. In our study, ovariectomised rabbits had the minimal increase in genital blood flow after pelvic nerve stimulation, whereas oestradiol and phytoestrogen treated groups had maximal changes. Interestingly, daidzein-treated animals showed very large increases in blood flow, which indicates that daidzein has a likely selective role in the maintenance of the endothelium and vascularity in female rabbit genitalia. Bone mineral density was highest in the red clover isoflavone-treated group thereby indicating the potential therapeutic benefits of this form of alternative treatment for prevention of osteoporosis. Pharmaceutical companies have been interested in the development of compounds that are selective oestrogen receptor modulators and alternatives to HT. The results from our investigation on phytoestrogen isoflavones indicate the beneficial and comparable effect of oestrogen mimics on some of the distressing menopausal impairments including sexual dysfunction and osteoporosis and provide the scientific evidence for their therapeutic potential in improving quality of life in aged women.

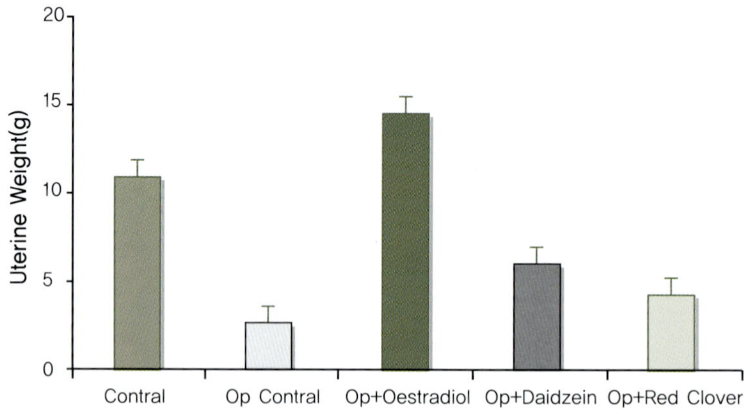

Figure 10. Uterine weight in experimental groups (n=6) showing significant increase in ovariectomised-oestradiol treated rabbits ($p < 0.05$)

V. Regulation of Commercially Available Medicinal Herbs

Singapore regulates drugs through the Poisons Act, Medicines Act, Sale of Drugs Act and the Medicines (Advertisements and Sale) Act and the Misuse of Drug Regulations. The Health Sciences Authority of Singapore (HSA) is the main regulatory body which is tasked to enforce health products' control for the population in Singapore. In this context, HSA also supervises the regulation of complementary medicines variously consisting of Chinese proprietary medicines, traditional medicines, homeopathic medicines, raw medicinal herbs and health supplements. Licensing requirements for these different categories vary only to a certain extent. Purity and absence of bacterial contamination together with documentary evidence of compliance to the HSA's requirements are needed from dealers intending to import any of these preparations into Singapore. In general, HSA does not impose licensing requirements for the import or local sale of raw medicinal herbs which are not sold as formulations comprising tablets, capsules or granules. As for the commercial labelling of alternative and complementary medicinal products over the shelf, any of the nineteen conditions or diseases listed under the Schedule of the Medicines (Advertisements and Sale) Act must not be mentioned in the packaging / labelling (see Table 2). In the area of sexual medicine, this restriction is found to apply to the proposed usefulness of any of these products for sexual function, impotency, frigidity and the allied indications such as infertility and contraception and pregnancy.

Table 2. Conditions and diseases listed under the first schedule of the medicines act

1	Blindness	11	Leprosy
2	Cancer	12	Menstrual disorders
3	Cataract	13	Paralysis
4	Drug addiction	14	Tuberculosis
5	Deafness	15	Sexual function
6	Diabetes	16	Infertility
7	Epilepsy or fits	17	Impotency
8	Hypertension	18	Frigidity
9	Insanity	19	Conception and pregnancy
10	Kidney diseases		

VI. Conclusions

In the recent years, there has been a conscious slant towards herbal medicine for various ailments accounting for their increased popularity and high volume global market. However, many of the purported claims have not been scientifically validated and very few of these plants in question have so far gone through proper scientific methodology in the identification of the constituents or delineation of effectiveness and modes of action. Since plant extracts contain a mixture of several active ingredients with variable potency as well as bioavailability, we often face considerable difficulties in titrating the dosage levels; this also accounts for the inter-individual variations in the pharmacokinetic characteristics. Additionally, there are limited evaluations of the real benefits as against the short-term market demands. These genuine concerns must be scientifically addressed to turn the promise of these medicinal preparations into a reality that benefits both human health and the commercial interests of product developers around the globe. It still remains to be seen as to how useful these phytochemicals may be in sexual medicine. Would they just remain as neutriceuticals or will they reach the stage of prescription medications? Will there be more effective structural analogs developed with industrial enthusiasm and support? Evidence-based studies and appropriate quality controls may have the answers to some or all of these queries.

REFERENCES

1. Wang B, Ma L, Liu T. 406 cases of angina pectoris in coronary heart disease treated with saponin of Tribulus terrestris. Zhong Xi Yi Jie He Za Zhi. 1990;10:85-7.
2. CHEMEXCIL. Tribulus terrestris Linn (N.O.-Zygophyllaceae). In: Selected Medicinal Plants of India (a monograph of identity, safety and clinical usage). Bombay: Compiled by Bharatiya Vidya Bhavan's Swamy Prakashananda Ayurveda Research Centre for CHEMEXCIL, Tata Press, 1992:323–326.
3. Dinchev D, Janda B, Evstatieva L, Oleszek W, Aslani MR, Kostova I. Distribution of steroidal saponins in Tribulus terrestris from different geographical regions. Phytochemistry 2008;69:176-86.
4. Ganzera M, Bedir E, Khan IA. Determination of steroidal saponins in Tribulus terrestris by reversed-phase high-performance liquid chromatography and evaporative light scattering detection. J Pharm Sci. 2001;90:1752-8.
5. Neychev VK, Mitev VI. The aphrodisiac herb Tribulus terrestris does not influence the androgen production in young men. J Ethnopharmacol. 2005;101:319-23.
6. Koumanov F, Bozadjieva E, Andreeva M, Platonva E, Ankov V. Clinical trial of Tribestan. Exper Med 1982;1:2-4.
7. Adimoelja A, Adaikan PG, Protodioscin from herbal plant Tribulus terrestris L. Improves male sexual functions possibly via DHEA. Int J Impot Res 1997;9:S64.
8. Adaikan PG, K Gauthaman, RNV Prasad. History of herbal medicines with an insight on the pharmacological properties of Tribulus terrestris. The Aging Male 2001;4:163-9.
9. Adaikan PG, Gauthaman K, Prasad RN, Ng SC. Proerectile pharmacological effects of Tribulus terrestris extract on the rabbit corpus cavernosum. Ann Acad Med Singapore 2000;29:22-6.
10. Gauthaman K, Ganesan AP, Prasad RN. Sexual effects of puncturevine (Tribulus terrestris) extract (protodioscin): an evaluation using a rat model. J Altern Complement Med 2003;9:257-65.
11. Gauthaman K, Adaikan PG, Prasad RN. Aphrodisiac properties of Tribulus Terrestris extract (Protodioscin) in normal and castrated rats. Life Sci 2002 9;71:1385-96.
12. Gauthaman K, Adaikan PG. Effect of Tribulus terrestris on nicotinamide adenine dinucleotide phosphate-diaphorase activity and androgen receptors in rat brain. J Ethnopharmacol 2005;96:127-32.
13. Tschesche R, Lüdke G, Wulff G. Steroid saponins with more than 1 sugar chain. II. Sarsaparilloside, a bisdesmosidic 22-hydroxy-furanostanol saponin. Chem Ber. 1969;102:1253-69 [Article in German].
14. Crombie L, Crombie W M L and Whiting D A. Structures of the oat root resistance factors to take-all disease, avenancins A-1, A-2, B-1 and B-2 and their companion substances J. Chem. Soc., Perkin Trans. 1986;1:1917 – 22.
15. Mitchell D. Nature's Aphrodisiacs: safe holistic approaches to intensified sexual responses and enjoyment. New York, USA: Dell Pub Co; 1999,1-213.
16. Cheek AO, McLachlan JA. Environmental hormones and the male reproductive system. J Androl 1998;19:5-10.
17. Sohoni P, Sumpter JP. Several environmental oestrogens are also anti-androgens. J Endocrinol 1998;158:327-39.
18. Ginsburg J, Prelevic GM. Lack of significant hormonal effects and controlled trials of phyto-oestrogens. Lancet 2000;355:163-4.
19. Brzezinski A, Debi A. Phytoestrogens: the "natural" selective estrogen receptor modulators? Eur J Obstet Gynecol Reprod Biol 1999;85:47-51.
20. Webb M, Glasier A. Phyto-oestrogens for the treatment of menopausal symptoms. IPPF Med Bull 2001;35:3.
21. Dornstauder E, Jisa E, Unterrieder I, Krenn L, Kubelka W, Jungbauer A. Estrogenic activity of two standardized red clover extracts (Menoflavon) intended for large scale use in hormone replacement therapy. J Steroid Biochem Mol Biol 2001;78:67-75.
22. Turner KJ, Sharpe RM. Environmental oestrogens - present understanding. Rev Reprod 1997;2:69-73.
23. Santti R, Makela S, Strauss L, Korkman J, Kostian ML. Phytoestrogens: potential endocrine disruptors in males.

Toxicol Ind Health 1998;14:223-37.
24. Stephens FO. Phytoestrogens and prostate cancer: possible preventive role. Med J Austr 1997;167:138-40.
25. Adlercreutz H, Mazur W. Phyto-oestrogens and western diseases. Ann Med 1997;29:95-120.
26. Wang GJ, Lapcik O, Hampl R, Uehara M, Al-Maharik N, Stumpf K, et al. Time-resolved fluoroimmunoassay of plasma daidzein and genistein. Steroids 2000;65:339-48.
27. Janning P, Schuhmacher US, Upmeier A, Diel P, Michna H, Degen GH, et al. Toxicokinetics of the phytoestrogen daidzein in female DA/Han rats. Arch Toxicol 2000;74:421-30.
28. Setchell KD. Phytoestrogens: the biochemistry, physiology and implications for human health of soy isoflavones. Am J Clin Nutr 1998;68:S1333-46.
29. Nicholls J, Lasley BL, Nakajima ST, Setchell KD, Schneeman BO. Effects of soy consumption on gonadotropin secretion and acute pituitary responses to gonadotropin-releasing hormone in women. J Nutr 2002;132:708-14.
30. Setchell KD. Soy isoflavones - benefits and risks from nature's selective estrogen receptor modulators (SERMs). J Am Coll Nutr 2001;20:S354-62.
31. Park K, Goldstein I, Andry C, Siroky MB, Krane RJ, Azadzoi KM. Vasculogenic female sexual dysfunction: the hemodynamic basis for vaginal engorgement insufficiency and clitoral erectile insufficiency. Int J Impot Res 1997;9:27-37.
32. Alexander LJ, Kotz K, Dennerstein L, Kutner SJ, Whallen K, Notelovitz M. The effects of menopausal hormone therapies on female sexual functioning: Review of double-blind randomized controlled trials. Menopause 2004;11:749-65.
33. Ostrzenski A, Ostrzenska KM. WHI clinical trial revisit: imprecise scientific methodology disqualifies the study's outcomes. Am J Obstet Gynecol 2005;193:1599-606.
34. Schonberg MA, Wee CC. Menopausal symptom management and prevention counseling after the Women's Health Initiative among women seen in an internal medicine practice. J Womens Health 2005;14:507-14.
35. Nelson HD, Vesco KK, Haney E, Fu R, Nedrow A, Miller J et al. Nonhormonal therapies for menopausal hot flashes: systematic review and meta-analysis. JAMA 2006;295:2057-71.
36. Tempfer CB, Bentz EK, Leodolter S, Tscherne G, Reuss F, Cross HS et al. Phytoestrogens in clinical practice: a review of the literature. Fertil Steril 2007;87:1243-9.
37. PG Adaikan, B Srilatha, AJ Wheat. Efficacy of red clover isoflavones in the menopausal rabbit model. Fertil Steril 2009;92:2008-13.
38. Berman J, McCarthy M, Kyprianou N. Effect of estrogen withdrawal on nitric oxide synthase expression and apoptosis in the rat vagina. Urology 1998;44:650-6.
39. Taddei S, Virdis A, Ghiadoni L, Mattei P, Sudano I, Bernini G et al. Menopause is associated with endothelial dysfunction in women. Hypertension 1996;28:576-82.

Chapter 10

Singapore Perspective II

Clinical Applications of Modern and Traditional Pharmacopoeias for Sexual Health in Singapore and Asia

Benny Tan K.H., Victor Ong Y.C., Peter Lim H.C.

I. Introduction

1. Factors in libido

Libido and sexual arousal in humans are complex processes, involving visual, olfactory, auditory, tactile, and temporal factors linked to psychological and physiological stimulation. These instincts in both men and women are strongly influenced by the male hormones, acting through the androgen receptor (AR). The clinical evidence supporting the pivotal role of AR is shown from published studies of hormone replacement therapy in perimenopausal and menopausal women in their climacteric. Whilst estrogen replacement therapy can stave off disorders such as osteopenia and osteoporosis, urogenital degeneration, mood swings and hot flushes, libido in these women remains attenuated. However, when androgen is included as part of their hormonal pharmacotherapy, a striking improvement in sexual interest can be detected in these women. These observations attest to the role that AR plays as a key transcriptional factor in the neurobiology of the female *eros*.

Similarly, male libido is primarily driven, at the hormonal level, by the AR. It is noted that androgen ablation in men from different causes, such as prostate cancer chemotherapy or chemical castration of male sex offenders, generally brings about severe curtailment of sexual interest (and penile erectile dysfunction). Attenuated male libido and virility that accompany andropause have

Benny Tan K.H., M.D., Ph.D.
Associate Professor of Department of Pharmacology, Yong Loo Lin School of Medicine, National University of Singapore, MD11, CRC Building, 10 Medical Drive, Singapore 117597. E-mail: phctankh@nus.edu.sg, benny_tan@nuhs.edu.sg

also been linked to impairment of AR. Hence, androgen replacement therapy, in combination with the pharmacotherapy of penile erectile dysfunction, is sometimes ascribed to senescent males, presenting with sexual hypofunction.

2. Biology of virility

Another basic attribute of male sexuality relates to virility. This is the capacity of a sexually aroused male to achieve and sustain penile tumescence till ejaculation takes place. The length of the refractory period between sexual response cycles, extent of penile rigidity and frequency of tumescence corresponding to each sexual response cycle (excitement, plateau, orgasmic and resolution stages) are descriptive patterns associated with male virility. One example of loss of male virility is erectile dysfunction (ED), commonly known as impotence - the inability of the male to achieve or sustain penile erection sufficiently for the copulatory act to be completed.

For tumescence to take place, the corpus cavernosum (spongy erectile tissue) of the penis must be filled with blood (Figure 1A). This is effected through relaxation of the cavernous arterial smooth muscle, mediated by a spike in intracellular cyclic guanosine monophosphate (cGMP) level. Nitric oxide (NO) released from the axons in the corpus cavernosum stimulates this increase in cGMP synthesis (Figure 1B). The concurrent suppression of the penile sympathetic nerves that normally control vasoconstriction ensures the development and maintenance of penile tumescence.

The association of androgens with the physiology of penile arterial inflow and associated penile tumescence has recently been reported in a number of clinical studies involving testosterone combination therapy to enhance penile erection through increased cavernous vasodilation (Aversa *et al*, 2000; Hwang *et al*, 2006).

Specifically, in one study, patients diagnosed with arteriogenic ED and decreasing response to PDE5 inhibitor (sildenafil) monotherapy, were co-administered transdermal testosterone in a combination treatment protocol. There were statistically significant improved outcomes on their penile flow and erectile function using scientific and clinical markers (Aversa *et al*, 2003).

Another study using IIEF and PADAM scores involved aging men with partial androgen deficiency (PADAM). It reported positive efficacy outcomes ($P<0.5$, paired t-test) in the group treated with a combination of sildenafil and testosterone (Shamloul *et al*, 2005).

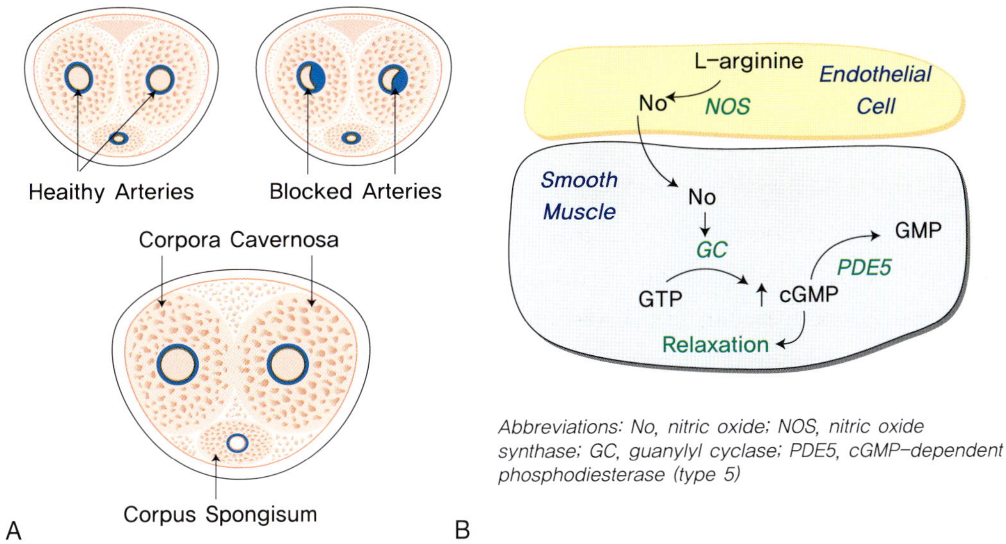

Figure 1. Mechanism of penile tumescence. A, Cross section of erectile penile tissues. B, Cavernous arterial dilation mediated by nitric oxide synthase and phosphodiesterase (PDE) type 5 through smooth muscle relaxation.

3. Sex hormone modulators from plant-derived ligands

Single plant extracts, containing thousands of phytochemicals, can modulate AR and the estrogen receptor isoforms, ER-α and ER-β. Furthermore, *in vivo* metabolism can result in an even greater number of metabolites, providing a wide range of pharmacological activities. Such sex hormone modulators provide broad and exciting prospects for the promotion of sexual health and/or treatment of sexual dysfunction.

4. Safety and toxicology of hormone modulators

The use of such modulators is not without some risk. Standard testosterone and estradiol hormone replacement therapies have been linked to statistically significant risks of gynaecologic and urologic cancers in patients of both genders. Hepatotoxicity is also an attendant risk factor with respect to androgen therapy, as evident from athletes with a history of anabolic steroid drug abuse. However, therapeutic agents that can boost sex steroid receptors, AR and ER, without the need for exogenous androgens or estrogens, would have less cancer risk. In fact, one of the adjunct benefits of activation of the ER-β is the anti-proliferative and pro-apoptotic effects on breast and prostate cancer cells.

5. Plant-derived products used as sexual medicines In Singapore and Asia

The male identity and sense of self-esteem, especially in Asia, are closely linked to sexual performance. Thus, sexual performance in the male has an unprecedented importance. Admitting to have ED is contra to the male ego, particularly if it occurs during midlife. It is reported that nearly 100 million people around the world live with ED (Kaiser, 1999). In diabetic patients, the incidence of ED is even more common. The number of diabetic patients is creasingly on the rise, with nearly 30% of ED in Singapore attributed to diabetes (Lim *et al*, 2002).

Only 10% of 100 million males with ED, i.e.10 million, seek scientifically-based Western style medical treatment (Kaiser, 1999). In Asia, the lower percentages of men with ED who seek treatment are 9% (in China) and 30% in Korea. Lim *et al* (2005) found that these lower figures can be attributed to the sensitivity and social stigma associated with ED. Hence, many patients self-medicate with local herbs and sex tonics.

Sexual herbs are eagerly consumed no matter how unappetizing or bizarre. In the continuous quest for better sex, Asians have ingested such diverse items as elephant tusks, lion blood, bull testicles, rhino horn, ram and ostrich penis, pig genitals and the dried remains of the Mediterranean Cantharis beetle, otherwise known as "Spanish Fly".

Popular in historic Singapore were "penis soup" and snake meat, whilst Surabaya in Indonesia is known for cobra meat and blood, which were claimed to improve erectogenic prowess. Animal testicles derived from bulls and wild boars contain an orchic substance that has been used to increase testosterone levels and sperm counts (Wang and Dahlen, 1994). In Singapore, testis soup has been very popular, and it remains so, in parts of China and Japan.

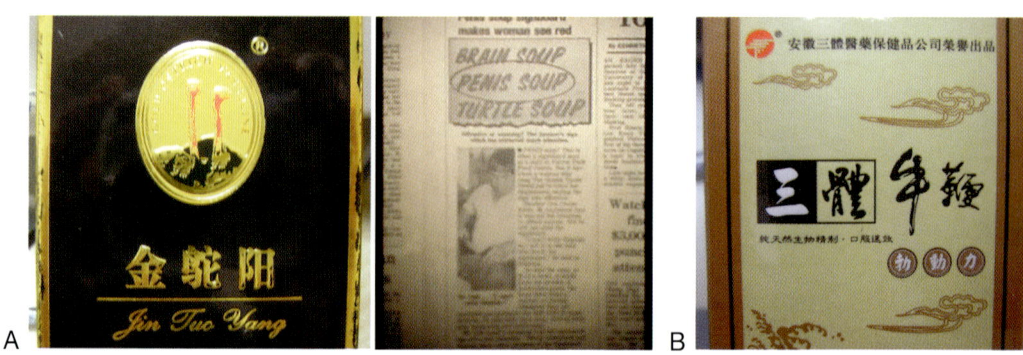

Figure 2. A, Ostrich Penis Powder. B, Cow Penis Powder

II. Simple Animal, Botanical and Pure Compound Formulations

1. Cervi pantotrichum (Deer antler)

This is probably the most popular sexual tonic used. In Chinese medical literature, kidneys are believed to control sexual function; hence foods and herbs that tonify the kidneys can improve impotence and infertility as well as increase semen production (Malo *et al*, 2005) (Figure 3).

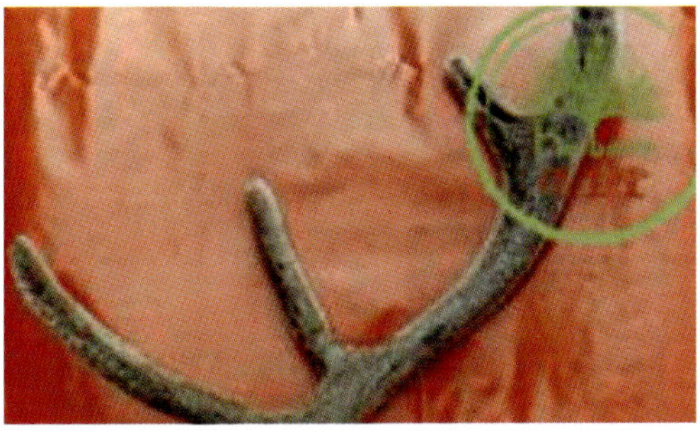

Figure 3. Deer antler

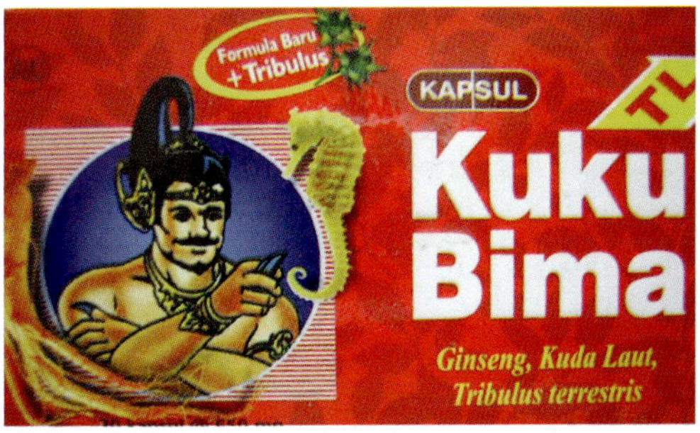

Figure 4. Kuku Bimat™ - an Indonesian product of powdered Sea Horse, mixed with other herbs

A B C

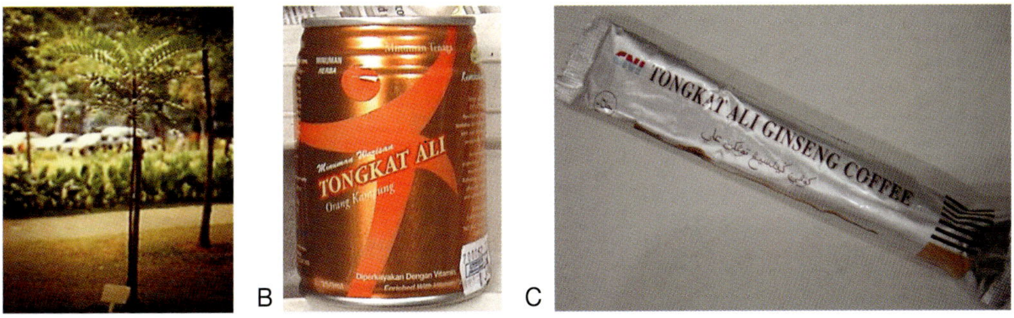

Figure 5. A, Eurycoma longifolia (Tongkat Ali™). B, Tongkat Ali: canned drink. C, Tongkat Ali: coffee mix

2. Hippocampus kelloggii (Seahorse)

This is used to prime the body's "yang," promote kidney function and normalize sexual activity. In Indonesia, it is usually used in powder form, and often packaged with other herbs e.g. "Kuku Bima" (Wang *et al*, 1994) (Figure 4).

3. Eurycoma longifolia (Tongkat Ali™)

This is a native plant found throughout Southeast Asia, that has been used as an aphrodisiac since 1996 (Ang *et al*, 2000). It has to be taken regularly and works by enhancing testosterone and cGMP production. Benefits are felt gradually over a period of time, mainly because it enhances the natural synthesis of testosterone. When this hormone level is increased, health and vitality are restored.

In mice studies, Tongkat Ali™ increased the frequency and duration of sexual performance by enhancing testosterone levels by up to 440%. In a recent study in humans, 62% of the subjects showed an increase in the free testosterone index, indicating its role in the biosynthesis of steroids. It has also been shown to increase sperm concentration and motility (Ang *et al*, 2000) (Figure 5).

4. Saccostrea species (Oyster)

Historically known as an aphrodisiac, oyster extract is excellent for men's reproductive health

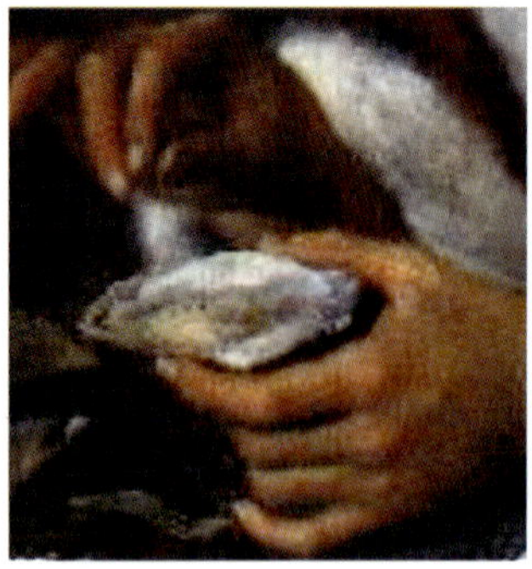

Figure 6. Oysters

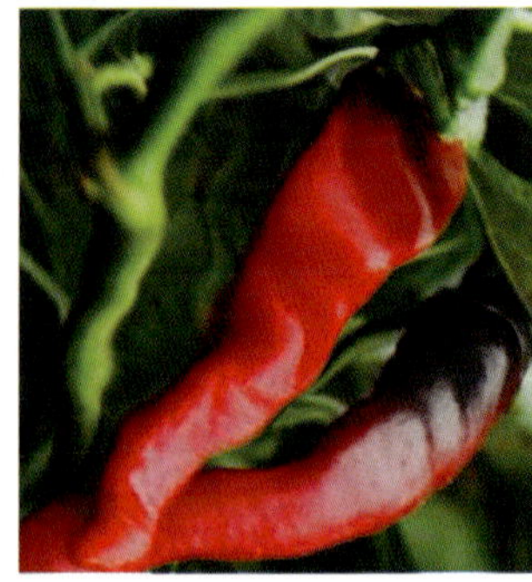

Figure 7. Fresh cayenne peppers (Capsicum annum)

and endurance. It is also a rich source for the amino acid, taurine, which has a cardio-protective effect and is involved in nerve transmission. The flavonoids in oyster flesh have been shown to stimulate the human reproductive system (Figure 6).

5. Capsicum annum (Cayenne)

Cayenne, also known as cayenne pepper, is a member of the *Capsicum* family of vegetables and plays a role in blood circulation (Rowland and Tai, 2003). When cayenne is ingested, it acts to dilate blood vessels, allowing blood flow to increase throughout the body, especially in the major organs. The male penis benefits greatly from the ingestion of cayenne. It is a widely held belief that cayenne aids in longer lasting erections, with stronger ejaculations and more intense orgasms (Figure 7).

6. Cuscuta chinensis

Cuscuta seed is a common component in tonic formulations designed to benefit *yin* and *yang*. It is a gentle tonic for the kidney *yin* and *yang* and also helps nourish *chi* (Wang and Dahlen, 1994; Rowland and Tai, 2003). It helps the kidney to consolidate the *chi* and is widely used to restore urogenital dysfunctions such as impotence, premature ejaculation, frequent urination and leucorrhoea, tinnitus and aching lower back, all symptoms which often accompany deficiency in kidney that is associated with sexual aesthenia (Figure 8).

7. Cordyceps sinensis

Cordyceps sinensis is one of the most popular, and expensive, herbs in the world, revered for thousands of years in the Orient. As a result of modern growing techniques, it is now available to everyone at a fraction of its traditional cost. According to traditional Chinese health theory, Cordyceps is used for the primary purpose of strengthening kidney function, which include sexual

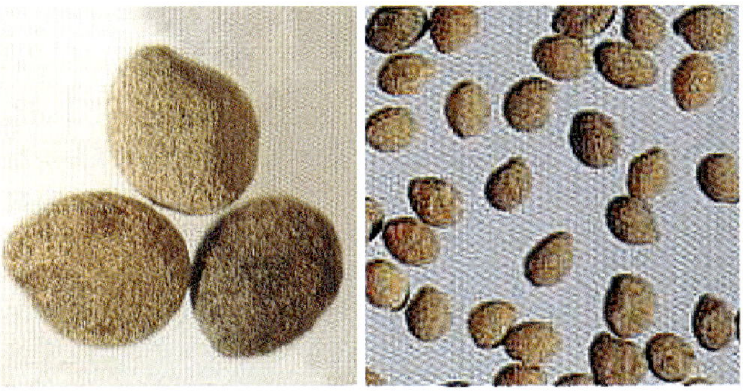

Figure 8. Dried fruits and seeds of *Cuscuta chinensis*

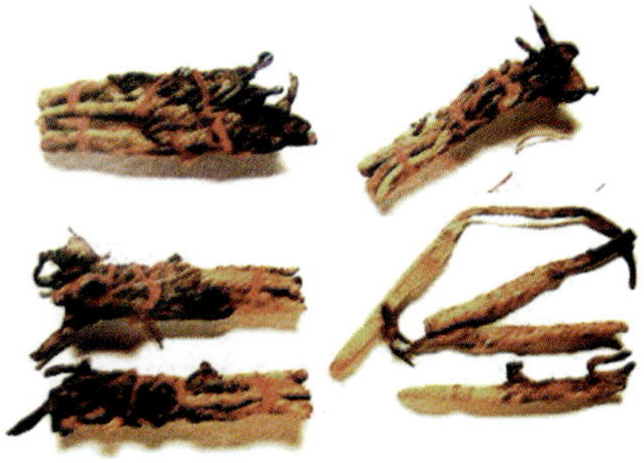

Figure 9. *Cordyceps sinensis*

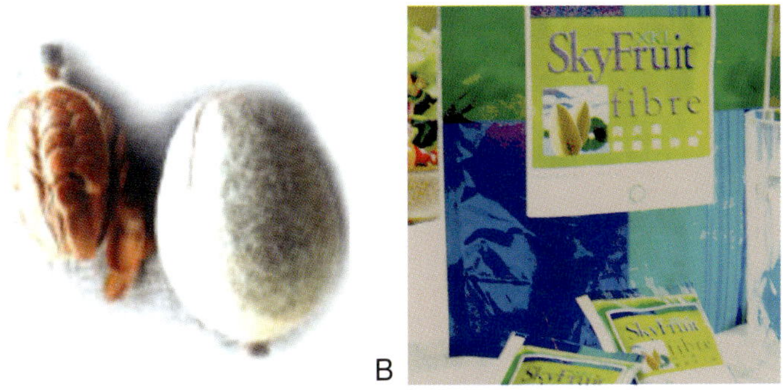

A B

Figure 10. Skyfruit. A, fresh fruit. B, Instant mix.

function, brain power, structural integrity and healing ability (Zhu *et al*, 1998) (Figure 9).

8. Swietenia macrophylla (Skyfruit)

This "Queen of plants" is mainly found in tropical areas in the South Pacific and in lesser quantity in other tropical areas of the world. The Malaysians with the help of their Government have produced from this another nitric oxide donor product which has become very popular.

The flavonoids found in Skyfruit interfere with the formation of atherosclerotic plaques, promote blood circulation and act as anti-oxidant as well as free radical scavenger. The saponins found in Skyfruit are recognised for their cancer prevention and capability to reduce body fats, enhance the immune system and improve vitality in giving better erections via its vascular effects. They can also reduce blood clotting and alleviate blood sugar levels (Figure 10).

9. Eucommia ulmoides and caprylic acid

The processed tree bark of duzhong [*Eucommia ulmoides*] (Figure 11A) is used in traditional Chinese medicine (TCM) to treat lumbago, osteopenia, osteoporosis and other musculoskeletal disorders associated with hypogonadal function. Interestingly, while it is a 'yin' herb, described as

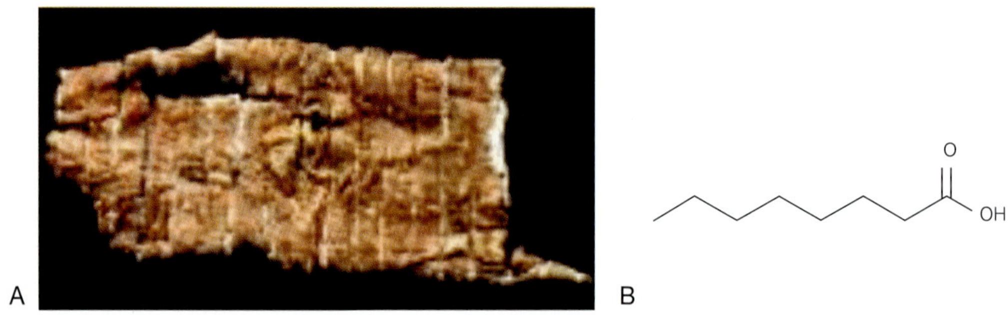

Figure 11. A, Dried cortex of *E.ulmoides*. B, Caprylic acid from *E. ulmoides*

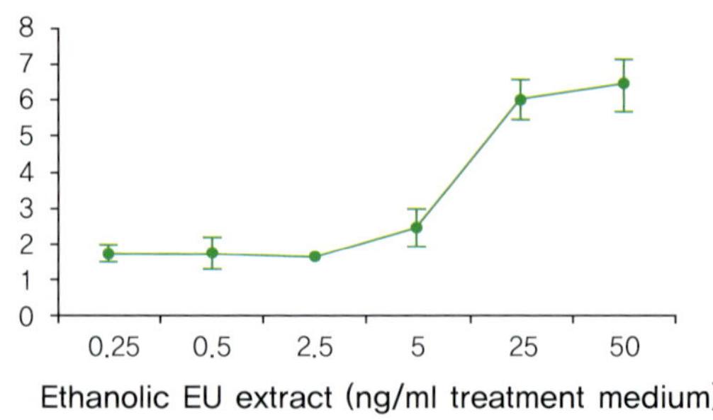

Figure 12. Phytoandrogenic activity of *E. ulmoides* extract

having a 'nourishing' effect on the kidneys in Chinese Materia Medica, its prescribed indications are anabolic and 'yang-like'. This paradox is resolved, because of the diverse pharmacologic actions of *E. ulmoides* at the molecular and cellular levels (Figure 11).

Novel phytoandrogenic activity in cortical extracts of *E. ulmoides* has been recently reported (Ong and Tan, 2007). However, the *E. ulmoides* agonist action on AR is weak [< 10% AR transactivation activity vis-à-vis 1nM dihydrotestosterone (DHT)] and mediated by triterpenoids, not steroids.

Most strikingly, previously unknown synergism between the AR, DHT and *E. ulmoides* lipidic compounds has been discovered, which can boost the *holo*-AR transactivational capacity by > 200%, benchmarked to the standard of 100% reporter gene (ARE-Luc) activation by the AR at saturating doses (≥10 nm) of DHT and testosterone (Figure 12).

Besides efficacy, the safety profile of *E. ulmoides* is well established, through its general use over millennia in China and parts of Asia, as a food tonic as well as specific inclusions in TCM prescriptions.

10. Eucommia ulmoides and phytoandrogens

The enriched fraction of E. ulmoides, which contains pharmacologically active

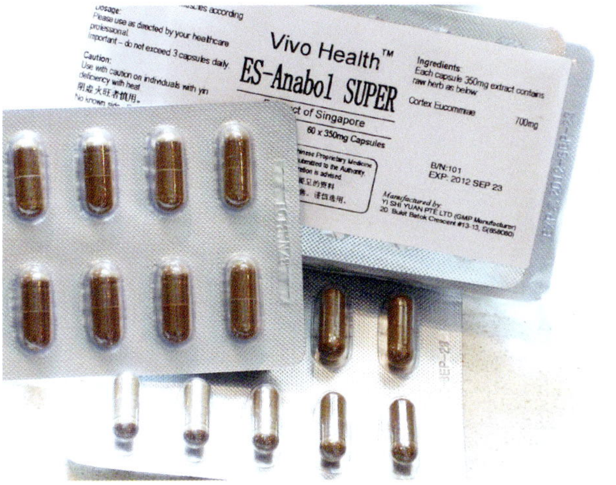

Figure 13. ES-Anabol SUPER for men and women

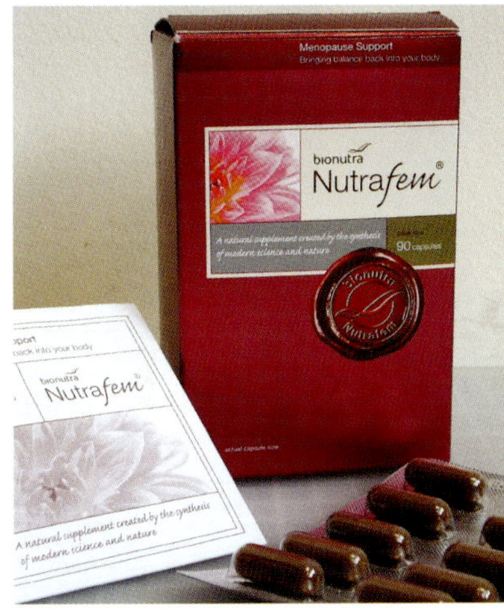

Figure 14. Nutrafem™ for women

phytoandrogens and suprahormonal lipidic augmenters (SuHLAs), can synergistically promote the anabolic and sexual milieu, in both men and women (Ong and Yong, 2005; Ong and Tan, 2007).

Dosage and Administration: In 2010, a specialised enrichment technique coupled to patented extraction methodology, has made phytoandrogens and SuHLAs clinically available - approved as the proprietary medicine ES-Anabol SUPER - from Vivo Health Centre for Integrative Weight-Healthcare (Figure 13). Recommended dosing regimen is 700 mg b.i.d., titrated up to t.i.d.; integrated into a weight-health programme, tailored to the individual patient's family and medical history, and a work-up of current clinical profile.

11. Eucommia ulmoides and Vigna radiata (Nutrafem™)

Nutrafem™ (Figure 14) is a dual bioassay-standardized formulation comprising the extracts of *E. ulmoides* and *Vigna radiata* (mung bean). It is recommended at daily dosages of 1,000 mg q.d. (for general healthcare) and 1,500 mg t.i.d. (for acute climacteric symptoms).

12. Pausinystalia yohimbe and arginine

Yohimbe (*Pausinystalia yohimbe*) is an evergreen tree native to West Africa, but is also present in Asia. It is the only herb listed in the Physician' s Index Reference for sexual function. The US FDA approved yohimbe as the first plant-derived drug for treating impotence long ago and was dubbed the "herbal viagra" in the February 1999 edition of Environmental Nutrition.

Alkaloids present in yohimbe such as isoyohimbine, allo-yohimbine, yohimbinine, yohimbane, yohimbenine and corynanthein block alpha-2 adrenergic activity leading to vasodilation. Yohimbine has a dual aphrodisiac function: it improves sexual function by displacing epinephrine

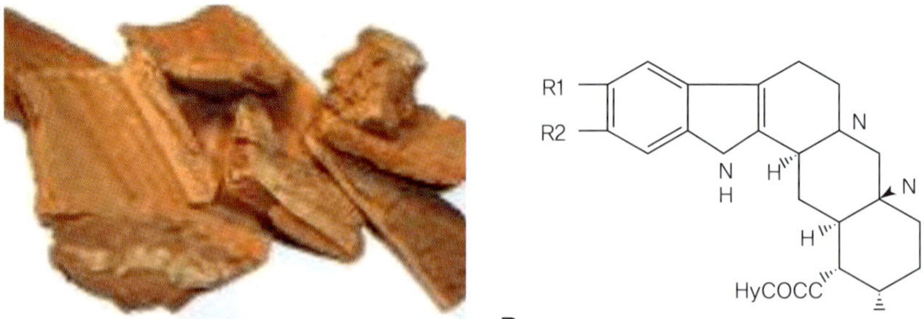

A B

Figure 15. *Pausinystalia yohimbe*. A, Dried cortex. B, Structure of yohimbine HCL.

from alpha-2 adrenergic receptors in the pelvic area and it increases proneness to arousal through supplying the epinephrine from the alpha-2 receptors to the central nervous system (brain) where it is active as a neurotransmitter. Side-effects include nervousness, anxiety, insomnia and mild hypertension (Carey and Johnson, 1996).

Yohimbine is an indole alkaloid isolated from the bark of the African evergreen tree, *Pausinystalia yohimbe* (Figure 15). In traditional African bush medicine, *P. yohimbe* extract was used as an aphrodisiac. Scientific studies have reported that yohimbine HCL and *P. yohimbe* extract have multiple mechanisms of action at the neurological and vascular levels. For instance, yohimbine is an antagonist of the α-adrenergic receptor and serotonin receptor sub-types, leading to excitation, vasodilation and smooth muscle relaxation at the physiological level. Nitric oxide release through an agonist action on endothelin β-receptor has also been reported.

A number of preclinical research work showed that yohimbine, a combination of yohimbine and arginine (amino acid substrate for nitric oxide generation) and extracts of *P. yohimbe* could stimulate sexual activity - increased mating behaviour and shorter refractory period. However, controlled clinical trials have reported only limited efficacy; only a subset of patients with ED respond to yohimbine pharmacotherapy while effectiveness in treating hyposexuality (low libido) is still anecdotal.

Acute safety is a major concern with yohimbine. Adverse side effects can include tachycardia, hypertension, vertigo, anxiety, irritability and nausea. Patients with cardiac, hepatic, renal or psychiatric disorders shoud not take yohimbine product. The complementary amino acid, arginine, can trigger painful herpes simplex (HSV) episodes, in carriers and aggravate severity of symptoms in infected patients; this adverse effect may be mitigated to some extent by the co-administration of lysine.

Dosage and Administration: Yohimbine HCL is available as a prescription drug for treating ED under various trade names such as Yocon™ and Procomil™. Recommended dosages are in the range of 5.4 mg to 6 mg t.i.d., while that of arginine is broad, from 3250 mg (for ED therapy, in combination with yohimbine) to the mega dose of 18 g (for bodybuilders). Arginine and

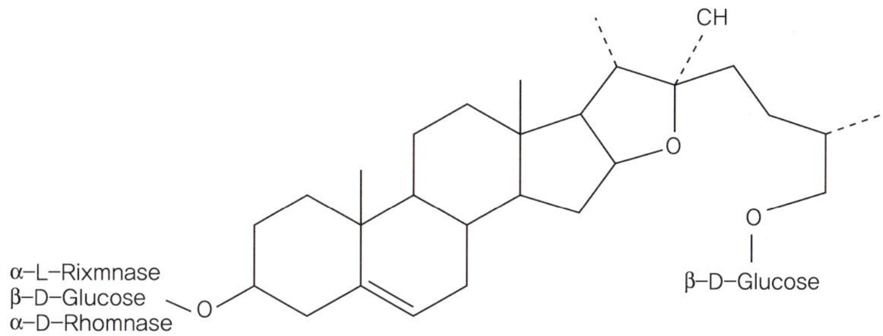

Figure 16. Structure of protodioscin

combinations of arginine, lysine and other amino acids are readily available in either generic versions or trademarked products such as GNC Pro Performance® L-Arginine L-Ornithine.

13. Tribulus terrestris

This has long been used as a folk medicine in several parts of Asia and most widely in Eastern Europe and Bulgaria for sexual deficiency (Rowland and Tai, 2003). In Bulgaria, the hormone-balancing effects of *Tribulus terrestris* are used for pre-menstrual and menopausal syndromes. The effects of this powerful herb have included increased sperm production, sexual endurance and testosterone levels (CHEMEXCIL, 1992).

There are three groups of active phytochemicals in *T. terrestris* viz. (1) dioscin- responsible for sexual energy by increasing the free testosterone level for men and modulating other sex steroids, including pregnenolone, progesterone and estrogen, (2) sterols, which protect the prostate from swelling and in combination with (3) the sex steroidal saponins, influence the immune system and also possess antiviral properties (possibly against herpes).

Protodioscin is a structural precursor of the weakly androgenic dehydroepiandrosterone (DHEA) (Figure 16) which is found in *T. terrestris*. At the same time, DHEA is a physiological precursor of the active androgens, testosterone and dihydrotestosterone (DHT). Since testosterone plays a significant role in men' s virility, the addition of this herb can prove to be very beneficial. Preclinical studies have reported a rise in serum levels of DHEA, testosterone and DHT in rodents, rabbits and primates, as well as improvements in sexual behaviour and penile erectile capacity of rats and rabbits given protodioscin (Adaikan *et al*, 2000; Gauthaman *et al*, 2003; Gauthaman and Adaikan, 2008).

Notably, *T. terrestris* is used ethnobotanically in both TCM and Ayurveda (traditional Indian medicine) as a prescription herb, not routinely consumed as a food tonic (Figure 17). Accordingly, daily lifelong use for maintaining sexual health may not be fully supported in terms of potential for chronic toxicity. In addition, given its reported pharmacological effect in raising serum androgens, long-term safety concerns regarding androgen replacement therapy and the attendant risk for

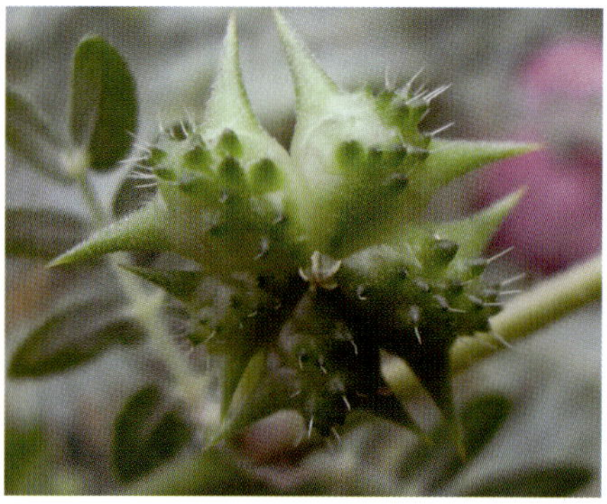

Figure 17. Fresh leaves and fruits of *Tribulus terrestris*

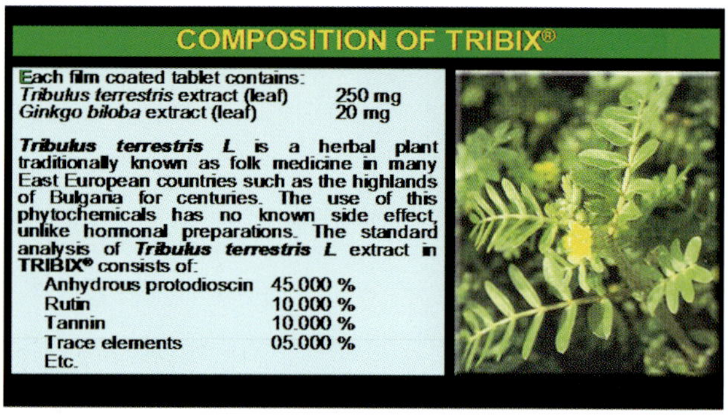

Figure 18. Tribix® - a *Tribulus terrestris* product

accelerating the growth of prostatic neoplasia will also apply to *T. terrestris* extract (Figure 17).

Dosage and administration: Mainstream nutraceutical companies with products manufactured from the leaf or fruit of *T. terrestris* for bodybuilding and improving sexual performance include Twinlab™ Tribulus Fuel and GNC™ Ultimate Nutrition Bulgarian Tribulus.

Libilov™, a combination of 250 mg leaf extract of T. terrestris, 20mg leaf extract of Ginkgo biloba and 250 mg arginine, has a product-specific clinical study carried out by the University of Sriwijaya, Indonesia, on its efficacy, with the report featured in the website of the Nutrica Inc company (Arsyad, 1996). Tribix™ is a combination of T. terrestris and G. biloba (Figure 18).

14. Panax ginseng and multivitamins

The dried and processed roots of *P. ginseng* have been prized over a few millennia, as a food tonic and curative panacea for many ailments, including sexual dysfunction in TCM, traditional Japanese medicine (Kampo) and traditional Korean medicine (TKM). Russian researchers termed it an adaptogen, with anti-cancer, anti-aging and other vitality-promoting properties. Extensive molecular, cellular, animal and clinical studies spanning decades have been published on ginseng and its pharmacological activities (see review in Ong and Yong, 2000).

Many of the therapeutic benefits of *P. ginseng* are attributed to ginsenosides, a class of related saponins found in both the Panax genus (*P. japonicus*, *P. vietnamensis*, *P. quinquefolius*) and Siberian ginseng (*Eleutherococcus senticosus*) (Figure 19). While each ginsenoside has its own pharmacodynamics (PD) and structure-activity relationships (SAR), a number of these saponins are also plant-specific (Figure 20).

However, ginsenosides are not agonists of the sex steroid receptors (Ong and Yong, 2005). Clinical studies that investigated penile hemodynamics and serum testosterone levels have also not detected any significant changes in these sex-specific parameters, while reporting improvements to

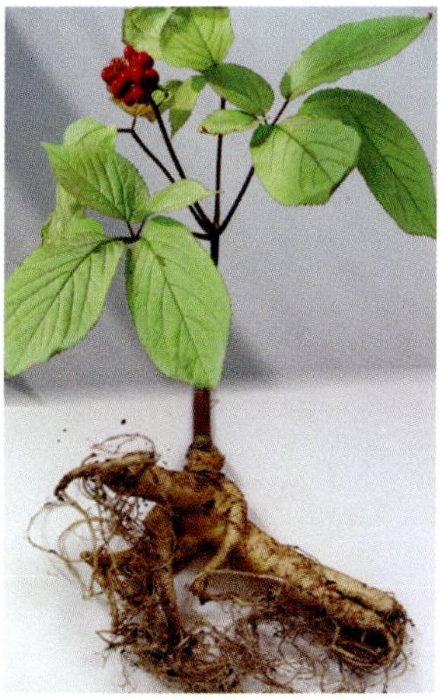

Figure 19. Fresh leaves, fruit cluster and roots of *Panax ginseng*

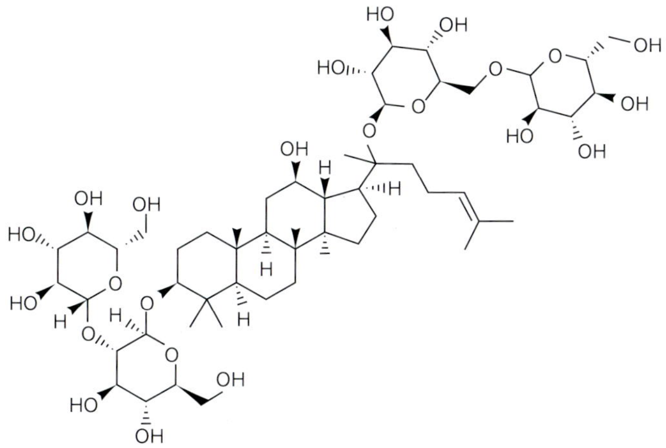

Figure 20. Structure of ginsenoside Rb1

both ED and psychometric clinical endpoints (Choi *et al*, 1995; Hong *et al*, 2002). Regarding the latter, ginsenosides' therapeutic effects on ED and other aspects of sexual health are likely to be due to improved general health and enhanced metabolic capacity (adaptogenic properties of ginseng), rather than to any specific mechanism of action that affects libido or virility.

Chronic deficiencies in vitamins and minerals can compromise general health, including sexual reproduction. Clinical studies investigating combinations of *P. ginseng* extract with multivitamins and multiminerals taken daily by the elderly have been reported to improve overall health and quality-of-life (Ong and Yong, 2000).

Dosage and administration: Standardized extracts contain 250 mg, 500 mg to 1,000 mg of ginsenosides. Once-daily multivitamin formulations containing standardized ginsenosides include Merck' s Seven Seas™ Multivitamins and Minerals with Ginseng, Pharmaton™ Complex and Vitaton™ Gold. The dosage of ginseng roots in traditional use range from 1 g to 5 g, administered as a decoction or infusion tea.

15. Epimedium species and Lepidium meyenii

'Yin Yang Huo' or Herba epimedii in TCM actually refers to the dried aerial parts of a group of plants belonging to the same genus - *Epimedium sagittatum*, *E. brevicornum*, *E. pubescens*, *E. wushanensis*, *E. koreanum*, and *E. grandiflorum* (Figures 21 and 22). *Epimedium* extract is referred to by the Chinese as '*Yin Yang Huo*', a 'licentious goat plant'; hence, its common name in many cultures is 'horny goat weed'. Phytochemicals that have been isolated include flavonoids, lignans, phenolic glycosides and ionones.

Scientifically, studies have shown that epimedium may restore low levels of both testosterone

A B C

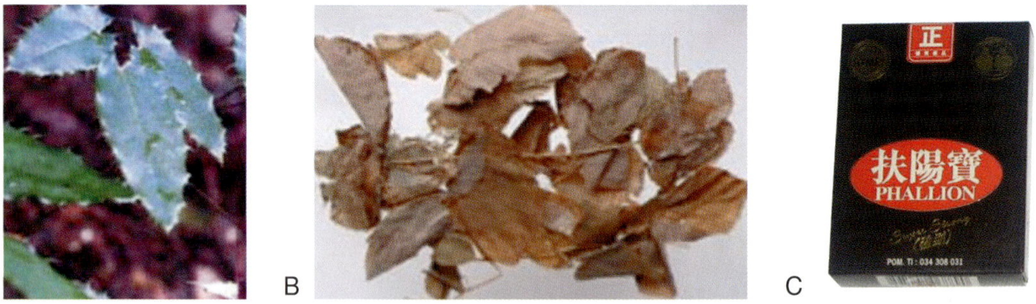

Figure 21. *Epimedium species.* A, *Epimedium* leaves. B, slices of *Epimedium* root. C, Phallion™ from China/Indonesia containing *Epimedium*.

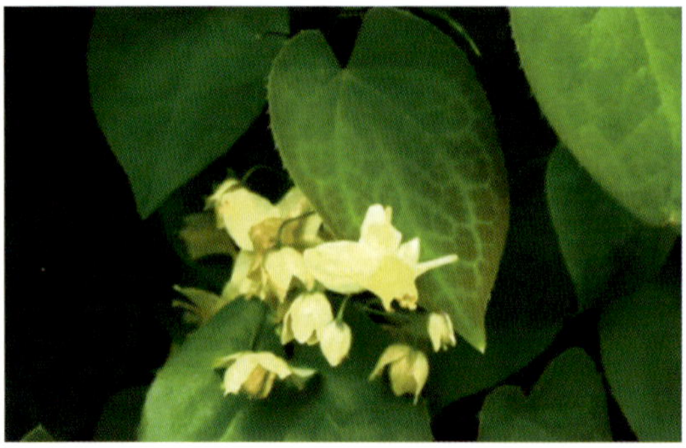

Figure 22. Fresh leaves and flowers of *Herba epimedii*

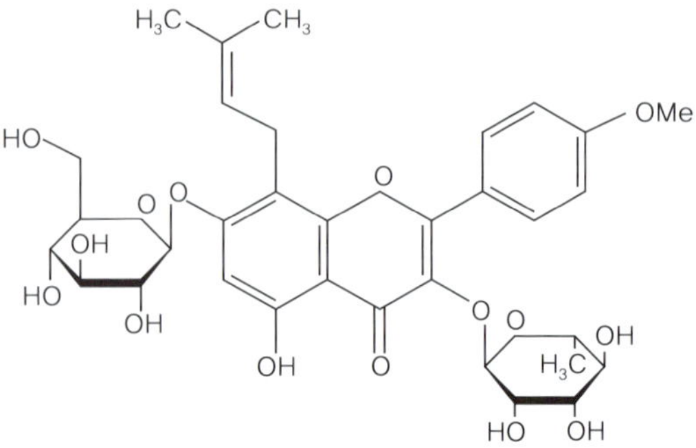

Figure 23. Structure of the *Epimedium* flavonol, icariin

and thyroid hormone. This may account for some of its benefits in improving sexual libido (Kuang *et al*, 1989). It reinforces the kidney 'Yang' and is used to treat impotence and weakness of limbs in ethnobotany. Interestingly, *Epimedium spp.* extracts are highly phytoestrogenic, activating both ER-α and ER-β. Icariin, a flavonol glycoside in *Epimedium*, has also been reported to increase serum testosterone level (Zhang and Yang, 2006). Prostatic and hepatic effects associated with testosterone replacement therapy are, therefore, long term safety concerns.

Epimedium species have been combined with *Lepidium meyenii* to produce an aphrodisiac for men and women, branded as Windmill™ Horny Goat Weed with Pure MACA, marketed by Walgreens Health Services, a United States company based in Chicago.

The common name for *L. meyenii* in the South American Andes is Maca; its dried roots are used in Peruvian folk medicine as an aphrodisiac and fertility aid. Maca belongs to the Brassica family, which include common vegetables such as cabbage, mustard and broccoli (Figure 24).

Rodent studies suggest that it can enhance sexual behaviour, with one recent clinical research involving healthy adults reporting that *L. meyenii* has efficacy in boosting male libido. In contrast, *in vivo* study using mice suggested that extract of *L. meyenii* may protect against androgen-induced prostatic hyperplasia.

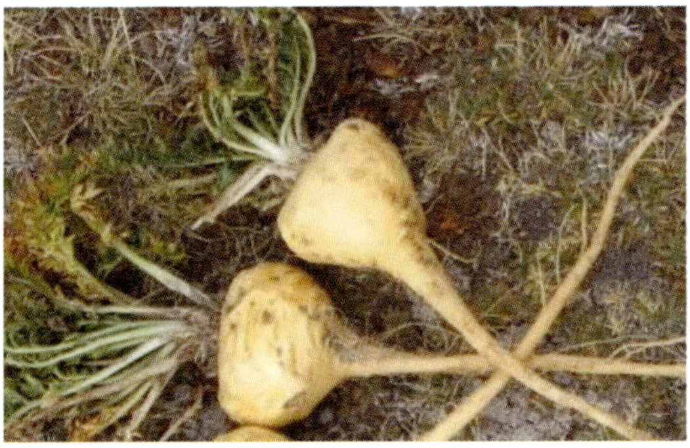

Figure 24. Fresh whole plant of *Lepidium meyenii*

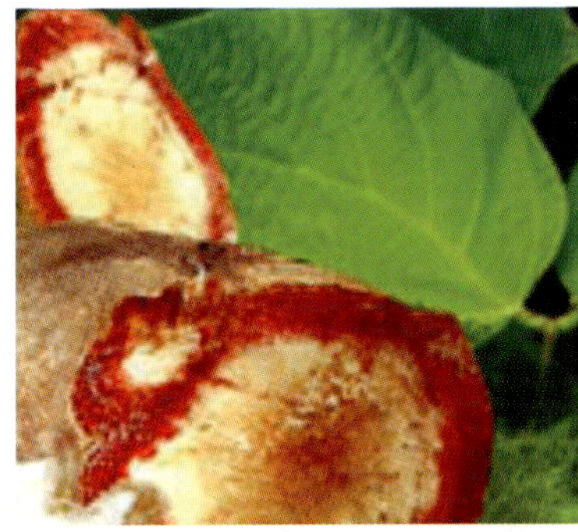

Figure 25. Fresh leaves and roots of *Butea superba*

The lack of coherent pharmacological data relating Maca' s efficacy to specific phytochemicals, pathways or target receptors currently limits its inclusion as a therapeutic agent in evidence-based healthcare. However, the positive preliminary data and its history of ethnobotanical use indicate that *L. meyenii* has good prospects for clinical use in the near future.

16. Butea superba

The tubers of *Butea superba*, known locally as *"red kwao krua"* in Thailand, are used in traditional Thai medicine for rejuvenation and sexual vigour (Figure 25). *B. superba* is a Southeast Asian forest plant with root tubers that contain flavonoids with PDE inhibitory activity.

There has been one randomized, double-blind, 3-month prospective clinical study (N = 39) conducted by Chulalongkorn University in Thailand examining its efficacy in treating ED, using self-administered IIEF-5 questionnaire. Improvements in the psychometric scores were statistically significant. For instance, 64.8% of pre-treated patients reported difficulty in maintaining erection to completion of sexual intercourse versus 29.50% post-treatment ($P<0.05$, n = 17).

On the other hand, an oral toxicological study using 90-day animal dosing reported adverse changes in hepatic function (increased levels of serum alkaline phosphatase and aspartate aminotransferase), the androgen milieu (decreased serum testosterone level) and enlarged spleen, with a dose-dependent effect, ranging from 0mg to 200 mg/kg BW/day.

Dosage and Administration: Human efficacy study suggests using daily oral dosages of 500 mg-2,000 mg dried tuber. Preclinical dose-response study in male rodents, using ethanol extract of *B. superba* roots indicate an optimal dose of 1mg/kg BW i.e. a man with a body weight of 80 kg will require 80 mg extract. An oral dosage form containing 200 mg extract (30:1) per capsule is available in North America, labeled as *Butea superba Premium Root Powder™*, and marketed by a Canadian company, Root of the Matter.

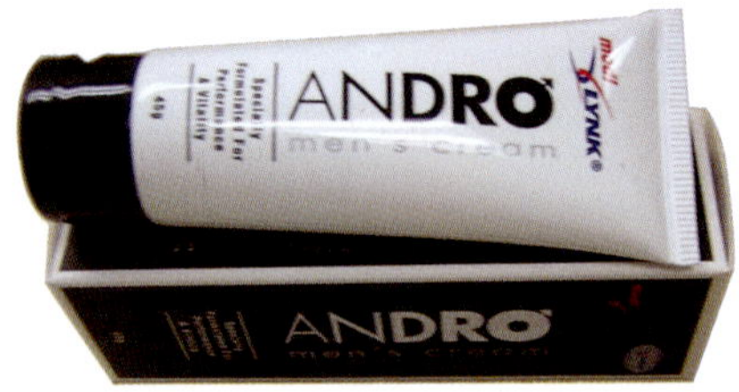

Figure 26. Medilynk™ Andro Men' s Cream

Addressing toxicity concerns, topical formulations of *B. superba* are now commercially available, such as Medilynk™ Andro Men' s Cream (10% w/w *B. superba* extract) (Figure 26), produced by the Singapore-based biotech company, Medilynk PL (Figures 26).

17. Complex herbal formulations

1) *Virilar*®

This is a formulated botanical complex for improving men' s health and sexual performance. It is a health supplement consisting of a proprietary blend of 27 natural ingredients in a single capsule made by a Singapore company, bioDYNE Labs, Inc. Spore and USA. Based on results from clinical studies done in the US and Indonesia, continuous therapy with the product was shown to be effective and safe in increasing erectile function and sexual desire in men with mild to moderate ED. As Virilar® (Figures 27) has a combination of many ingredients and compounds, multiple pathways and mechanisms of action might be involved.

Although the mechanisms of action are not completely understood, individual ingredients in Virilar® have been studied and reported by various laboratories. Several ingredients were shown to increase L-Arginine-Nitric Oxide (NO) pathway activity (important for penile smooth muscle relaxation and erectile function), while other studies were found to increase testosterone production (one of the important mechanisms to increase sexual desire). Other potentially relevant mechanisms include increasing angiogenesis, cardiovascular protection and anti-oxidative activities. The ingredients in Virilar® may act synergistically in multiple pathways to promote sexual function and desire. The pharmacokinetics of these botanical ingredients are mostly unknown. Future studies on pharmacokinetics of Virilar® are necessary to explain the 12-48 hour duration of the effect of Virilar®.

2) *Tongkat Ajimat Madura*™

In Madura, Indonesia, there is a formulation called Tongkat Ajimat Madura™ (Figures 28), used by mid-wives to reduce the vaginal laxity following childbirth. This has also been used by non-pregnant women just before sex to increase tone and narrow the vagina just before penetration to

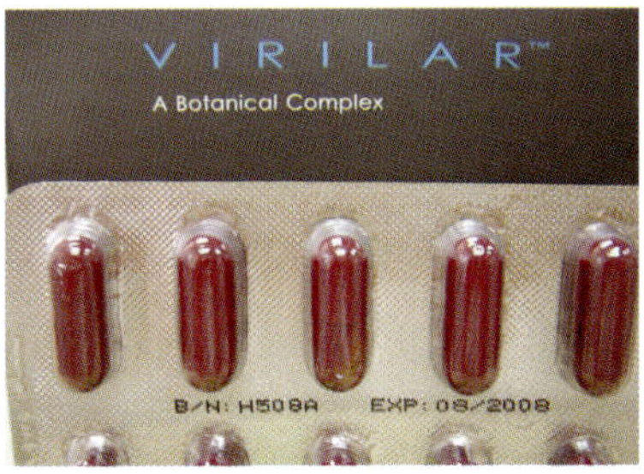

Figure 27. Virilar®

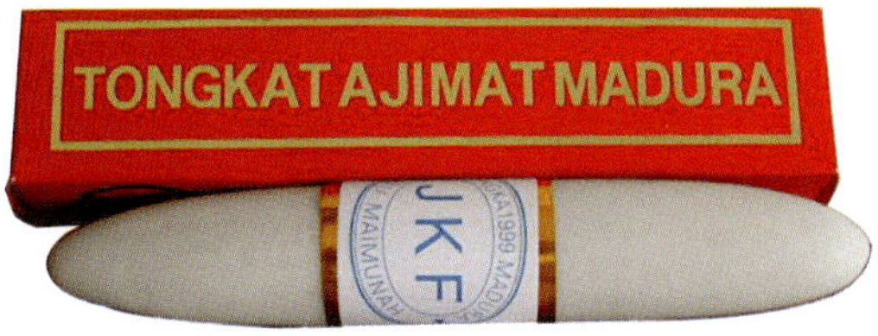

Figure 28. Tongkat Ajimat Madura™

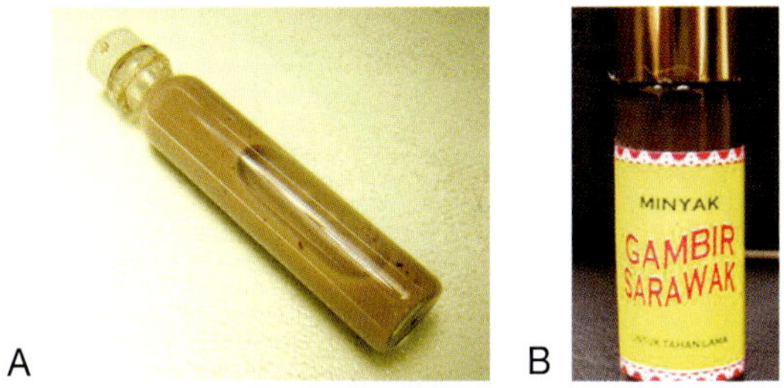

Figure 29. A, Powdered Gambir™. B, Gambir™ liquid.

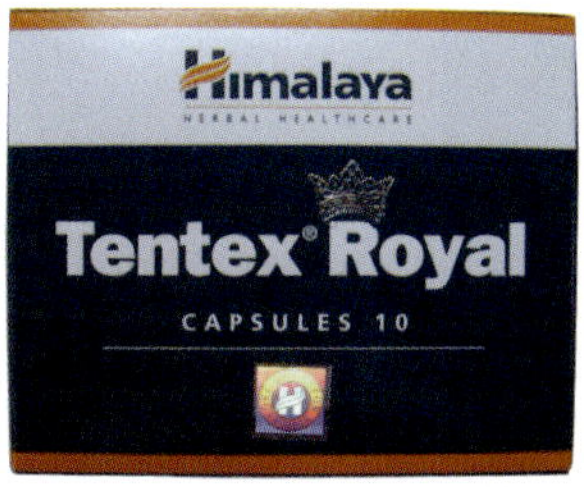

Figure 30. Tentex Royal™, a concoction of several herbs

increase sexual satisfaction for the male and female during the sex act.

3) *Gambir*™

Gambir™ (Figures 29) is a powdered medication, well-known in Singapore and Malaysia which, when applied on the surface of the penis, results in prolonged erection and declining premature ejaculation (Lunenfeld, 2006).

4) *Tentex royal*™

Tentex Royal™ (Figures 30), a concoction of several local Indian herbs, is made by the Indian company, Himalaya Herbal Healthcare in Makali, Bangalore, India. It can enhance sexual desire and performance, according to a clinical study (Sanjay, 2004).

III. Discussion

Apart from a small number of approved ethical drugs and their well-characterized pharmacology (namely sex hormones and their synthetic derivatives, and PDE inhibitors), how can herbs help with sex? In many instances, they probably act as "aphrodisiacs". An aphrodisiac (the word derives from Aphrodite, the Greek goddess of love and beauty) is anything that provokes sexual interest or desire. Indeed, many herbs can enhance sexual desire. Additionally, when it comes to sex, traditional medicines have been claimed to improve mood, increase sexual desire, drive and pleasure.

The sexual drive is perhaps the most fascinating of all the "bodily drives." True, its original purpose may have been to ensure the continuation of humankind. But the concept of procreation probably ranks much lower on most of our scales than a desire for plain, "old-fashioned" sexual enjoyment. Herbs thus provide the urge - the libido or desire or drive to have sex as often as we like. Lack of sexual drive can turn sex into more of a chore than a pleasure.

The herbs described in this discussion help put sexual desire and drive back into the patient' s life or back into the life of the person he/she loves.

Setting the mood and desire to have sex are certainly the first two key psychological steps to sexual enjoyment. At the physiological level, herbs help by initiating a change in the body' s internal milieu, such as increasing the body' s production of testosterone, the "male" hormone that functions in both men and women to create a sexual response. Because of this role, most of these herbs are more effective when taken consistently over a period of time. Within a few weeks, the patient will gradually begin to notice a change in sexual response, together with increasing sexual pleasure.

Furthermore, herbs have multiple properties that may also aid health conditions that might otherwise inhibit sex - (1) male problems of impotence, prostate problems and male menopause, (2) female problems of menopause and premenstrual syndrome, (3) chronic health problems such as arthritis or diabetes, (4) conditions that affect overall well-being, such as lack of energy or addiction to cigarettes, alcohol or drugs.

In the East, many herbal tonics and preparations are used to assist the aging male improve his sexual drive or ability to perform penetrative sex by increasing sexual stimulation, erectile, ejaculatory orgasmic and other responses for sexual function and satisfaction. The "energy-enhancing" herbs and tonics, such as ginseng (*Panax species*), may be useful to select patient subsets, such as the tired and fatigued male; possibly those suffering from sexual asthenia as well.

Apart from the benefits mentioned above, which pertain to potential aphrodisiac properties, a new generation of evidence-based botanical therapeutics is also emerging. For instance, the hydro-alcoholic extract of duzhong (*E. ulmoides*), with novel boosting action on sex steroid receptors, further extends the range of alternative and adjunct treatment options, in conjunction with current sex hormone replacement regimens, such as androgen replacement therapy.

Testosterone analogues and botanical "testosterone releasers" will have some impact on andropausal males. The caveat is that, male patients at risk of, or suffering from, prostate cancer, benign prostatic hyperplasia and/or elevated prostate-specific antigen (PSA) level, must be screened carefully, prior to prescription of such therapies.

Deer horn and antlers contain growth factors and androgenic precursors. Taking these may help improve nocturnal erections in the male with somatopause. On the other hand, dubious remedies such as "penis soup", the famous Indonesian cobra meat and cobra blood from Surabaya, also claim to have erectogenic prowess. Adding to these 'snake-oil' myths are sexual performance aids derived from the testicles of dog, wild boar, bull and ostrich; village witch-doctor remedies are still being practiced widely in some developing regions of Asia.

On the other hand, in China, the horny goat weed is popular and may have some scientific merit for enhancing sexual drive. Recently, the active phytochemical, icariin, was isolated from the foliage of the plant. The latter, better known as *Epimedii herba*, has the specific property of increasing erectile function with no influence on blood pressure. The mechanism of action for icariin is believed to be a cGMP-specific PDE5 inhibitor that increases cGMP level in the corpus cavernosum, whilst having no effect on the cAMP that influences systemic blood pressure. Hence, icariin, extracted from a herb used for centuries, could well be a safe and effective agent for the treatment of erectile dysfunction, in addition to the well-characterized PDE5 inhibitor class of ED drugs, namely - sildenafil, tadalafil and vardenafil.

Therefore, the future for herbals and tonics is promising, especially for selected folklore medicines that have rigorous scientific and clinical research, detailed toxicological data and high quality manufacturing (GMP) standards.

IV. Conclusions

Through the use of modern molecular tools coupled with animal and clinical studies, it is clear that ancient herbs found in traditional medicines such as TCM, Ayurveda, Jamu Melayu, African bush and South American rainforest ethnobotany will yield exciting pure compounds or drugs for therapeutic use by mainstream healthcare, in the years to come, especially in the field of sexual medicine.

The introduction of a new pharmaceutical category, Botanical Drug Products, by the USFDA in 2004 is a sign that holistic, traditional ethnobotany will eventually be transformed into modern, science-driven evidence-based medicine, for the good of all humanity.

● REFERENCES

1. Adaikan PG, Gauthaman K, Prasad RN, Ng SC. Proerectile pharmacological effects of *Tribulus terrestris* extract on the rabbit corpus cavernosum. Ann Acad Med Singapore. 2000 Jan; 29(1): 22-6.
2. Ang HH, Cheang HS, Yusof AP. Effects of *Eurycoma longifolia* (Tongkat Ali) in the initiation of sexual performance of inexperienced castrated male rats. J Exp Anim 2000; 49:35-8.
3. Arsyad KM. Effect of protodioscin on the quantity and quality of sperms from males with moderate idiopathic oligozoospermia. Medika 22 (8): 614-618 (1996).
4. Aversa A, Isidori AM, De Martino MU, Caprio M, Fabbrini E, Rocchietti-March M, Frajese G, Fabbri A. Androgens and penile erection: evidence for a direct relationship between free testosterone and cavernous vasodilation in men with erectile dysfunction. 2000 Oct; 53 (4): 517-22.
5. Bucci LR. Selected herbals and human exercise performance. Am J Clin Nutr 2000; 72: 624S-36S.
6. Carey MP, Johnson BT. Effectiveness of yohimbine in the treatment of erectile disorder: Four meta-analytic integrations. Arch Sex Behav 1996; 25:341-60.
7. CHEMEXCIL. *Tribulus terrestris* L. (N.O. Zygophyllaceae). Selected medicinal plants of India. A monograph of identity, safety and clinical usage. Tata Press: 1992. p. 323-6.
8. Cherdshewasart W, Nimsakul N. Clinical trial of *Butea superba*, an alternative herbal treatment for erectile dysfunction. Asian J Androl 2003 Sep; 5: 243-246.
9. Cherdshewasart W, Bhuntaku P, Panriansaen R, Dahlan W, Malaivijitnond S. Androgen disruption and toxicity tests of Butea superba Roxb., a traditional herb used for treatment of erectile dysfunction, in male rats. 2008 Jun 20;60(2):131-7. Epub 2008 Jun 12.
10. Choi HK, Seong DH, Rha KH. Clinical efficacy of Korean red ginseng for erectile dysfunction. 1995 Sep; 7(3):181-6.
11. Dording CM, Fisher L, Papakostas G, Farabaugh A, Sonawalla S, Fava M, Mischoulon D. A double-blind, randomized, pilot dose-finding study of maca root (L. meyenii) for the management of SSRI-induced sexual dysfunction. CNS Neurosci Ther. 2008 Fall; 14(3):182-91.
12. Gauthaman K, Ganesan AP, Prasad RN. Sexual effects of puncture vine (*Tribulus terrestris*) extract (protodioscin): an evaluation using a rat model. Altern Complement Med. 2003 Apr; 9(2):257-65
13. Gauthaman K, Ganesan AP. The hormonal effects of *Tribulus terrestris* and its role in the management of male erectile dysfunction--an evaluation using primates, rabbit and rat. Phytomedicine. 2008 Jan; 15(1-2):44-54.
14. Gonzales GF, Gasco M, Malheiros-Pereira A, Gonzales-Castaneda C. Antagonistic effect of *Lepidium meyenii* (red maca) on prostatic hyperplasia in adult mice. Andrologia. 2008 Jun;40(3):179-85.
15. Hong B, Ji YH, Hong JH, Nam KY, Ahn TY. A double-blind crossover study evaluating the efficacy of Korean red ginseng in patients with erectile dysfunction: a preliminary report. 2002 Nov; 168(5):2070-3.
16. Hryb DJ, Kahn MS, Romas NA, Rosner W. The effect of extracts of the roots of the stinging nettle (Urtica dioica) on the interaction of SHBG with its receptor on human prostatic membranes. Planta Med 1995; 61:31-2.
17. Hwang TI, Chen HE, Tsai TF, Lin YC. Combined use of androgen and sildenafil for hypogonadal patients unresponsive to sildenafil alone. Int J Impot Res. 2006 Jul-Aug; 18(4):400-4. Epub 2006 Jan 5.
18. Kaiser FE. In: The Medical clinics of North America: The aging male patient. Erectile dysfunction in the aging man. WB Saunders: PA; 1999.
19. Komesaroff PA, Black CV, Cable V, Sudhir K. Effects of wild yam extract on menopausal symptoms, lipids and sex hormones in healthy menopausal women. Climacteric 2001; 4: 144-50.
20. Lunenfeld B. Men' s health and aging: The 5th World Congress on the Aging Male. Taylor Francis 2006; 1:1-70.
21. Liang P, Li H, Peng X, Jiao J, Liu J, Ye Z. Effects of *Astragalus membranaceus* injection on sperm abnormality

in Cd-induced rats. Zhonghua Nan Ke Xue 2004;1 0: 42-5,48.

22. Lim PH, Li MK, Ng FC, Chia SJ, Consigliere D, Gooren L, et al. Clinical efficacy and safety of sildenafil citrate (Viagra) in a multi - racial population in Singapore. A retrospective study of 1520 patients. Int J Urol 2002; 9: 308-15.
23. Lim PH, Moorthy P, Tan RS. In: Aging men' s health - A case based approach. An overview of erectile dysfunction in aging men. Thieme: NY; 2005. p. 123-30.
24. Malo AF, Roldan EF, Garde J, Soler AJ, Gomendio M. Antlers honestly advertise sperm production and quality. Proc Biol Sci 2005; 272:149-57.
25. Ong YC, Tan BKH. Novel phytoandrogens and lipidic augmenters from *Eucommia ulmoides*. BMC Complement Altern Med. 2007 Jan 29; 7:3.
26. Ong YC, Yong EL. Panax (ginseng) - panacea or placebo? Molecular and cellular basis of its pharmacological activity. Ann Acad Med Singapore. 2000 Jan; 29(1):42-6.
27. Ong YC, Yong EL. A method for modulating steroidogenic activity. United States Patent No: US 6,905,714 B2. Jun 14, 2005. United States Patent and Trademark Office (USPTO). Priority claim of 60/185,757. Feb 29, 2000.
28. Rowland DL, Tai W. A review of plant-derived and herbal approaches to the treatment of sexual dysfunctions. J Sex Marital Ther 2003; 29:185-205.
29. Sanjay K Garg: Evaluation of Safety and efficacy of "Tentex Royal" in management of ED. Medicine Update (2004): 12(8), 51-55.
30. Shamloul R, Ghanem H, Fahmy I, El-Meleigy A, Ashoor S, Elnashaar A, Kamel I. Testosterone therapy can enhance erectile function response to sildenafil in patients with PADAM: a pilot study. J Sex Med. 2005 Jul; 2(4): 559-64.
31. Wang KY, Dahlen M. Chinese Herbal Medicine. Workman Press: Hong Kong; 1994.
32. Zhang ZB, Yang QT. The testosterone mimetic properties of icariin. Asian J Androl. 2006 Sep; 8(5):601-5. Epub 2006 Jun 5.
33. Zhu J, Halpern G, Jones K. The scientific rediscovery of a precious ancient Chinese herbal regimen: Cordyceps sinensis: Part II. J Alternat Complement Med 1998;4: 429-57.

● BIBLIOGRAPHY

1. Spector IP, Carey MP: Incidence and prevalence of the sexual dysfunction: a critical review of the empirical literature. Arch Sex Behav 1990; 19: 389-408.
2. Goldstein I, Lue TF, Padma-Nathan H, Rosen RC, Steers WD, Wicker PA: Oral sildenafil in the treatment of erectile dysfunction. Sildenafil Study Group. N Engl J Med. 1998; 338(20): 1397-404.
3. Porst H, Rosen R, Padma-Nathan H, Goldstein I, Giuliano F, Ulbrich E, Bandel T: The efficacy and tolerability of vardenafil, a new, oral, selective phosphodiesterase type 5 inhibitor, in patients with erectile dysfunction: the first at-home clinical trial. Int J Impot Res. 2001; 13(4):192-9.
4. Padma-Nathan H, McMurray JG, Pullman WE, Whitaker JS, Saoud JB, Ferguson KM, Rosen RC: IC351 On-Demand Dosing Study Group. On-demand IC351 (Cialis) enhances erectile function in patients with erectile dysfunction. Int J Impot Res. 2001; 13(1):2-9.
5. Shabsigh R: Therapy of ED: PDE-5 Inhibitors. Endocrine. 2004; 23(2-3):135-41.
6. Kalsi JS, Kell PD: Update on oral treatments for male erectile dysfunction. J Eur Acad Dermatol Venereol. 2004; 18(3):267-74.
7. Montorsi F, Verheyden B, Meuleman E, Junemann KP, Moncada I, Valiquette L, Casabe A, Pacheco C, Denne J, Knight J, Segal S, Watkins VS: Long-term safety and tolerability of tadalafil in the treatment of erectile dysfunction. Eur Urol. 2004 Mar; 45(3):339-44; discussion 344-5.
8. Pomara G, Morelli G, Pomara S, Taddei S, Ghiadoni L, Dinelli N, Travaglini F, Dicuio M, Mondaini N, Salvetti A, Selli C: Cardiovascular parameter changes in patients with erectile dysfunction using pde-5 inhibitors: a study with sildenafil and vardenafil. J Androl. 2004; 25(4): 625-9.

Chapter 11

Taiwan Perspective

Phytotherapy of Sexual Medicine in Taiwan

Han-Sun Chiang, Chun-Hou Liao

I. Introduction

The phytotherapy of sexual medicine in Taiwan could be derived from either traditional Chinese herbal medicine or present phytogen extract on market. Like other oriental societies, Taiwanese people is used to choose phytotherapy as an alternative therapy, or supplemental therapy for the sexual health. Even in the era of having effective oral medications for male erectile function, phytotherapy still has a place for the treatment of sexual dysfunction for our Taiwanese.

1. History

Most of the Taiwanese people was immigrated from mainland China and deeply influenced by the old Chinese culture. Chinese herbal medicine in belong to the old Chinese culture which lasted for more than 1500 years. It based on the old Chinese philosophy. One of the roots of this philosophy is said to go back to a legendary emperor "Shen Nong". "Shen Nong" is said to have introduced agriculture and tested hundred herbs so the art of medicine was born. Actually the Chinese herbal medical system was well-developed in the great Han dynasty, including the medical textbook and the medical therapy - in the point of modern medicine, it might rather be recognized as an old medical philosophy.

Han-Sun Chiang, M.D., Ph.D.
College of Medicine, Fu Jen Catholic University, No. 510, Chung Cheng Road, 24205 Hsin-Chuang, Taipei Hsien, Taiwan, Republic of China. Tel: +886-2-29053401, Fax: +886-2-29043387, E-mail: 053824@mail.fju.edu.tw, hansun@mails.fju.edu.tw, hansun@tmu.edu.tw

The old Chinese medical philosophy has the concept of "opposing natural force", and been established as the opposing and yet complementary and reciprocal "yin" and "yang" forces of nature, of all matter, of all action and thought, of all impetus. For example, men were yang, and women yin, and it was considered crucial that in the sexual union of the two the male must retain and conserve his vital and limited yang while absorbing as much as he could of the female' s supplies of yin essence. The male symptoms of sexual dysfunction were supposed to be lack of "yang", which was originated from the fatigue, depression, invigorate of the heart, kidney and other vital organ. The role of Chinese herbal medicine for the male sexual dysfunction played its part in a constant thrust for vitality in the form of herbal tonics which were taken to stimulate sexual potency and to fortify the weaker yang essence of the male. The effect of these medicine was not only for sexual function, but also for anti-aging. There are many references in the Han era and in later literature to men who had mastered the technique of ying-yang lined to the age of 150 or more.

The other principle of the Chinese herbal medicine follows the correlation and balance of force applied to diet and medicine. They were categorized according to the nature of their therapeutic value - "cold" foods reduce "heat" in the body, such as fruit and vegetables, "hot" high protein foods such as fatty meats, eggs and ingredients soaked in wine, taken to heat up and invigorate the system; were "supplementary" as an additional tonic and to strengthen the corresponding organ in the human body. According to this principle, most of Chinese herbal medicine tends to be a combination rather than single prescription. Among different medications, there exists several kinds of function, such as "re-enforce", "supplementary", or balance to prevent adverse effect.

2. Today

Recently, diet and traditional herbal medicine began to merge into "medicinal diets". It was used as a kind of nutritious food or "tonic" supplement. On the other hand, the Chinese herbal medicine was much more modernized. Some of the functional components was extracted, purified and some was combined with other effective phyto-medications. Many combinations had been commercialized. They were regulated to do practical applications of therapy. Such modern herbal medicines were made as a capsule, pill, extract essence, with clearly remark of the ingredients, produced and expired date, indications and contraindications. Even though they could be purchased without physician' s prescription, over-advertisement is not allowed. The customers' right are well-protected by the law.

3. Future trends

In the future, the traditional Chinese herbal medicine as well as other phytomedications will be more and more developed as a part of the complementary alternative medicine. In Taiwan, it is regulated by a special department of Health, Executive Yuan, Taiwan. The policy of Taiwanese government is going to modernize the herbal medications further two directions:

1. Looking for the evidence of the pharmacological effect with the modern technology. For example, the old Chinese herbal of Yin-yang huo, (Horny Goat Weed) is a renown product for male sexual function which was extracted from the plant. In vitro and in vivo studies were performed with the extract and some similar effect with that of the PDE5 inhibitor was detected. Such laboratory studies had been conducted by several graduate institutes' and sponsored by the govenment.

2. Clinical trials will be requested for the special effect of the phytomedications, such as the improvement of sexual function. The regulation will not be so strict as double blinded, placebo control, however, clinical efficacy and adverse effect should be evaluated more seriously for the license approval in the future.

4. Prevalence of sexual function in Taiwan

In Taiwan, results from a community-based survey gave the prevalence of ED among Taiwanese men older than 40 years as 17.7%[1]. In another cohort study, the prevalence of self-reported ED was 13.1% compared with 26.0% using the abridged, five-item version of the International Index of Erectile Function (IIEF-5) assessment[2]. Hwang et al[3]. also reported on the comparisons between sexual hormone levels in Taiwanese men with and without ED. A Taiwannese version of the QoL questionnaire, which included domain 1 (physical domain), domain 2 (psychological domain), domain 3 (social relationship domain), and domain 4 (environmental domain), was used to measure QoL. A significant association between low levels of serum cFT, Bio-T, and the severity of ED was found. In addition, abnormal erectile function was significantly associated with a low QoL level in all four domains.

II. The Phytotherapy Industry

1. Who are in the industry

In Taiwan, the pharmaceutic industries of the phytotherapy are usually different from the regular, modern pharmaceutic companies. Usually they are not so big, some of them is a kind of "family business" and develops secret prescription of herbal ingredient which is based on their own clinical experience. Phytotherapy or traditional Chinese herbs for sexual function is specially popular before the definitely effective oral medication as PDE5 inhibitors appeared on the market. Because "sex is taboo" and sexual dysfunction should be treated privately and most of the sexual medicine is our ancient society was belong to "secret prescription". The "secret prescription", might be a secret of a family with several generation of Chinese herbal physicians bases on their clinical experience. It is usually made from some precious material and only limited sales without a mass production by the industry.

2. Regulations

One modern development already alluded to is the production of patient herbal medicines refined from extracts of the crud herbs and they should contain effective essential ingredients. Quality control of the products is regulated, although not so strictly as that for the modern drug production. Industries as "Chinese herbal company" are not so many, however, all of the industries should be registered in the government.

3. Distribution channels

The traditional Chinese herbal medicine shop conveys a feeling that little has changed for thousands of years. Rows and rows of worn wooden drawers, a simple teak counter, crude balance scales, the ever present abacus, choppers and grinders identical to those depicted in the ancient scrolls and the age-old, natural varieties of herbs themselves. There is also a Chinese herbalist, who expertly prepares the mixture according to the herbal prescriptions written up by the physician in the clinic.

The well-prepared, well-packed herbal prescription can also be purchased from the herbal medicine shop. Some of these prescriptions could be found and bought from the internet. Even as a phytotherapy in sexual medicine, the complete informations of these prescriptions were exposed in the internet. Some prescriptions listed in the part II of this manuscript is either single prescriptions or combination prescriptions, which were made from Chinese herbs or other phyto-plants and distributed widely by the modern media.

III. The Herb Products

1. Property products (over the counter)

In general, the property products of the Chinese herbal prescriptions over the counter of Chinese herbal shop are natural products. They have now become scarce and quite expensive especially when the species is coming from the original place. For enhancement of the male sexual function or male potency, it is called "Tonics" of the Chinese herbs. "Tonics" are the most interesting - and by far the most expensive - items in the Chinese pharmacopoeia. They are directly linked to longevity because of their proven power to promote vital - hormone production - the "vital essence" of Chinese medical argot. Besides of the famous plant-derived herbs "Yin Yang huo" - "horny goat weed" (Epimedium Sagittatum), animal - derived medications are more prominent among the tonics. Such exotic items as rhinocerous horn, stag horn, the dried genitalia of male sea-lions and seals, the tails of red spotted lizards, dried sea- horses, gum of tortoise shell and wild donkey hide are all tonics. It is the thought that these items contain either high concentrations of male hormones or elements which promote the production of vital-essence. In the theory of traditional chinese medicine, they have natural affinity for the kidneys and related glands and have a general stimulating effect on the body' s vital primordial energies.

2. Prescribed products

When the prescription takes the form of broth, tea, wine or power, the mixed ingredients are taken home and prepared for consumption by the patient. Pills, pastes and other special forms must be prepared at the shop by the herbalist and usually require several days. The actual form of a herbal prescription takes depends upon the nature of the herbs used. Some herbs are only effective when ground to a talc-fine powder and mixed into pills, while others must be boiled or steamed to become medically active. Some herbal ingredients can be used in many different forms, such as in pills for internal use as well as in pastes for external use.

3. Product indications

One of the most characteristic thinking for the Chinese herbs medicine is a more variable indications and contraindications based on the theory of old, traditional Chinese medicine. For example, the various methods of preparing prescriptions differ in their concentrations of active ingredients and in their rates of absorption and distribution in the body. Weak or elderly patients are given gentler preparations which are absorbed slowly, while more robust patients can tolerate the stronger, faster-acting forms. The curative herbal cure the cause of disease by redressing the energy imbalances and tonifying the weak organs which permit disease to develop. When apply the curative herbal medication, it is vital not only to get the right tools for the job but also to be effective at the right time. Patients' diet and other daily routines should be adjusted and timed to the requirements of the cure, Chinese herbal medicine is so closely tied to food that the two are inseparable. As a kind of contraindication, some foods act as specific catalysts for certain herbal medications, while other foods completely neutralize them. Such foods are prohibited during treatment with Chinese herbs. Recently, as the requirement of Taiwanese FDA, special indication for the special prescription should be evidently based by adequate clinical trial. Over-advertisement is not allowed and will be punished by the regulations.

IV. Clinical Experience

1. Types of practitioners

Concerning the authorization of the prescription for the Chinese herbal medicine, modern "Chinese physician" is a specialist who is belong to a well-educated, well-trained with a special license approved profession. The "Chinese physician" must be graduated from the medical college, department of "Chinese medicine". Most of the course for the Chinese physicians is similar to that for the regular medical students. After a seven years courses, including 3 years practice, they should take national board examination for their license of "Chinese physician".

Chinese physicians can work in a big "Chinese hospital". They may also conduct a small "Chinese clinic", and some of them may work for a big Chinese herbal shop to prescribe the Chinese medicine as an old fashion. They combine some basic, modern medical diagnostic techniques, such as X-rays, blood pressure; blood and urine analysis, etc, with their own traditional diagnostic methods. The prescriptions of the authorized Chinese physicians can be totally reimbursed by the general government insurance in Taiwan.

2. Clinician regulations

If the Chinese herbal medicine is prescribed by the "Chinese physician", it can be reimbursed by the insurance and the safety and efficacy of the medication can be approved as well. The common regulations for the Chinese physicians are just the same as the regulations for other medical doctors in the modern medical fields.

Because the Chinese physicians also receive a formal medical training, so they also can do general medical practice in combination with some traditional medical therapy such as acupuncture and herbal medical prescriptions. They have their own medical association, and continued medical educations. Regulations for the medical practice of the Chinese physicians are well-established under their medical association. Mal-practice without authorization of these regulations will not be recognized as a legal medical practice.

● REFERENCES

1. Chen KK, Chiang HS, Jiann BP, et al. Prevalence of erectile dysfunction and impacts on sexual activity and self-reported intercourse satisfaction in men older than 40 years in Taiwan. Int J of Impot Res. 2004 Jun;16(3):249-255.
2. Wu CJ, Hsieh JT, Lin JS, et al. Comparison of prevalence between self-reported erectile dysfunction and erectile dysfunction as defined by five-item International Index of Erectile Function in Taiwanese men older than 40 years. Urology. 2007 Apr;69(4):743-7.
3. Hwang TI, Lo HC, Tsai TF, Chiou HY. Association among hypogonadism, quality of life and erectile dysfunction in middle-aged and aged male in Taiwan. Int J Impot Res. 2007 Jan-Feb;19(1):69-75.

Chapter 12

Thailand Perspective

Herbal Medicine in Thailand

Apichat Kongkanand, Kavirach Tantiwongse, Narisa Nakpairat

I. Background

1. Introduction

The herbal medicine in Thailand nowadays is not as popular as it had been in the old days. We are one of the ancient nations in Asia but it seems that we do not keep the herbal medicine as it was developed.

The herbal medicine for example if someone is seeking the treatment for stomachache, he will have a hard time looking for fresh herb as said works in the book, otherwise he must find one of the local doctors with a degree in herbal medicine (not MD).

Now it is much easier for us to see the doctors in Emergency rooms or buy the medicine over the counter for stomachache which most of them are westernized and there is limited number of physicians who specialized in herbal medicine.

Almost all of the herbal drugs in Thailand are sold over the counters and no prescription is needed. Herbal medicine is considered to be harmless and most of them are made in forms of capsules or tablets which would be registered by the Ministry of Public Health, Federal Drugs Administration (FDA).

Many of the drugs made from herbs such as tablet for cough or gas pain are manufactured by the Government Pharmaceutical Organization (GPO).

Apichat Kongkanand, M.D., FACS.
Department of Surgery, Bumrungrad International Hospital, 33 sukumvit soi 3 Bangkok Thailand 10110.
E-mail: dr_apichat@yahoo.com

2. Prevalence of erectile dysfunction in Thailand [1, 2]

In the year 1998, it was the first time in Thailand that there was a study in Erectile Dysfunction. Details of the study include risk factors, co-morbidity, exercise and previous surgery in general population.

There were also studies in the general population by interviewing face to face which outcomes were very good and found to be fundamental for studying men health in the country. The first study was found to have 38% ED in general population age 40-70 years old to which increased to 42% in the elderly in 2003, the second study of ED. The number was found to increase due to more people have come out to get help from the doctors.

There are numerous risks factors that contribute to the ED that includes;

- o Aging
- o Diabetic
- o Atherosclerotic
- o Hypertension
- o Smoking
- o Surgery

The risk factors and prevalence of ED in Thailand are not much different from our neighbor countries or from the rest of the world.

3. Phytotherapy in Thailand

There are many small companies in this field supplying small bottles of cream or some herbs claimed to work well, mostly filled with Butea or other type of herbs with good circulation in blood stream. They come in health food, not the medicine.

The Distributor comparison would be on the counter and can be easily bought by the consumers.

4. History

In the old days up until 200 years ago, the Thai called Siamese use old traditional medicine for our cheerful lives for good. Recently the Ministry of Public Health has set up one new department of traditional medicine so we could continue to depend and keep our culture and Thai herbal medicine. Herbal medicine in the ancient days could be mixed in food for good health and for increasing circulation through the blood stream. Today we could see many of these herbal plants in various kinds of recipe for Thai foods and some of them in the spa for aromatherapy or their traditional massage too.

Thai traditional massage is a kind of treatment applied famously as well as oral medicine, used as the treatment of fatigue both in muscular weakness[3], pain as well as postpartum, and for those who suffer from work of any kind; it can boost you physically and psychologically.

Thai herbal compresses, mixing all the following herbs and wrap the mixture in white cheesecloth formed into small balls then have them steamed. These balls are then used to compress around desired body areas such as joints or muscles to lessen pain and swelling or other parts of the body to increase circulation or for the treatment of pain and fatigue.

The heat will help circulation and makes the herb absorb into the inner layer of the skin.

Example of herbs use to make compressed balls

1. Plai	250 gm
2. Turmeric	50 gm
3. Lemon grass	100 gm
4. Bergamot skin "leech line"	10 gm
5. Camphor	15 gm
6. Salt	30 gm

5. Today

We are among one of the world's most leading countries in the spa industry. Mixing herbal and traditional massage together, this could help relax physical and mental condition by rejuvenating and relieving from stress and physical fatigue.

There are many herbal qualities;

1. Plumeria Alba known as white or red Rubra flower, has an appealing scent and is widely used to decorate in spas
2. Hibiseas flower and leaf extracts are used to moisturize the skin
3. Cape jasmine, Condemia jasmmoides, commonly known as Jasmine, a white color flower with a pleasant aroma scent
4. Champak; floating the flower inside the bowel of water, we use the water for aroma
5. Pandenas (leaves) for smelling, extraction from leaves are used to coat skin and hair

6. Spermatocyte decreasing agents[4, 5]

There are some herbs that should be widely noted for careful consumption.

The Chinese celery (Apiuns Graveolens) is a common vegetable, however if consumed everyday, could decrease male sperm and could be used as birth control in male.

Gossypium herbaceous (Chinese cotton) also has the same effect by decreasing the sperm to 0 and will return to the normal level when stop consuming the herb.

These 2 herbs should be used carefully, since it could be used in birth control or may decrease the male hormone for the consumer.

II. Phytoandrogen for the Treatment of Erectile Dysfunction[6, 7, 8]

There are several plants in Thailand believed to have androgenie effect and believed by Thai citizen and villagers from the ancient time. But in fact, after the modern medicine came into the Kingdom, the researchers investigated and there is only one or two that should be available for treatment of Erectile Dysfunction

1. Butea Superba [9,10]

Butea Superba is Thailand endemic species used as traditional medicine for tonic and rejuvenating effect. It is the big vine group in associated with the tree. The long underground tuberous root accumulated many phytochemical included mostly androgenic. It could produce vasodilatation especially at the penis. It can produce smooth muscle relaxation of corpora cavernosum.

Chemical properties; the results from the study of researchers and academics confirmed that these chemicals are non-mutagenic and could induce vasodilation especially at the penis with very similar reaction as did by Viagra but smoothly and thus elevate its erectile performance.

There are many Butea superba plant available for commercially used including gel, cream, and soaps.

Butea superba could be dangerous for the consumer if they consume or digest in overdose, so the manufacturers love to produce the form of cream or gel for consumer to apply.

Possible side effects are malaise feet pain, leg pain, scrotal skin thickening.

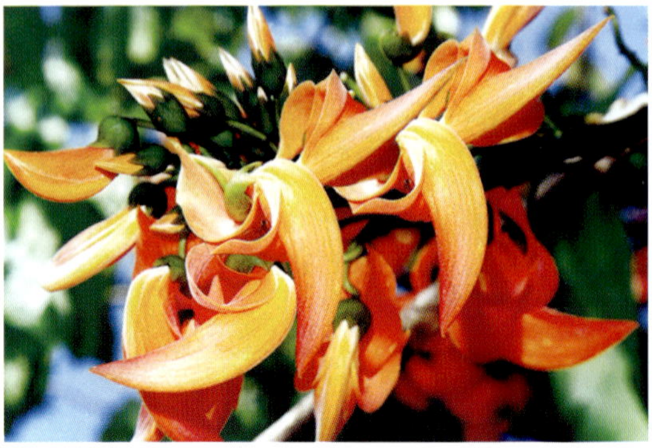

Figure 1. Butea superb flower

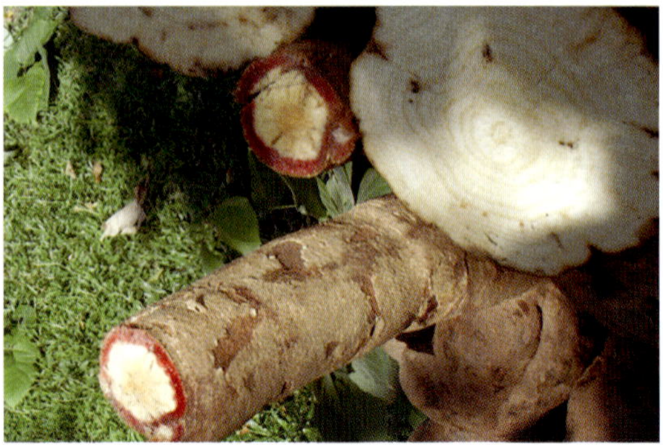

Figure 2. Root

Clinical Experience of Butea Superba (Red Kwao Kkreu or Red Gwao Geur) [10]: There is clinical trial on Human being Narong Nimsakul and Wichai Cherdshewasart did the study and presend at APSIR 2001 in Phuket meeting showing Butea Superba contain flavonoid and flavonoid glycoside with a cAMP phosphodiesterase inhibitory reaction, subchronic toxicity test in mice and rats exhibited no significant toxicity test in mice and rat extradited no significant toxic effect in physiology, blood chemistry and histology of vital organs including liver, kindney and testis.

Study in 47 Thai men with History of Diabetic hypertension and heart disease age 20-65 years for a period of 3 month was carried out. Overall results in 87% improvement for their sexual function.

2. Kachaidum or Zingileravear (Kaempferia panviflera)

Plant extract from underground roots ages 11-12 months old. They have good quality in mild vasodilatation and multiple effects, the 5-7 DMF flavonoid. They also have main other effect of vasodilation and antiplateletes quality.

In the ancient time, people used Kachaidum to treat abdominal pain and antiflatulence since they have mild effect of antibacterial.

How to use : Available in tonic or mix with honey or mix with alcohol. Then drink for good Health.

3. Black Sesame or Sesame Orientale

Sesame is rich in amino acid and sesame oil can be used for the treatment to lower Cholesterol. They are rich in Calcium, Iron, Magnesium, Vitamin B, etc.

They can help in promoting circulation systems. People in the ancient time believed this can help them in sexual stimulants.

How to use: Mix with food of any kind or consume by product foods.

● REFERENCES

1. Kongkanand Apichat and TEDES, "Prevalence of ED in Thailand". *International Journal of Andrology 23 supplement 2 (2000): 72-80.*
2. Permpogkosol Sompol et al, *"Increased Prevalence of ED:Result of the second epidemiology study on sexual activity and prevalence of ED in Thai male"*. Aging Male. Sep.2008, 11(3). 128-133.
3. Sithigariya. *Herbal medicine and alternative medicine.* Medical Science Research Institute. 1st ed. Chulalongkorn University Press, 2548.
4. *Natural Product Acting on Reproductive system.* Pharmaceutical department, Mahidol University. 2534.
5. Temsiri, Rungravee. *Herb Acting on Reproductive disease, Chronic disease.*
6. Choteanan, and colleague. Thai Herbal Medicine for Basic Public Health. 1st ed. DK Book distributors. 2551.
7. Chantorn, Pinij, and colleague. Therapeutic Herbal Medicine. 1st ed. Than Book Publishing. 2551.
8. Choteanan, and colleague. *Vegetable and Herb near you.* Sangdao Publishing Company. 2551.
9. Sophon Roengsumran et.al, *Flavonoid and Flavonoid glycoside from Butea superba Roxb. and their cAMP Phosphodiesterase Inhibitory Activity,* J. Sci. Res. Chula. Univ., Vol. 25, No.1 (2000).
10. *Asian Journal of Andrology June 2002;4 (2, suppl 1):1-130, ISSN 1008-682X,* 8th APSIR October 23rd-26th, Phuket, Thailand.

Chapter 13

The Necessity of Clinical Trial on Herbal Phytotherapy in the Field of Sexual Medicine

Je Jong Kim, Sung Won Lee

For the prevention and treatment of the disease, a variety of plants and materials from plants have been used throughout history in the countries over the world. The purposes of medicinal herbal use may vary with the different cultures of each individual society, but can simply be considered as being either for the promotion of health or the relief of ailments. People have a preconceived idea that the herbal phytotherapy is a panacea with a wide safety margin. It seems to be generous to apply traditional medicine to treat patients in most countries, because it had been used for a long time. However, some serious circumstances have been reported after using herbal phytotherapy. While herbs have been considered to be gentle, non-toxic and even harmless, mainly because of their natural origin, both adverse drug reactions and poisonings associated with the use of herbal medicines have increasingly been reported in last few years. Chinese herb nephropathy is well-known toxicity of the medicinal herb, and while it is not easy to clarify the causal relation between the herbs and side effect of them, other organ toxicities including cardiotoxicity, hepatotoxicity, hematotoxicity, neurotoxocity and even systemic toxicity induced by herbal consumption had been reported consistently. The cause of the side effect includes toxicities of herb itself and metabolites of herbs, contaminants such as residual pesticides, heavy metals, and adulterated toxic substances etc. Therefore, not only to keep the public health but also to maximize the plausible benefit of medicinal herbs, it is important to establish a system to control the medicinal herbs, including standardization of medicinal herb in producing and distribution, and a system to monitor developing toxicity of the medicinal herbs.

However, more basically, the actual effect of herbal phytotherapy in clinical field which is tending to be exaggerated or overestimated should be clearly investigated first. While prevailed favor belief on herbal phytotherapy, the scientific evidence supporting this belief is limited up to now. Furthermore, lack of regulation, easy accessibility, contamination and adulteration make it difficult to estimate the exact clinical role of herbal phytotherapy. If herbal phytotherapy shows significant benefit in specific health related issue as shown in other contemporary medicine, then it would be natural to turn the direction to finding the safe way in using this.

One of this issues which gained interest in herbal phytotherapy is maintenance of erectile function, or recovery from erectile dysfunction. However, in the area of erectile dysfunction, clinical trial design and conduct has been substantially developed and established. The successful conduct of several major drug development programs now affords us the ability to utilize referential standards. It is now widely recognized that validation of drug in sexual dysfunction requires a rational phased approach. It is appreciated that initial Phase 1 studies of novel therapeutics will explore safety, tolerability and pharmacokinetics. Phase 2 studies will assess preliminary evidence of clinical safety and efficacy and will explore arrange of doses. Phase 3 pivotal trials will confirm clinical efficacy of particular dose or dose range. Phase 4 studies can further investigate clinical safety and efficacy in subpopulations, can identify signals of previously unrecognized toxicity, and can identify new benefits of a marketed product. Besides, drug-drug interaction studies and studies in special populations are critical to the overall understanding of the safety and efficacy of a given drug for erectile dysfunction. From these erectile dysfunction experience, we recognize that results of clinical studies are only interpretable and generalizable when sensitive, reliable, validated outcome assessment instruments are consistently used as primary efficacy endpoints in adequate and well-controlled Phase 3 clinical trials and when these trials are conducted in clearly and consistently defined patient population.

These together give us the necessity of clinical trials using herbal phytotherapy in field of sexual function. Clinical trial on herbal phytotherapy in field of erectile dysfunction using this phased approach provides us the opportunity not only to validate the therapeutic advantage or disadvantage of it, but also to standardize it minimizing adverse events induced by over dosage or toxic component included. There is the development process for herbal drug to approve by the Korean FDA (Figure). Through these clinical trials, we can find a way to study the efficacy of the herbal phytotherapy, and suggest a guideline to how to use this safely. Nevertheless, "Seed-to-pill standardization" is an even greater challenge for botanical drugs that is less applicable to single-ingredient drugs.

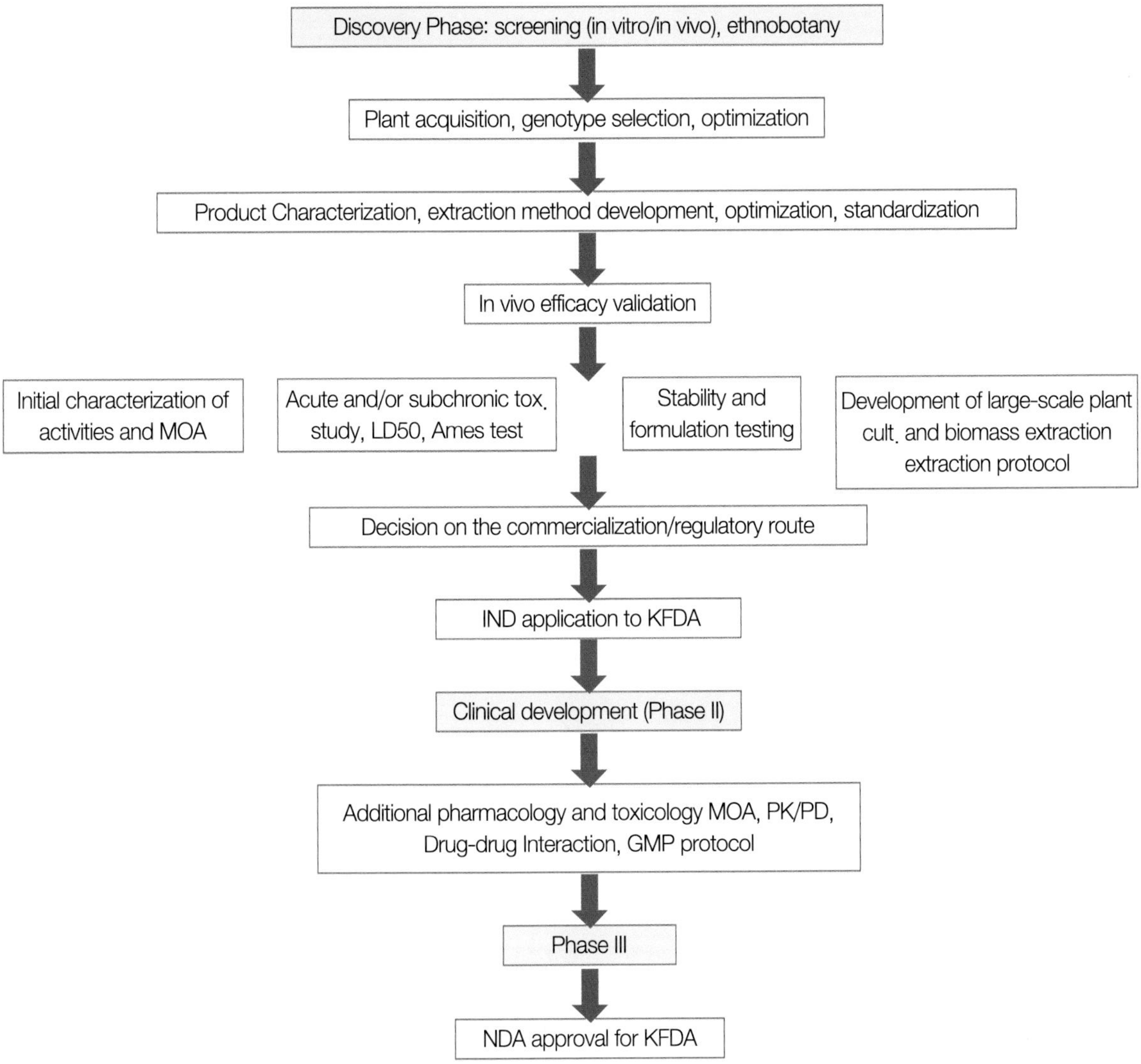

Figure 1. Development process for Herbal Medicine in Korea

(permitted by SK Sung, Seoul National University, Seoul, Korea)

Part II

The Commercially Available Medicinal Herb Products in Asia-Pacific Countries

Instruction for Part II Description

All information for profile structure, abbreviations and comments are as follows.

o Name of Medicinal Herb Product

CS	Chemical Structure This section provides information about chemical name and/or figure of chemical structure.
AA	Area of Application (Indications) The areas of application are described on the base of the permitted medical purpose by country FDA.
T	Type of Herb ☐ Tablet ☐ Cream ☐ Gel ☐ Powder ☐ Injection ☐ Patch ☐ Drink ☐ Others
S	How Supplies This section provides information about commercially available status of medicinal herb. (Examples) 1. Inboxes containing 5×2 gm bottles store under refrigeration. 2. *Sansuyu* Forte is supplied as brown, film coated, round ball shaped tables containing condensed sap of *Cornus officinalis* 88.95%, condensed sap of *Rubus coreanus* 10.0% and Arginine 1000 mg.
D	Dosage 1. The necessary quantity of medicinal herbs is indicated in grams; in addition, the teaspoon dosage is mentioned 2. For tea preparation, hot water is poured over the suggested quantity of medicinal herb and sieved after the proposed amount of time. (Example) 5 g/150mL, 10-15 min, 1 cup 3 times/day
A	Administration Instructions for the duration of application and the necessity of consulting a medical practitioner are suggested.
CP	Comments and Precautions This section provides information about the use of the herbs, their efficacy, and their safety, as well as particular risks. The traditional and/or folk medicinal use is mentioned in particular.
CI	Contraindications Serious contraindications are listed in this section.

AR	Adverse Reactions Important adverse reactions are listed and should be interpreted. Individual cases: without quantification
SC	Special Comment This section provides information about specially noticed additional information of medicinal herb.
I	Interactions Important and significant interactions are listed in this section.
M&D	Manufacturer and/or Distributor • Manufacturer Name and/or department of representative: Address: Tel: FAX: E-mail: Home-page: • Distributor Name and/or department of representative: Address: Tel: FAX: E-mail: Home-page:

Photograph of Medicinal Herb

1) Packaged box, sealed plate, bottle or container 2) Tablet or real photo of herb etc.

Chapter 1

Australian Products

Carolyn Earle

I. Commercially Available Phytotherapy Products for Female Sexual Medicine

1. Horny Goat Weed for Her

CS	Not stated
AA	Female Libido
T	Tablet
S	Herbal extracts equiv. dry Epimedium Sagittatum (Horny Goat Weed) Herb Top 1.5 g Liriosma Ovata (Muira-Puama) Root 1 g Turnera Diffusa (Damiana) Herb 1 g Panax Ginseng (Ginseng Korean) Root 500 mg Avena Sativa (Oats) Seed 500 mg Ginkgo Biloba (Ginkgo) Leaf 500 mg Standardised to contain: (Ginkgo flavonglycosides - 2.4 mg) (Ginkgolides and Bilobalide - 600 mcg) Asparagus Officinalis (Asparagus) Shoot 125 mg Vitex Agnus-Castus (Chaste Tree) Fruit 200 mg Angelica Polymorpha (Dong Quai) Root 250 mg Smilax Officinalis (Sarsaparilla) Root 100 mg

	Theobroma Cacao (Cocoa) Seed Powder 20 mg Pyridoxine Hydrochloride (Vitamin B6) 25 mg Cyanocobalamin (Vitamin B12) 50 mcg
D	One to two tablets daily, or as directed by a health practitioner.
A	Horny Goat Weed For Her should take effect in the first week.
CP	Always read the label. Use only as directed. If symptoms persist consult your healthcare professional. Vitamins can only be of assistance if the dietary intake is inadequate. Keep out of reach of children.
CI	Avoid if on heart or blood pressure medication. Avoid if on anticoagulants.
AR	The side effects are rare but may include insomnia, headaches, nausea and mild gastrointestinal complaints.
SC	You can take Horny Goat Weed For Her indefinitely though we recommend you take it every day for two months then take it only when you need to.
I	Not stated
M	Cat Media Pty Ltd trading as Naturopathica Address P.O. Box 154, Mona Vale, 1660, New South Wales, Australia Tel +1800 22 77 22 Email info@naturopathica.com.au Web www.naturopathica.com.au

2. Natural Desire for Women

CS	Not stated
AA	Promotes a healthy libido
T	Tablet - 48 per bottle
S	Each tablet contains: Herbal extracts equiv. to dry: Tribulus (tribulus terrestris) fruit 2,500 mg Tribulus (tribulus terrestris) root 2,500 mg Panax (Korean) ginseng root 500 mg Siberian ginseng (eleuthrococcus senticosus) root 500 mg Horny goat weed (epimedium sagittatum) leaf 1,500 mg Schizandra (schizandra chinensis) fruit 750 mg Green oats (avena sativa) herbal extract equiv. to fresh herb 750 mg. Contains: Gluten
D	Take one tablet twice daily or as advised by your healthcare professional
A	Not stated

CP	If symptoms persist consult your healthcare professional. Vitamins should not replace a balanced diet. Keep out of reach of children.
CI	The ingredients in this product can affect the way some prescription medications work, consult your doctor before use. Individuals taking anti coagulant and/or anti hypertensive medications should seek medical advice before taking this product.
AR, SC, I	Not stated
M	Australian Naturalcare Products Pty Ltd Address Unit 5, 5 Talavera Rd, North Ryde, New South Wales 2113 Australia Tel +61 2 8874 8100 Fax +61 2 8874 8111 Email myorder@ausnaturalcare.com.au Web http://www.ausnaturalcare.com.au/xxx.asp?ID=8622
Package	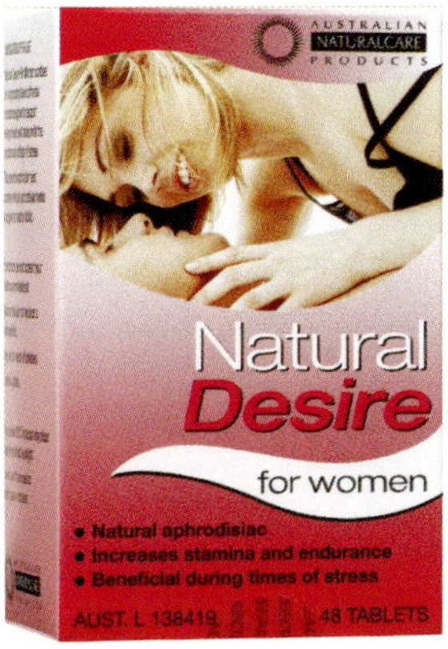

3. Nature' s Naturals Lifestyle Plus for Women

CS, AA, T, S, D, A, CP, CI, AR, SC, I	Not stated
M	Natural Pharmaceuticals Australia Pty Ltd Address PO BOX 8268, Sunnybank, Queensland, Australia Tel +61 7 3902 5100 Fax +61 7 3902 5199 Email info@naturesnaturals.com.au Web www.naturesnaturals.com.au

4. Super Horny Goat Weed for Her

CS	Not stated
AA	Enhance healthy sexual function and to heighten sexual desires.
T	Tablet - 300 per bottle
S	Each tablet contains concentrated extracts equivalent to dry : Ginkgo biloba (maiden hair) leaf 3,500 mg Tribulus terrestris root 750 mg Epimedium sagittatum (horny goat weed) leaf 1,000 mg Panax ginseng (Korean ginseng) root 350 mg Angelica polymorpha (Dong quai) root 500 mg Turnera diffusa (damiana) leaf 250 mg d-alpha tocopheryl acid succinate equivalent to natural Vitamin E 37 IU 30.3 mg Pyridoxine Hydrochloride (Vitamin B6) 15 mg Cyanocobalamin (Vitamin B12) 35 mcg Zinc amino acid chelate Equivalent zinc 5 mg - 25 mg
D	Adults Only: Take one (1) tablet 3 times daily with meals or as directed by a health care professional
A	Not stated
CP	Contains zinc which may be dangerous if taken in large amounts or for a long period. Do not use if cap seal is broken at time of purchase. Vitamins can only be of assistance if the dietary vitamin intake is inadequate. Information and statements regarding this dietary supplement have not been evaluated by the FDA (USA) and TGA (Australia) and should not be used to diagnose, treat, cure, or prevent any disease.
CI, AR	Not stated
SC	Store below 30°C in a dry place away from heat and direct sunlight.
I	Not stated
M	Enervite Pty Ltd Address 118/500 Centre Road, Bentleigh, Victoria, Australia 3204" Tel +61 3 9579 3322 Fax +61 3 9579 3323 Email Via "contact us" on their website Web www.enervite.com.au

5. WYLD Woman

CS	Not stated
AA	To enhance libido
T	Tablet
S	Each tablet contains : Herbal extracts equivalent to dry : Turnera diffusa herb (Damiana) 1,000 mg Eleutherococcus senticosus root (Siberian ginseng) 1,000 mg Tribulus terrestris fruit (Burra gokhru) 500 mg Gingko biloba leaf (Gingko) 3,000 mg Paullinia cupana seed (Guarana) 347.3mg containes caffeine 12.5 mg Thiamine nitrate (Vitamin B1) 12.5 mg Riboflavin (Vitamin B2) 12.5 mg Nicotinamide (Vitamin B3) 12.5 mg Pantothenic acid (Vitamin B5) as calcium pantothenate 12.5 mg Pyridoxine hydrochloride (Vitamin B6) 25 mg Cyanocobalamin (Vitamin B12) 25 mcg Folic acid 50 mcg Magnesium (as heavy magnesium oxide) 50 mg Calcium (as calcium carbonate) 100 mg Chromium (as chromium picolinate) 25 mcg
D	The recommended adult dosage is 1 tablet twice daily with food or as directed by your health care professional. Most women take a tablet in the morning and another mid afternoon to help maintain vitality throughout the day and into the evening.
A	"Most people experience an increase in their energy level within two to three weeks. However, this may differ based on individual workload and lifestyle factors."
CP	Please consult with your healthcare practitioner before using this product. This includes taking WYLD Woman in combination with any other health supplements or pharmaceuticals. Preferably ask a practitioner who specializes in natural medicines.
CI, AR, SC, I	Not stated
M	N-Hance Pty Ltd Address Suite 402, Lakeside Corporate Centre, 29-31 Solent Circuit, Baulkham Hills NSW 2153 Tel +1800 888 215 Email info@wyld.com.au Web www.wyld.com.au

Package and Tablet	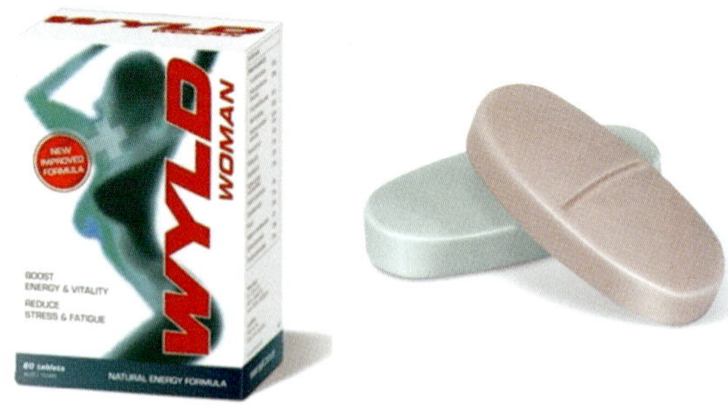

6. Sensu-L for Women

CS	Not stated
AA	Enhances libido
T	Tablets - 60
S	Each tablet contains : Herbal extracts equiv. dry Panax ginseng (Korean Ginseng) Root 750 mg Tribulus terrestris (Burra Gokhru) Fruit and Leaf 5 g Turnera diffusa (Damiana) Herb 2 g Ginkgo biloba (Ginkgo) Leaf 500 mg Thiamine Nitrate (Vitamin B1) 2 mg Riboflavine (Vitamin B2) 5 mg Nicotinamide (Vitamin B3) 10 mg Nicotinamide (Vitamin B3) 10 mg Pyridoxine Hydrochloride (Vitamin B6) 10 mg Cyanocobalamin (Vitamin B12) 100 mcg Copper (as Cupric Sulfate Anhydrous) 50 mcg Magnesium (as Magnesium Oxide Heavy) 25 mg Zinc (as Zinc Oxide) 2 mg
D	1 tablet daily for 1 week. Increase this dose by 1 tablet daily each week after this until you are taking 3 tablets daily. Do not take more than 6 tablets daily.
A	Should take effect within the first month.
CP	You should consult your health practitioner if you are on any heart, blood pressure or blood thinning medication. If you are taking other medications it is advisable that you check with your doctor to ensure it is acceptable to take the medicines concurrently.
CI	There is evidence that Sensu-L may reduce blood clotting, therefore if you suffer

	from bleeding disorders where clotting is not sufficient, or you are on medication that prevents blood clotting, you should speak with your medical professional before you start using it. If you are going to have surgery, you should tell the surgeon or anaesthetist that you are taking this complementary medicine.
AR	Side effects are rare but may include insomnia, headaches, nausea and mild gastrointestinal complaints.
SC, I	Not stated
M	Hershel-Beck Address 16 Jubille Avenue, Warriewood, New South Wales 2102, Australia Tel +1300 652 422 Fax +61 2 9997 1698 Email Via "contact us" on website Web www.hershel-beck.com.au

II. Commercially Available Phytotherapy Products for Male Sexual Medicine.

1. Aussie Super Sizzle

CS	Not stated
AA	Enhances sexual performance, increases stamina and endurance
T	Tablet - 60
S	Each tablet contains concentrated extracts equivalent to dry: Tribulus terrestris (fruit and root) 5,000 mg Epimedium sagittatum (leaf horny goat weed) 5,000 mg Liriosma ovata (root) muira puama (potency wood) 1,000 mg Ginkgo biloba (leaf maiden hair) equivalent flavonglycosides 4.9 mg - 1,000 mg Ginkgolides 620 mcg Bilobalide 580 mcg Withania somnifera (root) 300 mg Avena sativa (seed) 500 mg Turnera diffusa (leaf damiana eleeutherococcus senticosus (root and rhiz) siberian ginseng) 200 mg Panax ginseng (root) 100 mg Vitamin E (d alpha tocopheryl acid succinate) equivalent to natural vitamin E 501 U -

	41.38 mg Riboflavin (Vitamin B2) 10 mcg Nicotinic acid 15 mg Pyridoxine Hydrochloride (Vitamin B6) 20 mg Zinc amino acid chelate Equivalent zinc 5 mg - 25 mg
D	Adults Only: Take one to three (1 - 3) tablet(s) daily as required in the morning, after tea and before bed or as directed by a health care professional"
A	Not stated
CP	Do not use if cap seal is broken at time of purchase. Vitamins can only be of assistance if the dietary vitamin intake is inadequate. Information and statements regarding this dietary supplement have not been evaluated by the FDA (USA) and TGA (Australia) and should not be used to diagnose, treat, cure, or prevent any disease."
CI, AR	Not stated
SC	Store below 30°C in a dry place away from heat and direct sunlight.
I	Not stated
M	Enervite Health Supplements Address 118/500 Centre Road Bentleigh Victoria Australia 3204 Tel +61 3 9579 3322 Fax +61 3 9579 3323 Email Via "contact us" on website Web www.enervite.com.au

2. Australian Natural Deer Velvet

CS	Not stated
AA	Improves sexual function
T	Capsules
S	100% Australian Deer Velvet Powder
D	1 gram (2 capsules of 500 mg per day)
A, CP, CI, AR, SC, I	Not stated
M	Chinese Medicine National Aust Pty Ltd Address 16-20 Sultram Place, Adelaide, South Australia 5000 Tel +61 8 8211 9898 Fax +61 8 8231 6799

	Email heidi@chinesemedicineaust.com.au
	Web www.chinesemedicineaust.com.au
Package	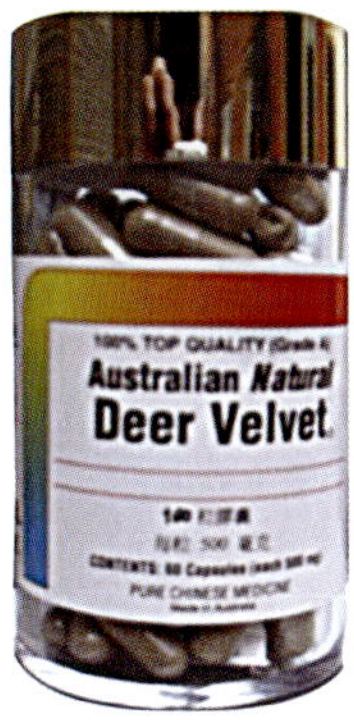

3. Biosis Horny Goat Weed Complex for Men

CS	Not stated
AA	Helps boost libido
T	Tablet - 60 per bottle
S	Epimedium sagittatum (Horny Goat Weed) leaf extracts equiv. to dry 5 g (5,000 mg) Tribulus terrestris (Burra Gokhru) fruit and root extracts equiv. to dry 3 g (3,000 mg) Liriosma ovata (Muira Puama) Root Wood extracts equiv. to dry 615 mg Eleutherococcus senticosus (Siberian Ginseng) Root equiv. to dry 300 mg Zinc Amino Acid Chelate 20% equivalent to elemental Zinc 35 mg
D	Adults only: Take one tablet twice daily with food or as directed by your healthcare practitioner
A, CP, CI, AR, SC, I	Not stated
M	Australia Natural Pharmaceutical Pty Ltd Address 18 Ferguson Avenue, Northgate Queensland 4013 Australia Tel +61 7 3216 6880 Fax +61 7 3216 6885 Email richard@naturalpharma.com.au Web www.naturalpharma.com.au/hornygoatweed.html

Package	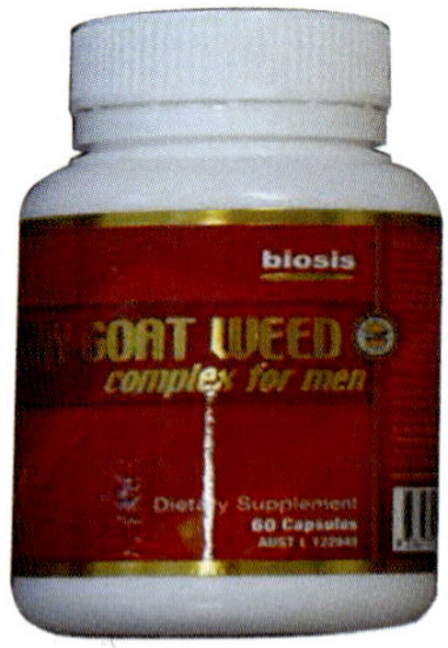

4. Blackmores Mens Performance Multi

CS	Not stated
AA	May assist with male sexual performance
T	Tablet
S	Each tablet contains : Vitamin B1 30 mg Vitamin B2 30 mg Nicotinamide 30 mg Vitamin B5 64.1 mg Vitamin B6 30 mg Vitamin B12 40 μg Vitamin C 100 mg Natural Vitamin E 50 IU Folic Acid 300 μg Inositol 25 mg Biotin 50 μg Calcium 50 mg Potassium Iodide 65.4 μg Magnesium oxide - heavy 63.1 mg Manganese amino acid chelate 20 mg Zinc amino acid chelate 75 mg Selenomethonine 64.6 μg Tumera diffusa 1 g (1,000 mg) Tribulus terrestris extract 6 g (6,000 mg) Ginko biloba extract 500 mg

	Milk Thistle 4 g (4,000 mg)
D	Take 1 tablet a day with a meal, or as professionally prescribed.
A, CP	Not stated
CI	This product contains selenium which is toxic in high doses. A daily dose of 150 μg for adults of selenium from dietary supplements should not be exceeded.
AR, SC, I	Not stated
M	Blackmores Address 23 Roseberry Street, Balgowlah New South Wales 2093, Australia Tel +61 2 9951 0111 Fax +61 2 9949 1954 Email Via "contact us" on website Web www.blackmores.com.au
Package	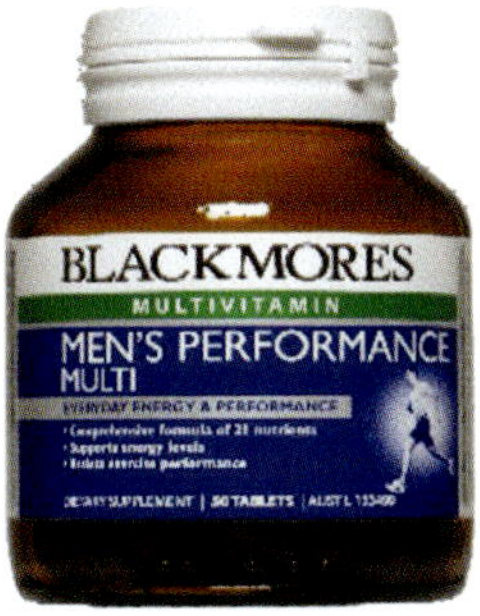

5. ErectOMax

CS	Not stated
AA	Aids poor sexual performance, lack of sexual desire, loss of libido
T	Tablet
S	Each tablet contains: Trigonella foenum graecum (Testofen) seed 9.9 g Urtica dioica (Stinging Nettle) leaf 1 g Dulacia inopiflora (Potency Wood) root 1 g Avena sativa (Oats) herb 1 g Magnesium Aspartate Dihydrate, Equiv. to Magnesium elemental 15.2 mg - 225 mg Zinc Amino Acid Chelate, Equiv. to Zinc elemental 15 mg - 75 mg Pyridoxine Hydrochloride (Vitamin B6) 6 mg
D	Take one tablet twice daily with main meals or as advised by your Health Care

	Professional
A	Not stated
CP	Contains Pyridoxine Hydrochloride (Vitamin B6) which may be dangerous when used in large amounts or for long periods of time,
CI, AR	Not stated
SC	Store below 30 degrees celsius in a cool dry place
I	Not stated
M	Totally Natural Products Address 13 - 14 Durian Place, Wetherill Park, New South Wales, 2164, Australia Tel +61 2 97560400 Fax +61 2 97560719 Email customerservice@tnp.com.au Web www.totallynatural.com.au
Package and Tablet	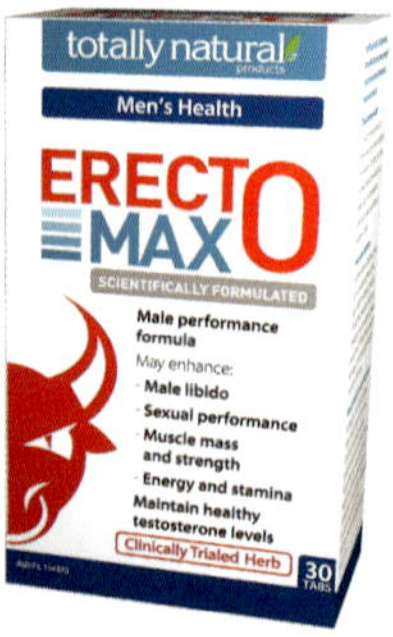 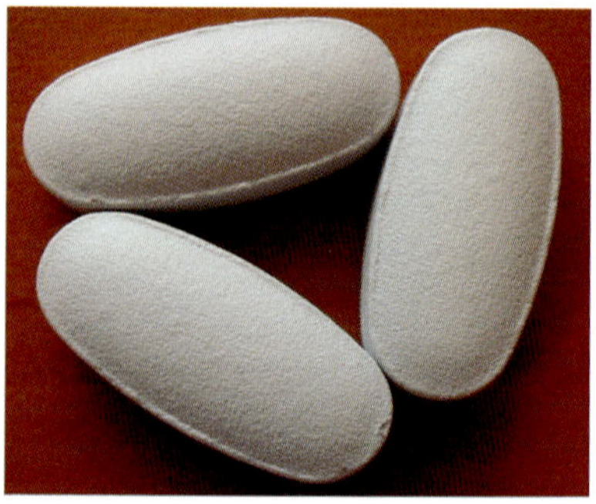

6. Ethical Nutrients Tribulus Performance Plus

CS	Not stated
AA	Balances and supports male function, performance and sexual desire
T	Tablets
S	Each tablet contains: Extracts equivalent to: Tribulus terrestris, herb dry (Tribulus) 4.8 g Mucuna pruriens, seed dry (Velvet Bean) 750 mg Withania somnifera, root dry (Indian Ginseng) 500 mg Nelumbium speciosum, seed dry (Sacred Lotus) 500 mg
D	Take 1 tablet twice daily with food or as directed by a healthcare professional
A, CP, CI, AR	Not stated
SC	Do not use if cap and/or bottle seals are missing or broken. Storage: Store below 30C.

I	Not stated	
M	Health World Limited	
	Address	Corner Nudgee and Toombul Roads, Northgate, Queensland, 4013, Australia
	Tel	+61 7 3117 3300
	Fax	+61 7 3117 3399
	Email	orders@healthworld.com.au
	Web	www.healthworld.com.au/ethicalnutrients

7. Fusion Health Tienchi Ginseng Tablets(same as Oriental Botanicals Tienchi Ginseng Tablets marketed as both brands)

CS	Not stated	
AA	Increases sexual stamina and endurance	
T	Tablet	
S	One 2,000 mg tablet is equivalent to: Panax notoginseng(Tienchi Ginseng) 2,000 mg	
D	Take 1-2 tablets once daily	
A	Not stated	
CP	Use only as directed. Always read the label. If symptoms persist, consult a healthcare practitioner	
CI, AR, SC, I	Not stated	
M	Global Therapeutics Pty Ltd trading as Oriental Botanicals	
	Address	5/93 Centennial Circuit, Byron Bay, New South Wales, 2481, Australia
	Tel	+1800 550 103
	Fax	+61 2 6680 7633
	Email	health@orientalbotanicals.com.au
	Web	www.orientalbotanicals.com.au/tienchiginseng.php
Package	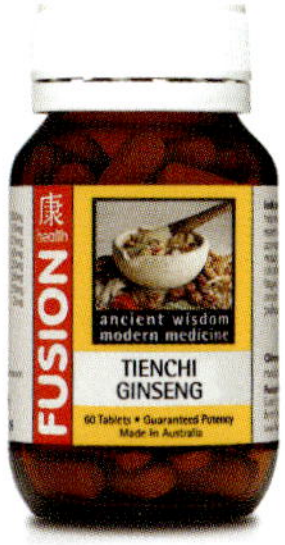	

8. Gen-Tec Ultimate Male Fuel

CS	Not stated
AA	Helps libido and male sexual performance
T	Liquid - 280 ml
S	Tribulus terrestris fruit 10 g Pyridoxine Hydrochloride (Vitamin B6) 10.5 mg Zinc Sulphate Monohydrate 30 mg - equiv 11 mg Zinc Magnesium 26.5 mg Magnesium gluconate 450 mg Epimedium saggittatum herb top 1 g Serenoa serrulata fruit 2 g Also, contains glucose, sodium, benzoate and sodium saccharin
D	Mix 10ml in pineapple juice 1 hour before bed. Cycle 4 weeks on 2 weeks off.
A, CP, CI, AR	Not stated
SC	Advised to consult medical practitioner prior to taking
I	None stated
M	Gen-Tec Nutrition Address GPO Box 1892, Adelaide, South Australia, 5001, Australia Tel +61 8 8186 4628 Fax +61 1 8186 4678 Email Via "contact us" on website Web www.gen-tec.com.au
Package	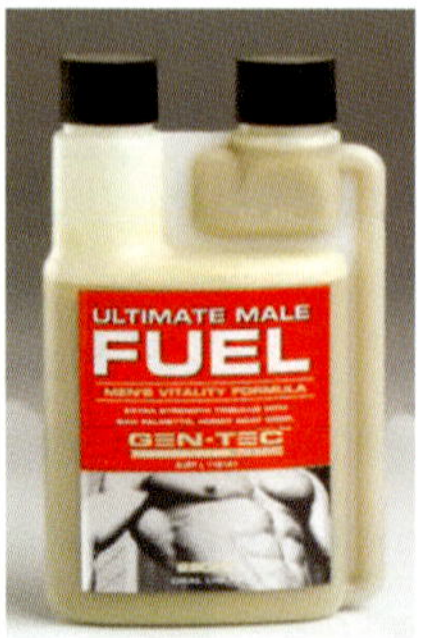

9. Golden Glow Enhance for Men with Horny Goat Weed

CS	Not stated
AA	To help maintain normal sexual function and libido
T	Tablet
S	Each tablet contains extracts equiv. dry: Tribulus terrestris (Burra Gokhru) total fruit and root (3 g) 3,000 mg, Epimedium sagittatum (Horny Goat Weed) leaf (3 g) 3,000 mg, Eleutherococcus senticosus (Siberian Ginseng) root 250 mg, Turnera diffusa (Damiana) leaf 250 mg, Pyridoxine Hydrochloride (Vitamin B6) 20 mg, Riboflavine (Vitamin B2) 20 mg, Nicotinamide (Vitamin B3) 20 mg, d-alpha Tocopheryl acid succinate 41.3mg equiv. Natural Vitamin E 50IU, Choline Bitartrate 121.69 mg equiv. Choline 50 mg, Histidine 50 mg, Zinc (as Amino Acid Chelate) 7 mg.
D	Adults: Take one tablet twice daily with food, or as recommended by your healthcare professional.
A	Not stated
CP	Use only as directed. If symptoms persist, consult your healthcare professional. Always read the label. Vitamin supplements should not replace a balanced diet.
CI	Not to be taken in any acute phase of illness. Contraindicated with androgen sensitive tumors, anti-androgen agents and cholestasis.
AR	Not stated
SC	If taking Thyroxine, this product must be taken 4 hours away from the Thyroxine dosage. Caution with digoxin and patients with benign prostatic hyperplasia.
I	Not stated
M	Queensland Biochemics Pty Ltd Trading as Symbion Consumer Address Reply Paid 45, Virginia BC Queensland 4014, AUSTRALIA Tel +61 7 3246 4411 Fax +61 7 3865 8677 Email info@goldenglow.com.au Web www.goldenglow.com.au

Package and Tablet	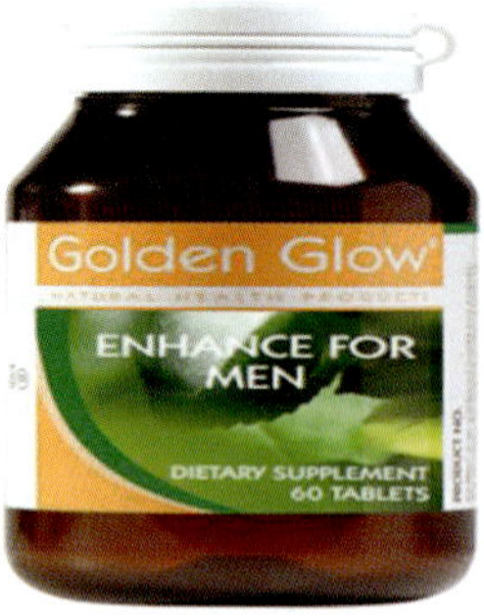 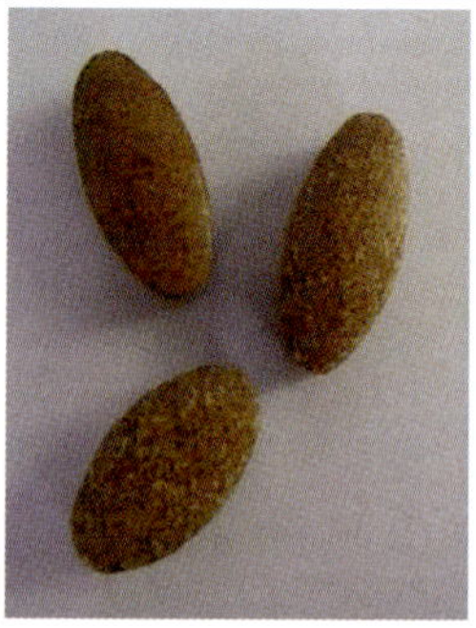

10. Herb Valley Korean Ginseng 1000 mg

CS	Not stated
AA	May facilitate penile erection
T	Tablet - 50
S	Korean Ginseng (Panax Ginseng) exact concentrate 333 mg Equivalent to dry herb 1,000 mg
D	Take 2 tablets daily with food.
A	Not stated
CP	If symptoms persist consult your healthcare practitioner. Vitamin, mineral, and herbal supplements are not intended to replace a balanced diet. Always read the label. Take only as directed.
CI	Ginseng may decrease the effectiveness of warfarin. Panax ginseng may lower blood glucose. Please consult your medical practitioner if you are using oral hypoglycaemic, or using insulin for the treatment of diabetes. Please consult your medical practitioner if taking any other prescribed medications.
AR	Not stated
SC	Free from artificial colouring, flavouring and preservatives. Store below 30 degrees C in a dry place away from sunlight.
I	As mentioned above
M	Essential Nutrients Address 107A Ledger Road, Beverly, South Australia, 5009, Australia Tel +61 8 82686122 Fax +61 8 82688552 Email info@essentialnutrients.com.au Web www.esssentialnutrients.com.au

Package and Tablet	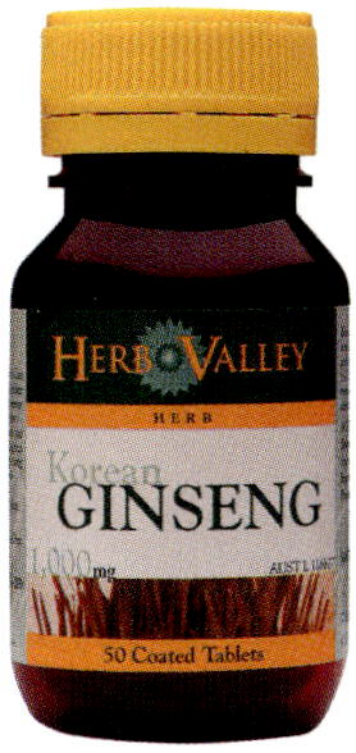	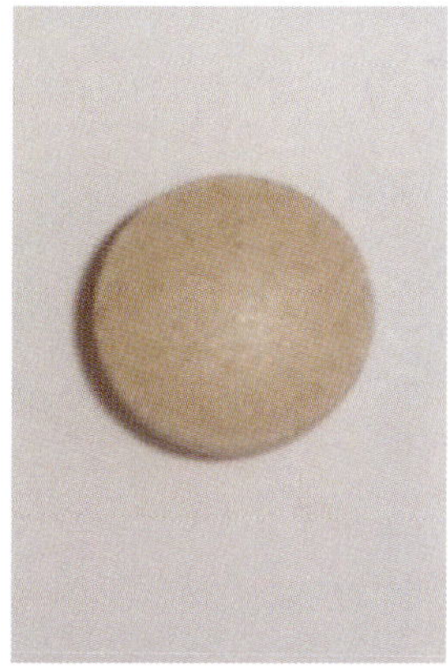

11. Horny Goat Weed Plus

CS	Not stated	
AA	Enhances libido and supports male sexual function	
T	Tablets	
S, D, A, CP, CI, AR, SC, I	Not stated	
M	Cat Media Pty Ltd trading as Naturopathica	
	Address	P.O. Box 154, Mona Vale, 1660, Victoria, Australia
	Tel	+1800 22 77 22
	Email	info@naturopathica.com.au
	Web	www.naturopathica.com.au

12. Mediherb Tribulus Forte (Aerial Parts)

CS	Not stated
AA	To maintain healthy physiology
T	Tablets
S	Each tablet contains : Tribulus terrestris (Tribulus) extract equivalent to dry herb (aerial parts) standardised to contain furostanol saponins as protodioscin 110 mg - 9.0 g
D	1 tablet 1-3 times daily.
A	Not stated
CP	Steroidal saponin-containing herbs such as Tribulus are best kept to a minimum in

	patients with pre-existing cholestasis. Discontinue 7 days prior to general anaesthesia.
CI, AR, SC, I	Not stated
M	MediHerb Pty Ltd Address PO Box 713, Warwick Queensland, 4370, Australia Tel +61 7 4661 0700 Fax +61 7 4661 0788 Email webmaster@mediherb.com.au Web www.mediherb.com.au

13. Medimist Natural Oral Spray Male Enhancer

CS	Not stated
AA	Enhances male sexual function and increases libido
T	Sublingual spray
S	Each 1 ml contains herbal extracts equivalent to dry: Horny Goat Weed (Epimedium sagittatum) leaf 2.0 g Tribulus (Tribulus terrestris) fruit 1.2 g Tribulus (Tribulus terrestris) root 800 mg Ginkgo (Ginkgo biloba) leaf 500 mg Oats (Avena sativa) seed 500 mg Siberian Ginseng (Eleutherococcus senticosus) root and rhizome 50 mg Panax ginseng (Korean ginseng) root 50 mg Zinc (as sulphate heptahydrate) 1 mg
D	Shake well before use. Spray under the tongue. Male adults: 3 sprays (390ul) twice a day or as advised by your healthcare practitioner.
A, CP, CI, AR, SC, I	Not stated
M	MCH Research Pty Ltd Address PO Box 366 Maroochydore, Queensland, 4558 Australia Tel +61 7 5479 5600 Fax +61 7 5479 5601 Email info@mchhealth.com.au Web http://medimist.mchhealth.com.au

Package	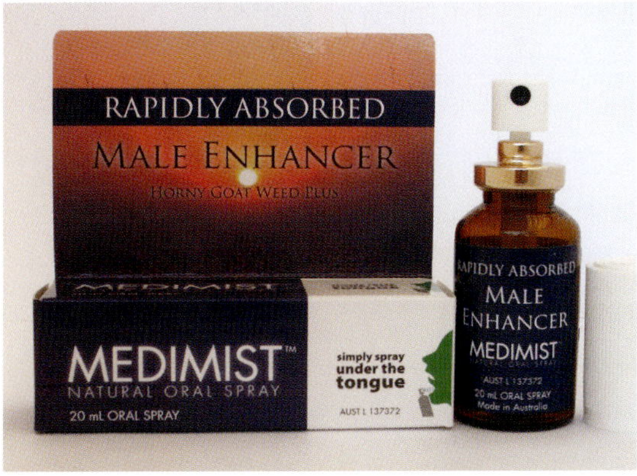

14. Metagenics Tribulus Synergy

CS	Not stated
AA	To support male sexual health
T	Tablets
S	Each tablet contains : Tribulus fruit 10:1 extract (Tribulus terrestris) (containing saponins) 250 mg Ashwagandha Root 5:1 extract (Withania somnifera) (containing withanolides) 200mg Cowage seed 10:1 extract (Mucuna pruriens) (containing naturally occurring levodopa) 50 mg
D	Take one twice daily or as directed by your healthcare provider
A, CP, CI, AR, SC, I	Not stated
M	Health World Limited Address Corner Nudgee and Toombul Roads, Northgate, Queensland, 4013, Australia Tel +61 7 3117 3300 Fax +61 7 3117 3399 Email orders@healthworld.com.au Web www.metagenics.com.au

15. Natural Perform Plus for Men

CS	Not stated
AA	To improve libido, while supporting male sexual function including sexual stamina in healthy individuals.
T	Tablet - 48 per bottle
S	Each tablet/capsule contains : Herbal extracts equiv to dry: Tribulus (Tribulus terrestris) fruit. (2.5 g) 2,500 mg Standardised to Furostanol saponins calc. Protodioscin.75 mg Tribulus (Tribulus terrestris) root.(2.5 g) 2,500 mg Horny Goat Weed (Epimedium sagittatum) leaf.(1.5 g) 1,500 mg Korean Ginseng (Panax Ginseng) root.500 mg Siberian Ginseng (Eleutherococcus senticosus) root.500 mg Schizandra (Schizandra chinensis) fruit.750 mg Green Oats (Avena sativa) extract equiv to fresh herb.750 mg
D	Take 1 tablet twice daily, or as directed by your healthcare professional
A	Not stated
CP	Vitamin Supplements should not replace a balanced diet. If symptoms persist consult your healthcare professional.
CI	The ingredients in this product can affect the way some prescription medications work, consult your doctor before use. Individuals taking anti coagulant and/or anti hypertensive medications should seek medical advice before taking this product.
AR, SC, I	Not stated
M	Australian Naturalcare Products Pty Ltd Address Unit 5, 5 Talavera Rd, North Ryde, New South Wales 2113 Australia Tel 61 2 8874 8100 Fax 61 2 8874 8111 Email myorder@ausnaturalcare.com.au Web http://www.ausnaturalcare.com.au
Package	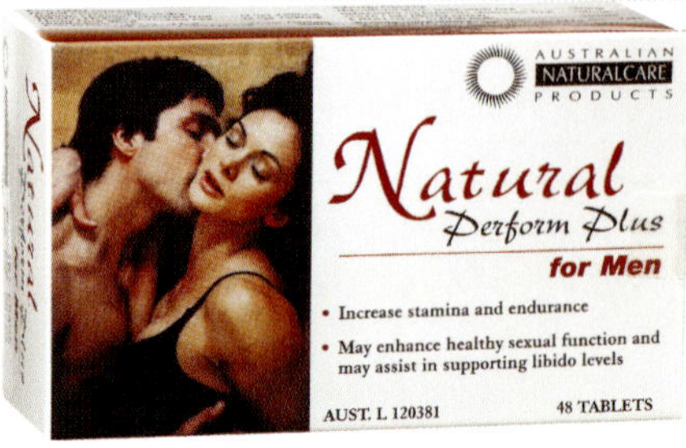

16. Nature' s Naturals Libido Plus for Men

CS, AA, T, S, D, A, CP, CI, AR, SC, I	Not stated	
M	Natural Pharmaceuticals Australia Pty Ltd	
	Address	PO BOX 8268, Sunnybank, Queensland, 4109, Australia
	Tel	+61 7 39025100
	Fax	+61 7 39025199
	Email	info@naturesnaturals.com.au
	Web	www.naturesnaturals.com.au

17. Natures Sunshine Damiana

CS	Not stated	
AA	To support sexual function	
T	Capsules - 100 per bottle	
S	Each 'preservative free' capsule contains 350 mg of Turnera diffusa leaf powder.	
D	For adults: take two capsules with a meal three times daily.	
A	Not stated	
CP	Always read the label. If symptoms persist consult your healthcare practitioner.	
CI	Damiana may affect blood sugar levels and may stimulate intracellular receptors for progesterone cells.	
AR, SC, I	Not stated	
M	Nature' s Sunshine Products of Australia	
	Address	19 Brookhollow Avenue, Baulkham Hills, New South Wales 2153
	Tel	+61 2 9894 0111
	Fax	+61 2 9894 2422
	Email	Via "contact us" on website
	Web	www.naturessunshine.com.au

Package

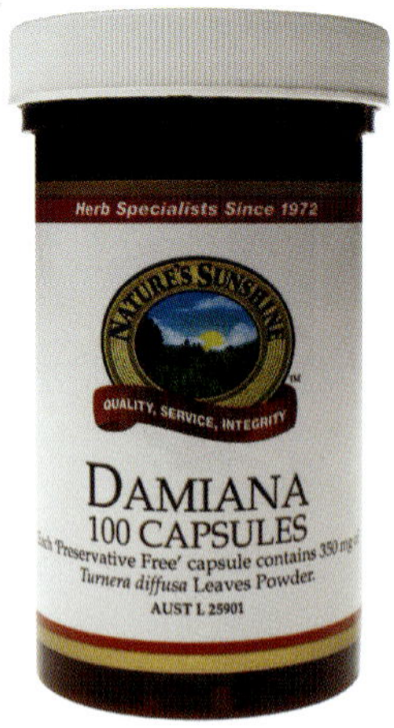

18. Nature' s Way Mens Energy Multi-Vitamin

CS	Not stated
AA	Improves sexual function and libido
T	Tablet - 60
S	Betacarotene 3 mg
	Vitamin B1 30 mg
	Vitamin B2 30 mg
	Vitamin B3 50 mg
	Folic Acid 200 mcg
	Vitamin B5 50 mg
	Vitamin B6 30 mg
	Vitamin B12 30 mcg
	Vitamin C 150 mg
	Vitamin D3 200 IU
	Vitamin E 50 IU
	Biotin 50 mcg
	Calcium 54 mg
	Copper 1 mg
	Magnesium 50 mg
	Manganese 2 mg
	Iodine 50 mcg
	Potassium 10 mg
	Selenium 26 mcg

	Zinc 20 mg Bioflavonoids 40 mg Choline Bitartrate 25 mg Inositol 25 mg Panax Ginseng 250 mg Saw Palmetto 360 mg
D	Adults only: Take 1 capsule daily with the morning meal.
A	Not stated
CP	Vitamin supplements should not replace a balanced diet. This product contains selenium, which is toxic in high doses. A daily dose of 100mcg of Selenium from dietary supplements should not be exceeded. Products containing Selenium are not suitable for children under 15 years of age.
CI, AR, SC, I	Not stated
M	Natures Way Address 16 Jubilee Avenue, Warriewood New South Wales 2102, Australia Tel +61 2 9997 1466 Fax +61 2 9979 1696 Email labpharm@pharmacare.com.au Web www.naturesway.com.au/docs/vitamin.asp

19. Nutrition Care Gingkoseng Ginkgo Biloba and Panax Ginseng Complex GG

CS	Not stated
AA	Erectile Dysfunction
T	Tablet
S	Each tablet contains : Ginkgo biloba (maidenhair tree) leaf 2 g Equiv. Gingkoflavonglycosides 9.6 mg Equiv. Ginkgolides and Bilobalide 2.4 mg Panax ginseng (Korean ginseng) root 150 mg
D	Take one tablet three times a day or as directed by a healthcare professional
A	Treatment must be continued for 4 to 6 weeks before beneficial effects can be expected
CP	None stated
CI	If supplementation is accompanied with a high caffeine intake (more than 4 cups of coffee/day), this should be reduced otherwise over-stimulation may occur.

AR	No serious side effects - In rare cases, some mild gastrointestinal complaints, headache and allergic reactions have been reported.
SC	It is recommended that the product is used for a few weeks at a time, followed by a break of approximately one week
I	None stated
M	Nutrition Care Pharmaceuticals Pty Ltd Address 25-27 Keysborough Avenue, Keysborough, Victoria, 3173, Australia Tel +61 3 9769 0811 Fax +61 3 9769 0822 Email enquiries@nutritioncare.com.au Web www.nutritioncare.com.au
Package	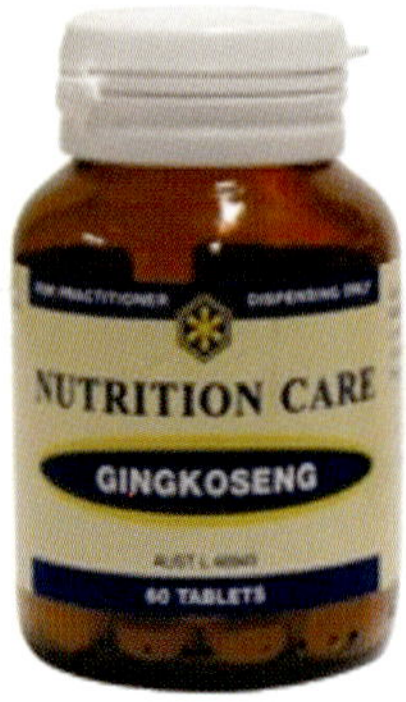

20. Oriental Botanicals Tienchi Ginseng Tablets(same as Fusion Health Tienchi Ginseng Tablets - marketed as both brands)

CS	Not stated
AA	Increases sexual stamina and endurance
T	Tablet
S	One 2,000 mg tablet is equivalent to: Panax notoginseng(Tienchi Ginseng) 2,000 mg
D	Take 1-2 tablets once daily
A	Not stated
CP	Use only as directed. Always read the label. If symptoms persist, consult a healthcare practitioner
CI, AR, SC, I	Not stated
M	Global Therapeutics Pty Ltd trading as Oriental Botanicals

	Address 5/93 Centennial Circuit, Byron Bay, New South Wales, 2481, Australia Tel +1800 550 103 Fax +61 2 6680 7633 Email health@orientalbotanicals.com.au Web www.orientalbotanicals.com.au/tienchiginseng.php
Package	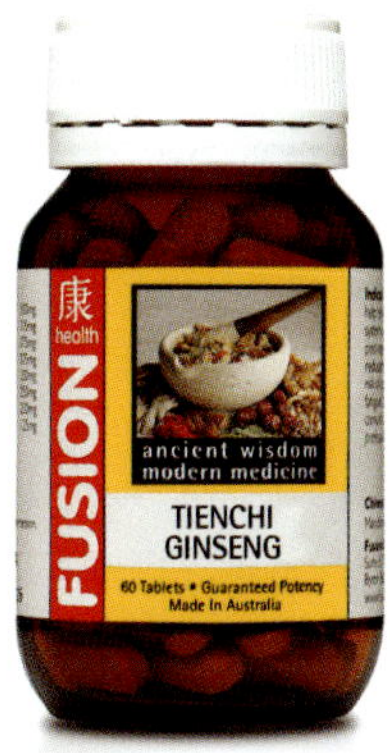

21. RedBak Xtra Hard Performance and Libido Booster

CS	Not stated
AA	Promotes sexual desire (aphrodisiac), improves sexual function and stimulates blood flow.
T	Capsules 60 or 120
S	Each capsule contains herbal extracts equivalent to dry: Tribulus terrestris Whole Plant(12,000 mg)12 g Epimedium sagittatum Leaf (Horney Goat Weed)(2,000 mg) 2 g Liriosma ovata Leaf(Muria Puama) (1,000 mg) 1 g Ginkgo biloba Leaf(Ginkgo) (2,000mg) 2 g Zinc 15 mg Selenium 8.6 mcg
D, A, CP, CI, AR, SC, I	Not stated
M	International Health Investments Pty Ltd trading as RedBak. Address 29 Millennium Circuit, Helensvale , Queensland 4212, AUSTRALIA Tel 1800 733 225 Fax 61 7 5529 7984 Email inquiries@ihiaustralia.com Web www.redbak.net

22. Royal Jelly

CS	Not stated
AA	Plays a role in sexual function
T	Capsules 1,000 mg x 60
S	Royal Jelly Lyophilized Powder 183.3 mg
D	1 capsule per day
A	Not stated
CP	If you have allergies, please contact a medical practitioner before taking.
CI, AR	Not stated
SC	Store in a cool place and avoid direct sunlight
I	Not stated
M	Panax Pharmatec Pty Ltd Address 20/198 - 222 Young Street, Waterloo, New South Wales, 2017, Australia Tel +61 2 9319 7700 Fax +61 2 9319 7711 Email info@panaxpharm.com Web www.panaxpharm.com

23. Shen Qi Da Bu Wan

CS	Not stated
AA	Low Libido
T	Capsules - 300 per bottle
S	Each pill contains herbal extract of panax ginseng 85 mg and astragalus membanaceus 85 mg.
D	8 capsules, three times a day.
A	Not stated
CP	Be cautious with excess heat patterns, Yin deficiency with hyperactivity of yang, damp-heat patterns.
CI, AR, SC, I	Not stated
M	Cathay Herbal Laboratories Address 5/5-15 Dunning Ave, Rosebery NSW 2018 Australia? Tel +61 2 8345 6588 Fax +61 2 8345 6577

	Email enquiries@cathayherbal.com Web www.cathayherbal.com
Package and Capsule	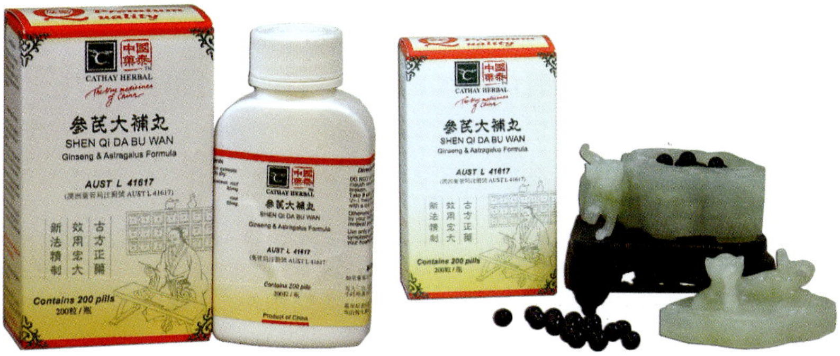

24. Super Horny Goat Weed for Him

CS	Not stated
AA	May enhance sexual performance and healthy sexual function, increase sexual desires and support erectile function in men.
T	Tablet - 100
S	Each tablet contains concentrated extracts equivalent to dry: Ginkgo biloba (maiden hair) leaf 3,500 mg Tribulus terrestris root 1,250 mg Epimedium sagittatum (horny goat weed) leaf 1,000 mg Panax ginseng (Korean ginseng) root 700 mg Ginkgolides 620 mcg Bilobalide 580 mcg Withania somnifera (root) 300 mg Turnera diffusa (damiana) leaf 175 mg d-alpha tocopheryl acid succinate equivalent to natural Vitamin E 37 IU -30.3 mg Pyridoxine Hydrochloride (Vitamin B6) 15 mg Cyanocobalamin (Vitamin B12) 35 mcg Zinc amino acid chelate Equivalent zinc 10 mg - 50 mg
D	Adults Only: Take one (1) tablet 3 times daily, with meals or as directed by a healthcare professional
A	Not stated
CP	Contains zinc which may be dangerous if taken in large amounts or for a long period.

	Do not use if cap seal is broken at time of purchase. Vitamins can only be of assistance if the dietary vitamin intake is inadequate. Information and statements regarding this dietary supplement have not been evaluated by the FDA (USA) and TGA (Australia) and should not be used to diagnose, treat, cure, or prevent any disease.
CI, AR	Not stated
SC	Store below 30°C in a dry place away from heat and direct sunlight.
I	Not stated
M	Enervite Health Supplements Address 118/500 Centre Road Bentleigh Victoria Australia 3204 Tel +61 3 9579 3322 Fax +61 3 9579 3323 Email Via "contact us" on website Web www.enervite.com.au

25. TestOroid

CS	Not stated
AA	Enhances libido and sexual performance
T	Tablet
S	Each tablet contains: Trigonella foenum graecum (Testofen) 9.9 g - 9,900 mg Urtica dioca (Stinging nettle) 1,000 mg Dulacia inopiflora (potency wood) 1,000 mg Avena sativa (Oats) 1,000 mg Magnesium aspartate 15.2 mg Zinc amino acid chelate 15 mg Pyridoxine Hydrochloride (Vitamin B6) 6 mg
D	2 tablets daily
A	Not stated
CP	Caution: Take at least one hour away from all other medications
CI, AR, SC, I	Not stated
M	Totally Natural Products Address 13 - 14 Durian Place, Wetherill Park, New South Wales, 2164, Australia

	Tel +61 2 97560400 Fax +61 2 97560719 Email customerservice@tnp.com.au Web www.totallynatural.com.au
Package and Tablet	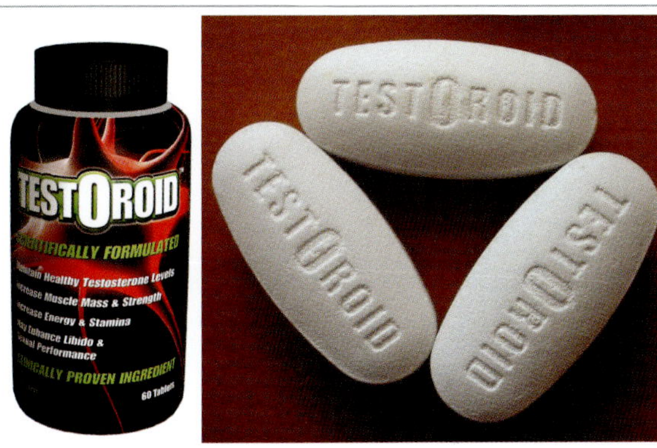

26. Tribulus Maximus

CS	Not stated
AA	Elevates male stamina, performance and sex drive
T	Tablets - 50
S	Each tablet contains: Herbal extracts equivalent to dry: Tribulus Terrestris (Burra Gokhru) Fruit 5,000 mg; Panax Ginseng (Ginseng Korean) Root 500 mg; Pyridoxine Hydrochloride 25 mg; Ascorbic acid 45 mg; Copper (as copper gluconate) 1.5 mg; Magnesium (as Magnesium oxide) 100 mg; Zinc (as Zinc oxide) 25 mg.
D	Take one to two tablets daily with food
A	Not stated
CP	Contains zinc which may be dangerous if take in large amounts of for a long period.
CI	Consult your healthcare professional if on heart and blood pressure medication including blood thinners. Should be avoided if suffering from any prostate problems such as BPH.
AR, SC, I	Not stated
M	Cat Media Pty Ltd Trading as Naturopathica

Address	P.O. Box 154, Mona Vale, 1660, New South Wales, Australia
Tel	+1800 22 77 22
Email	info@naturopathica.com.au
Web	www.naturopathica.com.au

27. Viril-X

CS	Not stated
AA	Assists healthy sexual function and gives you back your sex drive
T	Tablets
S	Tribulus Terrestris (Burra Gokhru) Fruit 5 g Ginkgo Biloba (Maidenhair Tree) Leaf 1.5 g Dulacia Inopiflora (Muira-Puama) Root 1.5 g Panax Ginseng (Korean Ginseng) Root 500 mg
D	Dosage may vary from person to person. We recommend you start by taking 1 tablet daily for 1 week. Increase this dose by 1 tablet daily each week after this until you are taking 3 - 4 tablets daily.
A	Men have reported positive changes after two to four weeks of daily use, and optimal results after 12 weeks, however individual results may vary.
CP	CAUTIONS: If symptoms persist, consult your healthcare practitioner. Store below 30C.
CI	You should consult your health practitioner if you are on any heart, blood pressure or blood thinning medication.
AR, SC, I	Not stated
M	Hershel-Beck Address 16 Jubille Avenue, Warriewood, New South Wales 2102, Australia Tel +1 300 652 422 Fax +61 2 9997 1698 Email Via "contact us" on website Web www.hershel-beck.com.au

28. WYLD Man

CS	Not stated
AA	Drives libido
T	Tablet - 60
S	Each tablet contains : Herbal extracts equivalent to dry : Tribulus terrestris fruit (Burra gokhru) 3,000 mg Epimedium sagittatum leaf (Horny goat weed) 3,000 mg Ginkgo biloba leaf (Ginkgo) 3,000 mg Schizandra chinensis fruit (Chinese magnoliavine) 750 mg Panax ginseng root (Korean ginseng) 500 mg Paullinia cupana seed (guarana) 347.3 mg contains caffeine 12.5 mg Zinc (as Zinc amino acid chelate) 6 mg
D	1 tablet twice daily with food or as directed by your healthcare professional.
A	Most people experience an increase in their energy level within two to three weeks. However, this may differ based on individual workload and lifestyle factors.
CP, CI, AR, SC, I	Not stated
M	N-Hance Pty Ltd Address: Suite 402, Lakeside Corporate Centre 29-31 Solent Circuit, Baulkham Hills, New South Wales, 2153, Australia. Tel: +1800 888 215 Email: info@wyld.com.au Web: www.wyld.com.au
Package and Tablet	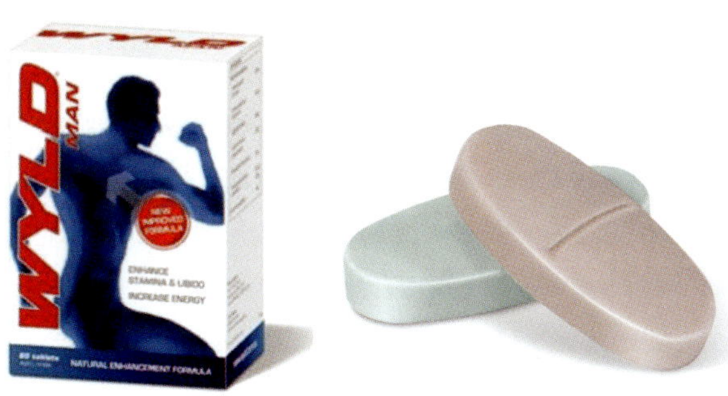

III. Commercially Available Phytotherapy Products for Both Male and Female Sexual Medicine

1. Fusion Health Libido Tablets

CS	Not stated	
AA	Enhance sexual desire and sensitivity and promotes vitality in men and women.	
T	Tablet - 60 per bottle	
S	Each 2,800 mg tablet contains Tribulus terrestris 800 mg Epimedium sagittatum (Horny Goat Weed) 700 mg Curculigo orchioides 400 mg Morinda officinalis 400 mg Schizandra chinensis 400 mg Zizyphus jujuba 100mg Contains No colours, flavours, yeast, wheat, gluten, sugar, dairy or animal products	
D	1-2 tablets once or twice daily	
A	Not stated	
CP	Best taken an hour away from food. Not suitable during pregnancy	
CI	Not recommended if an androgen sensitive tumour is present or warfarin is being taken.	
AR	Not stated	
SC	May take 2-4 tablets one hour before sexual intimacy	
I	Not stated	
M	Global Therapeutics Pty Ltd trading as Fusion Health	
	Address	5 / 93 Centennial Cr, Byron Bay, NSW PO Box 1999 Byron Bay, NSW 2481, Australia
	Tel	+61 2 6680 7622
	Fax	+61 2 6680 7633
	Email	health@fusionhealth.com.au
	Web	www.fusionhealth.com.au

Package	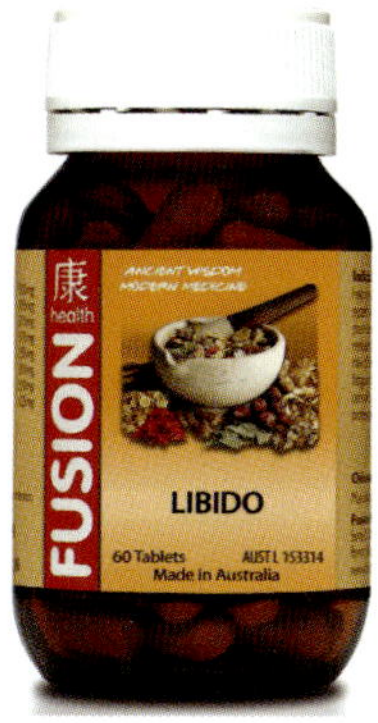

2. Performance Max Tribulus

CS	Not stated	
AA	Enhances sexual function and libido in both males and females	
T	Capsules - 60 or 180	
S, D, A, CP, CI, AR, SC, I	Not stated	
M	Top Nutrition Pty Ltd	
	Address	Unit 14, 7 Anella Ave, Castle Hill New South Wales 2154 Australia
	Tel	+61 2 4957 8949
	Fax	+61 2 4957 8949 (same as telephone)
	Email	sales@topnutrition.com.au
	Web	www.topnutrition.com.au

3. Xcitement Plus

CS	Not stated
AA	Aids male and female sex drive
T	Tablets - 30 or 60
S	Each Tablet Contains: Active ingredients. Each tablet contains: Concentrated Herbal Extracts Equiv. Dry: Tribulus terrestris (Tribulus) fruit and root 10 g Standardised to protodioscin 80 mg Epimedium sagittatum (Horny Goat Weed) leaf 3 g Panax Ginseng (Korean Ginseng) root 1 g

	Liriosma ovata (Potency Wood) root 1.5 g Avena sativa (Oats) herb (equiv. to fresh) 1 g Zinc amino acid chelate (equiv. Zinc 15 mg) 75 mg
D	Take one tablet daily with food or as advised by your healthcare Professional.
A, CP	Not stated
CI	Caution in individuals taking anti-platelet and anticoagulant medications Contraindicated with MAO inhibitors
AR	Not stated
SC	Take one hour away from other medications
I	Not stated
M	Totally Natural Products Address 13-14 Durian Place, Wetherill Park, New South Wales, 2164, Australia Tel +61 2 9756 0400 Fax +61 2 9756 0719 Email customerservice@tnp.com.au Web www.tnp.com.au
Package and Tablet	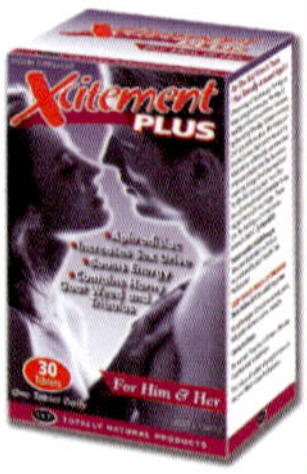 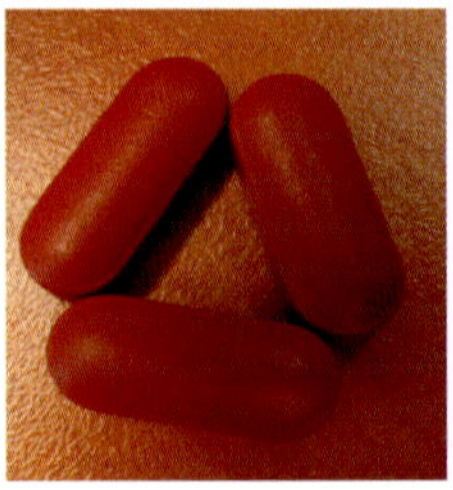

Chapter 2

Chinese Products

Zhong-cheng Xin

1. Zuogui Wan

CS	Not stated
AA	Enhancement of the Kidney -Qi and Yin
T	Pill
S	Zuogui Wan is packed as bottles of 600 pills, and each pill contains 0.1 g mixture of such crude drugs as prepared rehmannia root , cuscuta seed, radix achyranthis bidentatae, colla carapacis et plastri testudinis, deerhorn glue, Chinese yam, asiatic cornelian cherry fruit and barbary wolfberry fruit.
D	The usual adult dose is 18 g/day orally in 2 divided doses before or between meals. The dosage may be adjusted according to the patient's age, body weight and symptoms.
A	Duration of application for effectiveness may differ individually.
CP	Zuogui Wan is indicated for the relief of the symptoms of kidney-yin deficiency, waist soreness, feeble knee, night sweat , fatigue and thirst.
CI	Pregnant women, children, and patients allergic to this medicine should nottake it.
AR	Not stated
SC	When this product is used, oily food should be avoided; Patients with colds should not take this medicine; If the symptoms and the situation of patients do not get better in 2 weeks, or even get worse, the patients should stop the administration of this medicine; If the quality of medicine is changed, the medicine must not be administered.

I	Not stated
M	Henan Wanxi Pharmaceutical Co., Ltd. Address Binhexilu Road 1888#, Nanyang City, Henan Province, China Tel +86-0377-63536666 Fax +86-0377-63536888 Email ey360kf@ey360.cn Web http://www.wanxi.com
Package and Pill	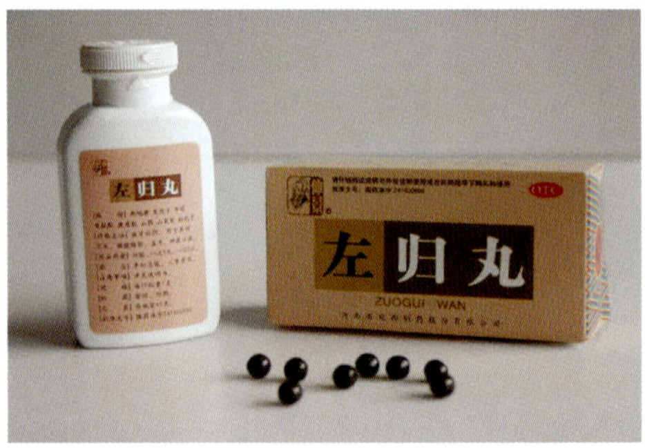

2. Yougui Pill

CS	Not stated
AA	Enhancement of the vital-gate-fire and Kidney-Yang
T	Pill
S	Yougui Pill is packed as bottles of 200 pills, and each pill contains 9.0 g of extract of such mixed crude drugs as prepared rehmannia root, aconite root, cassia, Chinese yam, asiatic cornelian cherry fruit, cuscuta seed, deerhorn glue, barbary wolfberry fruit, angelica root, eucommia bark.
D	The usual adult dose is 27.0 g/day orally in 3 divided doses before or between meals. The dosage may be adjusted according to the patient's age, body weight and symptoms.
A	Duration of application for effectiveness may differ individually.
CP	Yougui Pill is indicated for the relief of the following symptoms of those patients with deficiency of kidney-yang and decline of vital gate-fire, weakness of Qi and Shen because of illness or aging, chilly limbs, flabbiness of waist and knees, impotence and premature ejaculation, azoospermia, poor appetite, and et al.
CI	Patients with renal deficiency and turbid damp should not take this medicine.
AR	Not stated
SC	If the patient has a decline of Yang and Qi combined , the Yougui Pill and Ginseng

	can be taken together; Psoralea fruits and Yougui pill can be used together to tonify kidney to arrest spontaneous emission; Chinese magnoliavine fruit, muscade and Yougui pill can be used together to prevent the leakage of Kidney-qi; Radix Morindae Officnalis, caulis cistanchis and Yougui pill can be used together to invigorate the kidney and strengthen yang;
I	Not stated
M	Beijing Tongrentang Group Co., Ltd. Address Xihuannanlu Road 8# ,Economic and Technological Development Zone, Beijing, China Tel +86-10-67186699 Fax +86-10-36575980 Email gfbgs@tongrentang.com Web http://www.tongrentang.com
Package	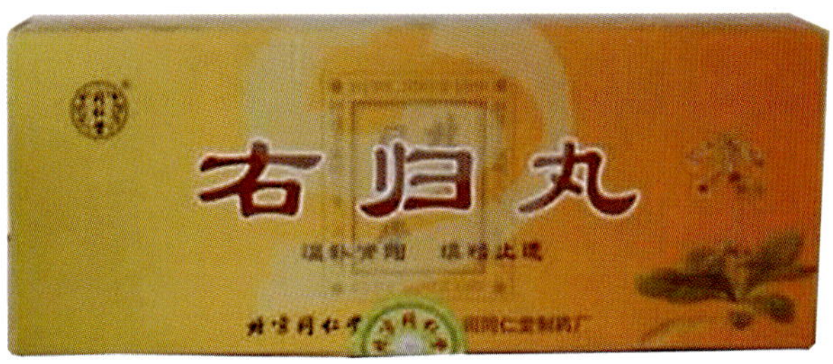

3. Xiaoyao Wan

CS	Not stated
AA	Dispersing the depressed liver-energy, invigorating the spleen, regulating menstruation and supporting blood.
T	Pill
S	Xiaoyao Wan is packed as bottles of 200 pills, and each pill contains 9.0 g of extract of such mixed crude drugs as bupleurum root, angelica root, white peony root, atractylodes macrocephala, tuckahoe, peppermint, ginger and licorice root.
D	The usual adult dose is 18.0 g/day orally in 2 divided doses before or between meals. The dosage may be adjusted according to the patient's age, body weight and symptoms.
A	Duration of application for effectiveness may differ individually.

CP	Xiaoyao Wan is indicated for the relief of the following symptoms of those patients with depression of liver qi, irregular menses, chest pain and hypochondrium, dizziness, and anorexia.
CI	Patients allergic to this medicine should not take it.
AR	Not stated
SC	When this product is used, oily and cold food should be avoided; Pregnant patients should take this medicine only on doctor's advice; Patients with a cold or menorrhagia should not take this medicine; Patients with usually normal menstrual blood volume ,who exhibit symptoms such as low menstrual blood volume or postponed menstruation or irregular vaginal bleeding should see their doctor; If the symptoms and the situation of patients does not get better in 2 weeks or gets worse the patients should stop the administration of this medicine; If the quality of medicine is changed the medicine must not be administered.
I	Not stated
M	Henan Wanxi Pharmaceutical Co., Ltd. Address Binhexilu Road 1888# , Nanyang City, Henan Province, China Tel +86-0377-63536666 Fax +86-0377-63536888 Email ey360kf@ey360.cn Web http://www.wanxi.com
Package	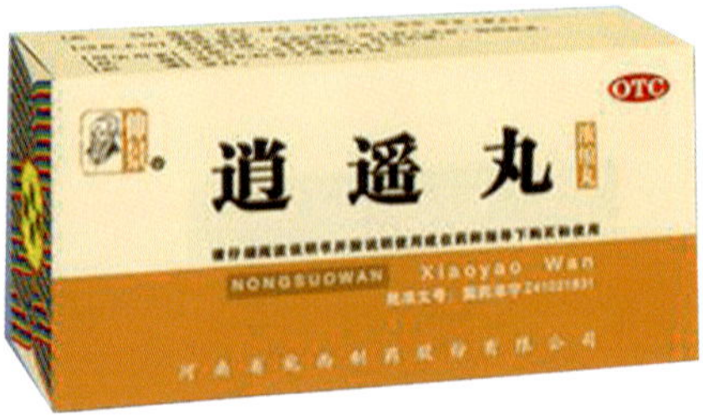

4. Jingui Shenqi Wan

CS	Not stated
AA	Enhancement of the Kidney-yang
T	Pill
S	Jinguishenqi Pill is packed as bottles of 10 pills, and each pill contains 6.0 g of extract of such mixed crude drugs as rehmannia, tuckahoe, Chinese yam, asiatic

	cornelian cherry fruit, moutan cortex, alisma rhizoma, ramulus cinnamomi, radix achyranthis bidentatae, isapgol, aconite root.
D	The usual adult dose is 12.0 g/day orally in 2 divided doses before or between meals. The dosage may be adjusted according to the patient's age, body weight and symptoms.
A	Duration of application for effectiveness may differ individually.
CP	Yougui Pill is indicated for the relief of the following symptoms of those patients with renal deficiency and edema , flabbiness of waist and knees, difficulty in micturition and chilly limbs. Avoid sexual intercourse , anger, and cold meal or drink during the use of medication.
CI	Pregnant women must not take this medicine. Patients with yin deficiency generating intrinsic heat should pay more caution to this medicine.
AR, SC, I	Not stated
M	Beijing Tongrentang Group Co., Ltd. Address Xihuannanlu Road 8# ,Economic and Technological Development Zone, Beijing, China Tel +86-10-67186699 Fax +86-10-36575980 Email gfbgs@tongrentang.com Web http://www.tongrentang.com
Package	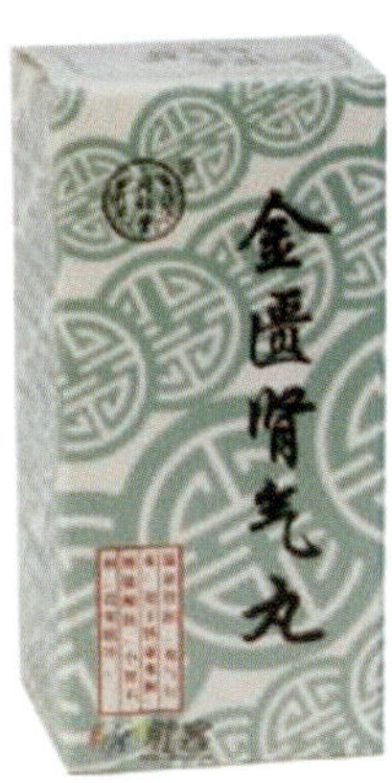

5. Xuefu Zhuyu Keli

CS	Not stated
AA	Promoting blood flow and qi circulation to relieve pain
T	Granule
S	Xuefu Zhuyu Keli is packed as packs of 5.0 g of extract of such mixed crude drugs as peach seed, safflower, angelica, chuanxiong, rehmannia dride rhizome, paeoniae radix, achyranthis radix, Chinese thorowax root, aurantii fructus, the root of balloon flower and licorice root.
D	The usual adult dose is 15.0 g/day orally in 3 divided doses. The dosage may be adjusted according to the patient's age, body weight and symptoms.
A	Duration of application for effectiveness may differ individually.
CP	Xuefu Zhuyu Keli is indicated for the relief of the following symptoms of those patients with headache , chest pain , insomnia and dreamful sleep and restlessness.
CI	Pregnant women must not take this medicine.
AR	Not stated
SC	When this product is used, cold food and drink should be avoided.
I	Not stated
M	Guizhou Liansheng Pharmaceutical Group Co., Ltd. Address No 1 Huai he Road, Economic and Technological Development Zone, Zunyi, Guizhou Province,China Tel +86-852-8672330~333 Fax +86-852-8672908 Email lianshengyaoye@vigourmed.com Web http:\\www.vigourmed.com
Package	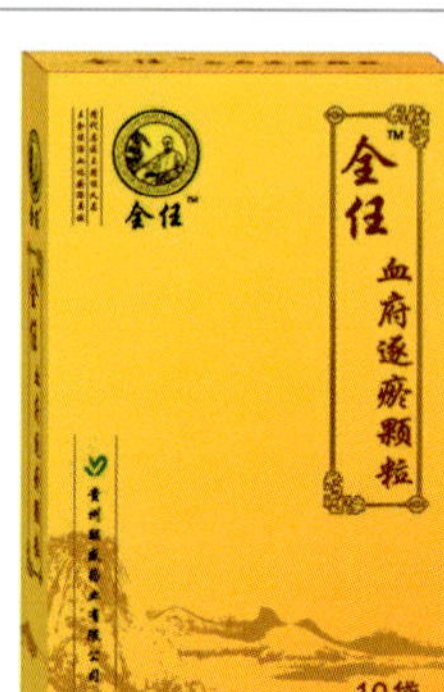

6. Shengjing Capsule

CS	Not stated
AA	To invigorate the Kidney, enhance the Kidney-yang, increase Jing and Yin
T	Capsule
S	Shengjing Capsule is packed as packets of 24 capsules, and each capsule contains 0.4 g of extract of such mixed crude drugs as hairy deerhorn , Chinese caterpilar fungus, solomonseal rhizome, cuscuta seed, barbary wolfberry fruit, ginseng, flatstem milkvetch seed, epimedium, fleece flower root, mulberry fruit, psoralea fruits, rhizoma drynariae, Rhizoma Curculiginis, chrokee rose fruit, blaeberry, eucommia bark, sargentgloryvine stem, European Verbena Herb, ginkgo leaf.
D	The usual adult dose is 4.8 g/day orally in 3 divided doses before or between meals. The dosage may be adjusted according to the patient's age, body weight and symptoms.
A	Duration of application for effectiveness may differ individually.
CP	Shengjing Capsule is indicated for the relief of the following symptoms of renal deficiency patients with flabbiness of waist and knees, dizziness and acratia , aspermatism , nonliquefaction of semen, and et al. Avoid sexual intercourse , anger and cold meal or drink when taking this medication.
CI	Patients with asthenic yin causing excessive pyrexia must not take this medicine.
AR	Some patients may feel dizzy and nauseated after taking this medicine .
SC, I	Not stated
M	Chongqing Tonghai Co., Ltd. Address Yifeng Building, B stand, 31 floor, Taoyuan Road 89# ,South Bank Economic and Technological Development Zone, Chongqing, China Tel +86-800-8078808 Fax +86-023-62837004 Email CQ_tonghai@126.com Web http://www.cqthyy.com
Package	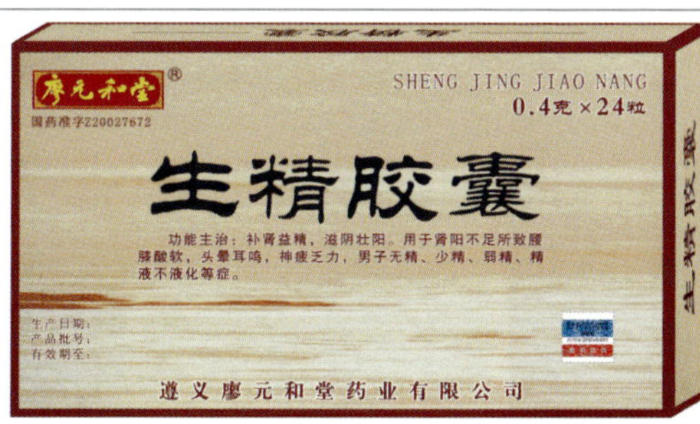

Chapter 3

Indonesian Products

FX Arif Adimoelja, Johannes Soedjono

1. Virilar TM

CS	Not stated
AA	Sexual Performance enhancer
T	Tablet
S	This product contains 27 different plant chemical extracts packed in blisters of 10 red capsules each. Panax Ginseng, Noto ginseng, Tribulus, Cordicep, Polygonum, Epimedium, Cistanche, Gastrodia, Pinella, Limonium, Gingko, Astragalus, Psoralea, Angelica Sinensis, Wild Yam, Marinda, Rehmania, Carthamus, Ginger, Ginger, Eurycoma Longifolia, Niacinamid, Guarana and L-Arginine.
D	2 capsules daily on an empty stomach for 4 weeks
A, CP, AR, SC, I	Not stated
CI	None
M	Manufactured by bioDyne Labs, Inc. Reno, Nevada, USA Distributed by bioDyne Labs Group of Companies, Singapore.
Tablets	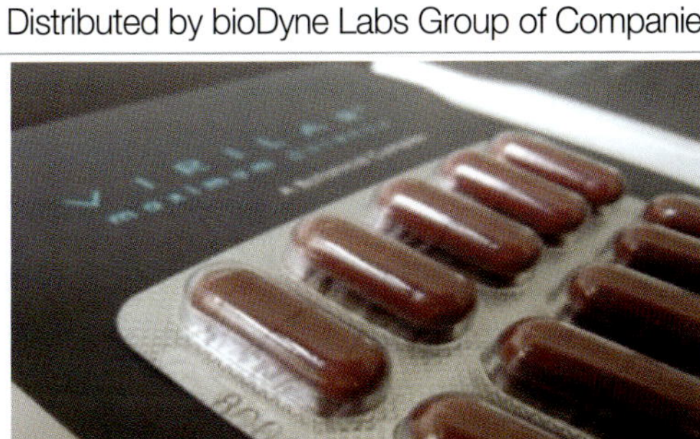

2. Tribestan®

CS	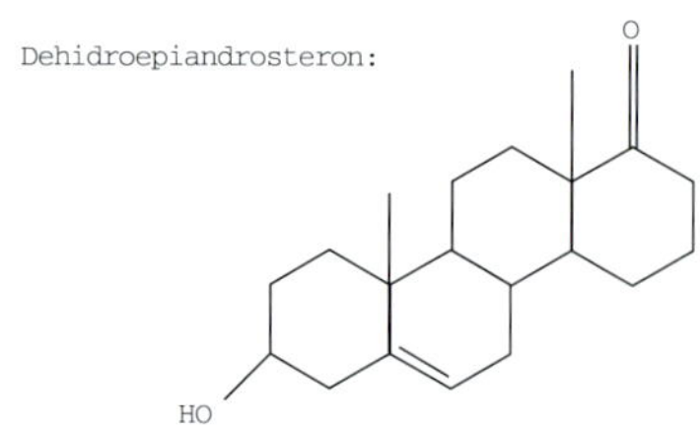 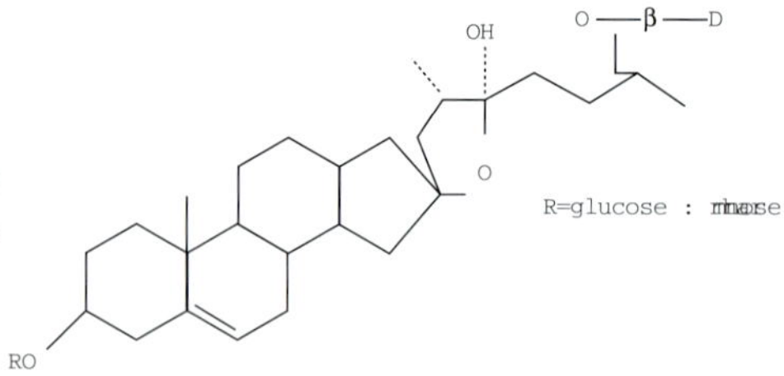 PROTODIOSCIN DHEA
AA	Men: Maintain Men's health, infertlity, enhance sexual functions
T	Tablet
S	5 blisters of 4 red film-coated tablets in one box (20 tablets/box of 250 mg/tablets) Tribulus terrestris L
D	Men: 1-2 tablets for 30-40 days Women: 1-2 tablets. 3 x/day for 30-40 days
A, CP, AR, SC, I	Not stated
CI	None
M	P.T. TEGUHSINDO LESTARITAMA Address Jl. Kebayoran Lama 225 JAKARTA, Indonesia
Package	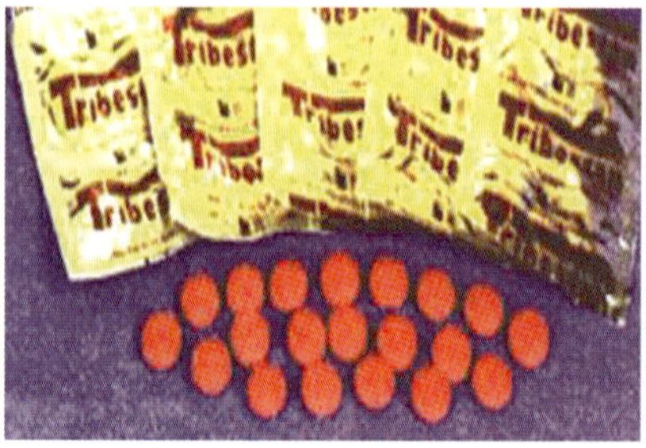 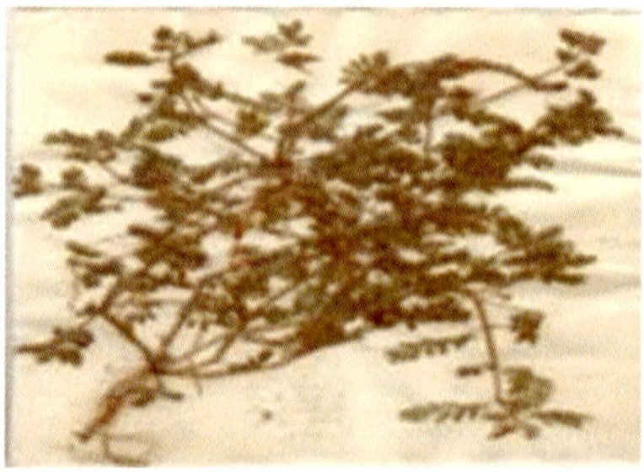

3. Ratax®

CS	Not stated
AA	Improve vitality and treatment of sexual Dysfunctions.
T	Tablet
S	20 red capsules/box (2 blisters of 10 capsules) Panax Ginseng 45 mg, Cordiceps 15 mg

	Herba Epimedii 60 mg, Vit. E 10 mg, Vit B1 1.4 mg Vit. B2 1.6 mg, Vit.B6 2.2 mg, Vit B12 3 mg., Nicotinamid 18 mg, Zinc sulfate 15 mg.
D	One capsule daily, 2 hours before meal, 3 hours before/after taking any other medication. Maximum 3 capsules daily. (Take all at once, on an empty stomach).
A, CP, CI, AR, SC, I	Not stated
M	Manufactured by PT. PYRIDAM FARMA Tbk. Address Jakarta, INDONESIA
Package and Tablet	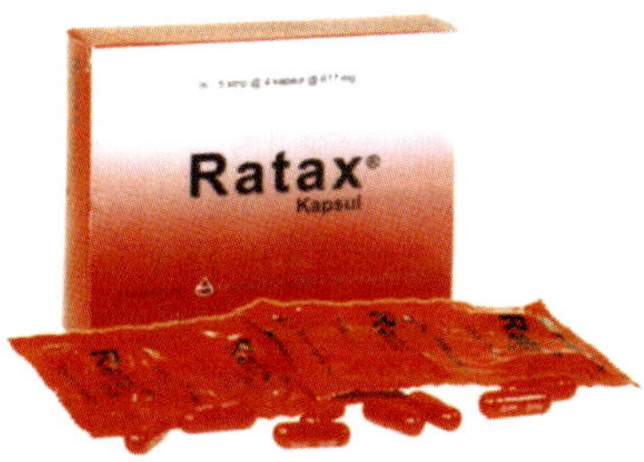

4. (Manuka Honey) MGO™

CS	$C_3H_4O_2$ (metylglyoksal)
AA	Enhance the body's immune system by virtue of its antibacterial activity : • 8x more potent against H.Pylori • 2x more effective against E Coli. • Streptococcuspyogenes,Pseudomonas sp and Staphylococcus aureus, • Haemofilus influenzae • Mycobacterium tuberculosis • Salmonella typhi • Shigella sp • virus hepatitis, etc...
T	Liquid
S	In bottles containing UMF (Unique Manuka Factor) MGO™ 100-900
D	Stomach troubles: 1-2 teaspoon 3x/day (MGO 400) Stamina and Health promotion: 1-2 teaspoon 3x/day
A, CP, CI, AR	Not stated
SC	Active ingrdient Metylglyoksal Unique to New Zealand MGO™ Manuka honey

	obtained from **Leptospermum scoparium**. (Plant grown in Newzeeland)
I	Not stated
M	Distributed by PT Citra Bening Berseri, Jkt. Indonesia
Package	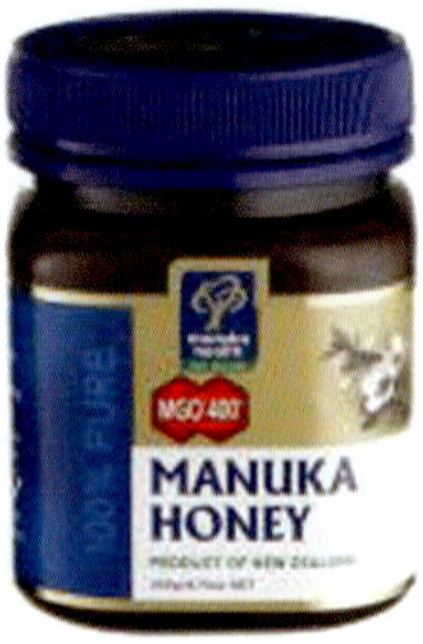

5. Kyolic 107

CS	Not stated
AA	Reduce risk of heart disease
T	Tablet
S	In boxes of 80 capsules. Aged Garlic extract™ 300 mg Phyto-sterol 200 mg Gelatin, Cellulose, Silica andMagnesium Stearate (Vegetable Source)
D	2 Capsules daily Sold as food supplement
A	Not stated
CP	Product is free of: Sodium, Yeast, Dairy, Preservatives, Sugar, Gluten, Artificial Colours, or Flavour.
CI, AR, SC, I	Not stated
M	Manufactured by Wakanuga Nutritional Supplements USA Distributed by Natural Farm Indonesia

Package	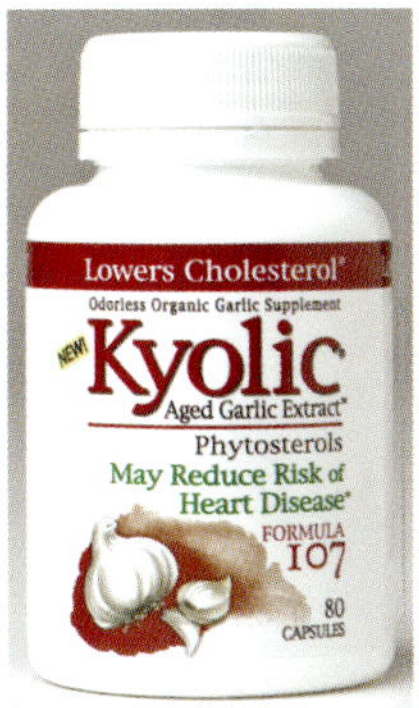

6. Sun Recome

CS	Not stated
AA	Cancer treatment as adjuvant
T	Powder
S	Extract Ganoderma powder in boxes of 10 sachets
D	3 sachets / day, to be dissolved in warm water or as advised
A, CP, CI, AR, SC, I	Not stated
M	Manufactured by Shanghai Green Valley Holding Co, Ltd. Shanghai, China. Imported by Teguhsindo Farma Indonesia Address Graha Kencana Block EF-EG, Jl. Raya Pejuangan 88, Jakarta Barat, Indonesia
Package	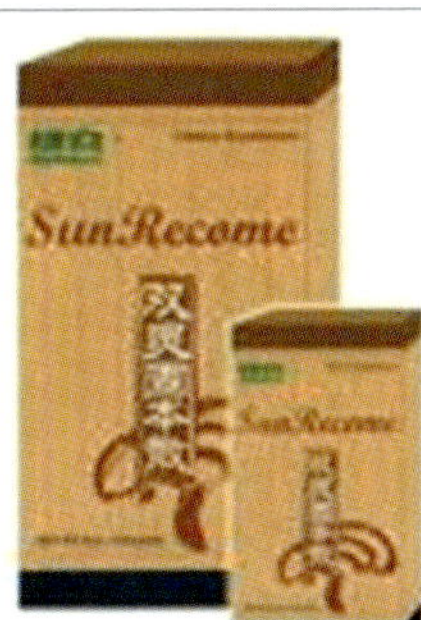 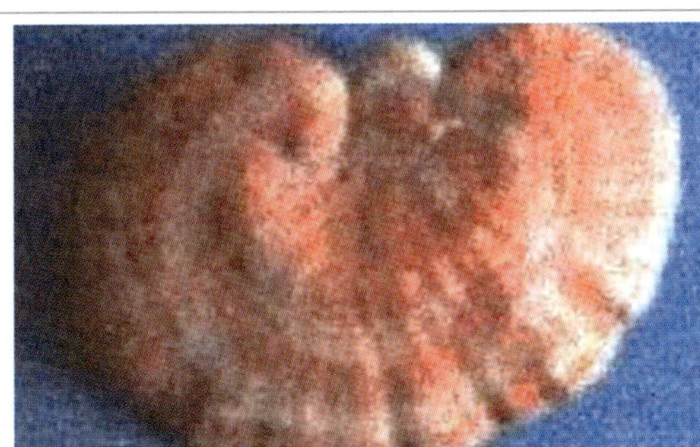

Chapter

4 Japanese Products

Yasushi Miyagawa, Akihiko Okuyama

1. Hachimijiogan TJ-7
- TSUMURA Hachimijiogan Kampo Extract Formulation for Prescription, Tsumura and Co.

CS	Not stated
AA	Hachimijiogan is indicated for patients with severe fatigue or malaise, decreased urinary output or increased urinary frequency, dry mouth, alternating heat and cold sensations in the extremities presenting the following symptoms or conditions: nephritis, diabetes mellitus, impotence, sciatica, low back pain, beriberi, cystorrhea, prostatic hypertrophy and hypertension.
T	Extract formulation
S	Hachimijiogan is packaged as 500g bottles, 5 kg boxes (500g × 10 bottles), 2.5 g × 42 packets, or 2.5 g × 189 packets. 7.5 g of TSUMURA Hachimijiogan contains 4.0 g of dried extract of the following mixture of crude drugs: Rehmannia rhizome .... 6.0 g Cornus fruit .... 3.0 g Dioscorea rhizome .... 3.0 g Alisma rhizome .... 3.0 g Poria sclerotium .... 3.0 g Moutan bark .... 2.5 g

	Cinnamon bark .... 1.0 g Processed Aconite root (powdered).......... 0.5 g
D	The usual adult dose is 7.5 g/day orally in 2 or 3 divided doses before or between meals. The dosage may be adjusted according to the patient' s age, body weight and symptoms.
A	Duration of administration is not specified. Precaution must be exercised before administration to the following patients: (1) Patients with a strong constitution (adverse reactions and aggravation of symptoms are more likely to occur.) (2) Patients with sensitivity to heat, tendency towards hot flush and red face (palpitation, hot flush, numbness of the tongue, nausea, etc. may occur.) (3) Patients with an extremely weak digestion (poor appetite, gastric distress, nausea, vomiting, abdominal pain, diarrhea, constipation, etc. may occur.) (4) Patients with anorexia, nausea or vomiting (these symptoms may be aggravated).
CP	Important basic precautions (1) When this product is used, the patient' s "SHO" (constitution/symptoms) should be taken into account. The patient' s progress should be carefully monitored, and if no improvement in symptoms/findings is observed, treatment should be discontinued. (2) When this product is concomitantly administered with other Kampo formulations (Japanese traditional herbal medicines), caution should be observed against interactions of duplicating crude drugs. Special care should be exercised when this product is coadministered with formulations containing aconite root to prevent toxicity by exceeding the suggested maximum dosage of aconite. SHO: The term "SHO" refers to Kampo diagnosis which matches a particular pathological state with a Kampo prescription. SHO is further categorized according to the patient's constitution, symptoms, abdominal diagnosis, etc. Kampo formulations should be prescribed after the SHO of the patient has been clearly identified.
CI	Not stated
AR	Adverse effects This product has not been investigated (drug use investigations, etc.) to determine the incidence of adverse reactions; therefore, the incidence of adverse events remains unknown.

Symptoms	Unknown Rate of Incidence
Hypersensitivity	Rash, redness, pruritus, etc.
Liver	Hepatic dysfunction (elevation of AST (GOT), ALT (GPT), total bilirubin levels, etc.)

Gastrointestinal	Anorexia, gastric distress, nausea, vomiting, abdominal pain, diarrhea, constipation, etc.
Others	Palpitation, hot flushes, numbness of the tongue, etc.

* NB: Discontinue administration if any of the above symptoms occur.

SC Precautions

1. Geriatric Use

Since elderly patients often have reduced physiological functions, careful monitoring and appropriate dose adjustments are recommended.

2. Pregnancy and Lactation

The use of this product in women who are pregnant or possibly pregnant is not recommended. (Moutan bark contained in this product may cause premature birth or abortion due to its strong blood-activating and stasis-removing functions. Also, adverse reactions from powdered processed aconite root contained in this product are more likely to occur).

3. Pediatric Use

This product should be administered with care in children (as this product contains powdered processed aconite root).

Pharmacological effects

1. Anti-diabetic action

Oral administration of Hachimijiogan to rats inhibited streptozotocin-induced increases in blood glucose levels, water intake, urine volume, and food intake. Immunohistochemical observation revealed that the product inhibited decrease in the number of pancreatic B cells due to streptozotocin[1)].

2. Effects on circulatory system

(a) Coadministration of Hachimijiogan with a high cholesterol diet to rabbits inhibited the decrease of elastic modulus in the blood vessels[2)].

(b) Coadministration of Hachimijioga with a high cholesterol diet to rats, inhibited the increase of calcium and collagen levels in the aorta[3)].

3. Effects on bone metabolism

(a) Oral administration of Hachimijiogan to ovariectomized rats inhibited decrease in the levels of calcium in the tibia[4)].

(b) Oral administration of Hachimijiogan to rats inhibited decrease in femoral mass under the low-estrogen conditions caused by a GnRH agonist, and increased bone formation rate (BFR) of the tibia[5)].

4. Effects on spermatogenic function

(a) Oral administration of Hachimijiogan to immature or castrated mature rats increased prostatic thymidine kinase activity[6].

(b) Oral administration of Hachimijiogan to mice improved spermatogenic dysfunction caused by adriamycin[7].

5. Diuretic effect

Oral administration of Hachimijiogan to older rats increased urine volume and urinary sodium excretion[8].

6. Anti-hypertensive action

(a) Oral administration of Hachimijiogan to introductory-MHR (rats under the induction phase of hypertension induced by metyrapone and heat stress-loading) inhibited increase in blood pressure[9].

(b) Coadministration of Hachimijiogan with high sodium diet and to Dahl salt-sensitive rats inhibited increase in blood pressure[10].

7. Effect on the kidneys

Hachimijiogan, which was mixed with salt-loaded diet and administered to Dahl salt-sensitive rats, inhibited decrease in the glomerular filtration and Improved injuries of the glomerular and the renal vascular tissues[10].

8. Mechanism of action

The mechanisms of Hachimijiogan' s pharmacological effects are the following:

(a) Inhibition of aldose reductase (AR) activity

Hachimijiogan inhibited AR activity of rat lenses (in vitro)[11].

(b) Effect on spermatogenic function

Oral administration of Hachimijiogan to rats increased testosterone levels in the testis[12].

REFERENCES

1) Luo, W. Q. et al. Biomed. Res. 1998, 19(2), p.127.
2) Amagaya, S. et al. J. Med. Pharm. Soc. WAKAN- YAKU. 1986, 3(3), p.338.
3) Haranaka, R. et al. J. Med. Pharm. Soc. WAKAN- YAKU. 1986, 3(1), p.51.
4) Sassa, S. et al. Recent progress of KAMPO MEDI-CINE in obstetrics and gynecology No.10. Shindan to Chiryosha, 1993, p.46.
5) Kaneko, H. et al. J. Jpn. Menopause Soc. 1995, 3(2), p.225.
6) Sakamoto, S. et al. Recent progress of KAMPO MEDICINE in obstetrics and gynecology No.4. Shin-dan to Chiryosha, 1987, p.98.
7) Sudou, K. et al. J. Med. Soc. Of Toho University. 1991, 38(4), p.476.
8) Haranaka, R. et al. Proc. Symp. WAKAN-YAKU. 1982, 15, p.15.
9) Tei, M. et al. J. Med. Pharm. Soc. WAKAN-YAKU. 1989, 6(3), p.416.
10) Uehara, Y. et al. Prog. Med. 1994, 14(6), p.1761.

11) Aida, K. et al. Clin. Endocrinol. 1985, 33(12), p.75.

12) Usuki, S. et al. J. Med. Pharm. Soc. WAKAN-YAKU. 1986, 3(3), p.362.

I	Not Stated.
M	Manufactured and distributed by: Tsumura and Co.

Address	2-17-11 Akasaka, Minato-ku, Tokyo 107-8521, Japan
Tel	+81-3-6361-7176
Fax	+81-3-5574-6662
Email	kudou_kazuho@mail.tsumura.co.jp
Web	www.tsumura.co.jp

Package

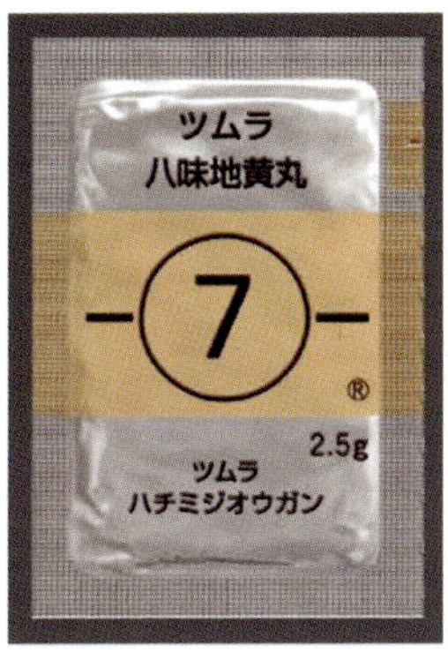

Product

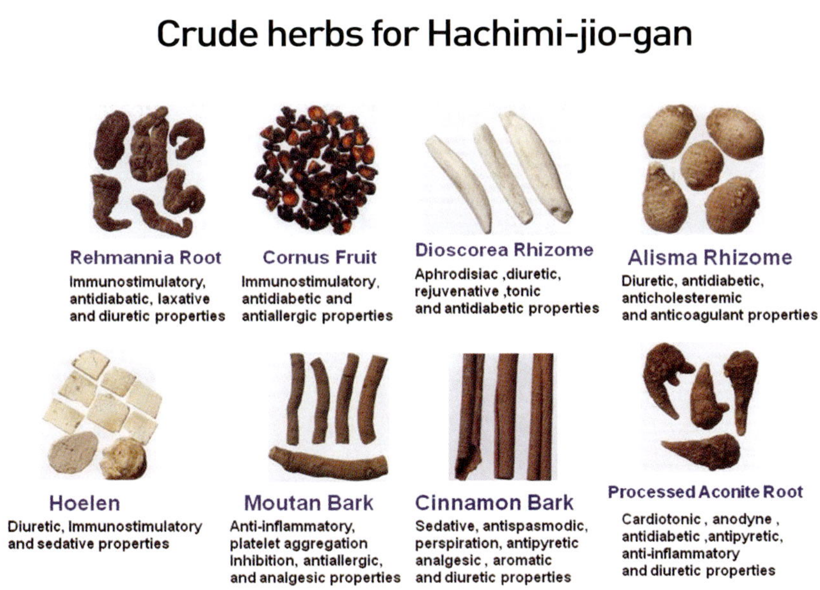

2. Saikokaryukotsuboreito TJ-12
- TSUMURA Saikokaryukotsuboreito, Kampo extract formulation for prescription, Tsumura and Co.

CS	Not stated
AA	Saikokaryukotsuboreito is indicated for patients with a relatively strong constitution, palpitation, insomnia, irritability and other psychiatric symptoms presenting the following symptoms or conditions: Hypertension, arteriosclerosis, chronic renal disease, neurasthenia, neurotic palpitation, epilepsy, hysteria, childhood night terror, and impotence.
T	Extract formulation
S	Sasikokaryukotsuboreito is packaged as 500g bottle, 5kg box (500g × 10 bottles), 2.5 g × 42 packets or 2.5 g × 189 packets. 7.5 g of TSUMURA Sasikokaryukotsuboreito contains 4.5 g of dried extract of the following mixture of crude drugs: Bupleurum root .... 5.0 g Pinellia tuber .... 4.0 g Cinnamon bark .... 3.0 g Poria sclerotium .... 3.0 g Scutellaria root .... 2.5 g Jujube fruit .... 2.5 g Asian ginseng root .... 2.5 g Oyster shell .... 2.5 g Dragon bone .... 2.5 g Ginger rhizome .... 1.0 g
D	The usual adult dose is 7.5 g/day orally in 2 or 3 divided doses before or between meals. The dosage may be adjusted according to the patient' s age, body weight and symptoms.
A	The duration of administration is not specified.
CP	Important basic precautions (1) When this product is used, the patient' s "SHO" (constitution/symptoms) should be taken into account. The patient' s progress should be carefully monitored, and if no improvement in symptoms/findings is observed, treatment should be discontinued. (2) When this product is concomitantly administered with other Kampo formulations, caution should be observed against interactions of duplicating crude drugs. SHO: The term "SHO" refers Kampo diagnosis which matches a particular

	pathological status of a patient with a Kampo prescription. SHO is further categorized according to the patient's constitution, symptoms, abdominal diagnosis, etc. Kampo formulations (Japanese traditional herbal medicines) should be prescribed after the SHO of the patient has been clearly identified.
CI	Not stated
AR	Adverse reactions: This product has not been investigated (drug use investigations, etc.) to determine the incidence of adverse reactions. Therefore, the incidence of adverse reactions is not known. (1) Clinically significant adverse reactions a) Interstitial pneumonia: If fever, cough, dyspnea, abnormal pulmonary sound (fine crackle), etc. are observed, administration of this product should be discontinued, examinations such as X-ray should be performed immediately and appropriate measures such as administration of adrenocortical hormones should be taken. The patient should be advised to discontinue this product immediately and to contact the physician in the event of fever, cough, dyspnea, etc. b) Hepatic dysfunction and jaundice: Hepatic dysfunction and/or jaundice with elevation of AST (GOT), ALT (GPT), Al-P and γ-GTP or other symptoms may occur. The patient should be carefully monitored for abnormal findings. Administration should be discontinued and appropriate therapeutic measures should be taken, if abnormalities are observed. (2) Other adverse reactions

	Related symptoms (rate of occurrence is unknown)
Hypersensitivity	Rash, redness, pruritus, urticaria, etc.
Gastrointestinal	Gastric distress, etc.

SC	Precautions 1. Geriatric Use Since elderly patients often have reduced physiological function, careful supervision and measures such as reducing the dose are recommended. 2. Pregnancy and Lactation The safety of this product in pregnant women has not been established. Therefore, the product should be used in pregnant women, women who may possibly be pregnant only if the expected therapeutic benefits outweigh the possible risks associated with treatment. 3. Pediatric Use The safety of this product in children has not been established (insufficient clinical data.)

Pharmacological effects

1. Hypotensive actions
   (a) Rabbits fed on diet pretreated with Saikokaryukotsuboreito demonstrated inhibition of noradrenalin-induced vasoconstriction and elevation of blood pressure[1).
2. Antiarteriosclerotic effect
   (a) Oral administration of Saikokaryukotsuboreito to spontaneously hypertensive rats attenuated the progression of aortic intimal thickening[2).
   (b) Concomitant administration of Saikokaryukotsuboreito with high carbohydrate, high salt, low protein diet pretreated with heat to rabbits suppressed the elevation of aortic wave velocity (PWV) and resulted in unremarkable histological changes of the thoracic aortic media[3).
   (c) Administration of high cholesterol diet pretreated with Saikokaryukotsuboreito to rats following carotid endarterectomy inhibited vascular endothelial thickening and proliferation of vascular smooth muscle cells[4).
3. Antipsychotic effect
   (a) Pretreatment of E1 mice with diet containing Saikokaryukotsuboreito decreased motor activity level (improved spontaneous locomotor hyperactivity?) and prolonged sodium pentobarbital-induced sleep during the light periods[5).
   (b) Oral administration of Saikokaryukotsuboreito to chronically stressed rats from water-immersion and restraint improved motor activity level as measured by the rotarod behavior[6).
4. Anti-convulsive effect
   (a) Oral administration of Saikokaryukotsuboreito to mice shortened the duration of clonic cramps induced by electric stimulation and prolonged the interval until death induced by pentetrazol or picrotoxin treatment[7).
5. Mechanisms of action

   The mechanisms of Saikokaryukotsuboreito' s pharmacological effects are the following:

   (a) Antiarteriosclerotic actions
   - When a high cholesterol diet was fed to mice for 12 months with Saikokaryukotsuboreito dissolved in drinking water, hepatic triglyceride and phospholipid levels, and cardiac phospholipid levels decreased[8).
   - Administration of a high cholesterol diet containing Saikokaryukotsuboreito to rabbits with hereditary hypercholesterolemia decreased the plasma levels of total cholesterol and LDL, and increased apoE and LDL receptor mRNA levels in the liver. In addition, Saikokaryukotsuboreito inhibited atherosclerotic

lesions in the thoracic aortic arch[9].

- Saikokaryukotsuboreito inhibited the intracellular synthesis of cholesterol ester and triglyceride and decreased the secretion of apoB of human hepatocellular carcinoma cell line, Hep G2 cells (in vitro)[10].

(b) Antipsychotic actions

- Oral administration of Saikokaryukotsuboreito to chronically stressed rats from water-immersion and restraint inhibited adrenal gland weight gain and improved attenuation of the glucocorticoid negative feedback[11].
- Oral administration of Saikokaryukotsuboreito to chronically stressed rats from water-immersion and restraint improved decreased release of serotonin and dopamine from the prefrontal cortex[6].

REFERENCES

1) Okano, H. et al. in vivo. 1999, 13(4), p.333.
2) Yamada, T. et al. The Journal of Japan Atherosclerosis Society. 1986, 3(2), p.71.
3) Hasegawa, M. et al. NIKKEI MEDICAL (supplementary). 1996, 25(4), p.31.
4) Chung, H. -J. et al. Biol. Pharm. Bull. 2003, 26(1), p.56.
5) Iizuka, S. et al. Meth. Find. Exp. Clin. Pharmacol. 1998, 20(1), p.19.
6) Mizoguchi, K. et al. Pharmacol. Biochem. Behav. 2003, 75, p.419.
7) Itoh, T. et al. Kampo to saishin chiryo. 1992, 1(3), p.274.
8) Haranaka, R. et al. J. Med. Pharm. Soc. WAKAN- YAKU. 1986, 3(1), p.51.
9) Yoshie, F. et al. Pharmacol. Res. 2001, 43(5), p.481.
10) Furukawa, S. et al. J. Traditional Med. 1994, 11(3), p.236.
11) Mizoguchi, K. et al. Life Sci. 2002, 72(1), p.67.

I	Not Stated.
M and D	Manufactured and Distributed by Tsumura and Co. Address 2-17-11 Akasaka, Minato-ku, Tokyo 107-8521, Japan Tel +81-3-6361-7176 Fax +81-3-5574-6662 Email kudou_kazuho@mail.tsumura.co.jp Web www.tsumura.co.jp

Package

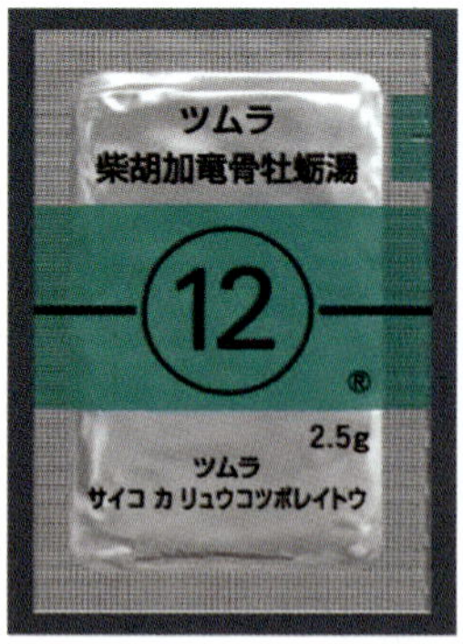

Product

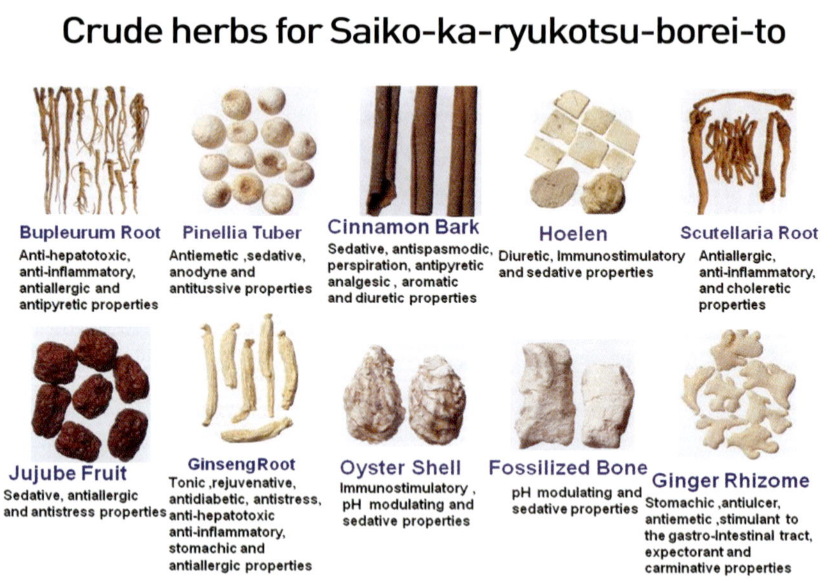

3. Keishikaryukotsuboreito (TJ-26)
- TSUMURA Keishikaryukotsuboreito Kampo Extract Formulation for Prescription, Tsumura and Co.

CS	Not Stated
AA	Keishikaryukotsuboreito is indicated for patients with tightness of lower abdominal rectus muscles and relatively weak constitution presenting the following symptoms or conditions: Nocturnal enuresis in childhood, neurasthenia, sexual neurasthenia, nocturnal emission and impotence
T	Extract formulation

S	Keishikaryukotsuboreto is packaged as 500 g bottles, 5 kg boxes (500 g×10 bottles), 2.5 g×42 packets or 2.5 g×189 packets. 7.5 g of TSUMURA Keishikaryukotsuboreito contains 3.25 g of dried extract of the following mixture of crude drugs: Cinnamon bark .... 4.0 g Peony root .... 4.0 g Jujube fruit.......... 4.0 g Oyster shell .... 3.0 g Dragon bone.......... 3.0 g Chinese licorice root.......... 2.0 g Ginger rhizome.......... 2.0 g
D	The usual adult dose is 7.5 g/day orally in 2 or 3 divided doses before or between meals. The dosage may be adjusted according to the patient' s age, body weight and symptoms.
A	The duration of administration is not specified. Careful administration by the clinician is needed.
CP	Important basic precautions (1) When this product is used, the patient' s "SHO" (constitution/symptoms) should be taken into account. The patient' s progress should be carefully monitored, and if no improvement in symptoms/findings is observed, treatment should be discontinued. (2) When this product is concomitantly administered with other Kampo formulations, caution should be observed against interactions of duplicating crude drugs. SHO: The term "SHO" refers Kampo diagnosis which matches a particular pathological status of a patient with a Kampo prescription. SHO is further categorized according to the patient's constitution, symptoms, abdominal diagnosis, etc. Kampo formulations (Japanese traditional herbal medicines) should be prescribed after the SHO of the patient has been clearly identified.
CI	Not stated
AR	Adverse reactions: This product has not been investigated (drug use investigations, etc.) to determine the incidence of adverse reactions; therefore, the incidence of adverse reactions is not known. (1) Clinically significant adverse reactions a) Pseudoaldosteronism: Symptoms of pseudoaldosteronism such as hypokalemia, increased blood pressure, retention of sodium and body fluid, edema, increased body weight, etc. may occur. Serum potassium level should be carefully monitored, and if any abnormality is observed,

	administration should be discontinued and appropriate interventions such as administration of potassium should be employed. b) Myopathy: Myopathy may occur as a result of hypokalemia. The patient should be carefully monitored, and if any abnormality such as weakness, convulsion or paralysis of limbs, etc. occur, administration should be discontinued and appropriate interventions such as administration of potassium should be employed. (2) Other adverse reactions a) Hypersensitivity: If symptoms of hypersensitivity such as rash, redness, or pruritus occur, administration of the drug should be discontinued.
SC	Precautions 1. Geriactric Use Since elderly patients often have reduced physiological function, careful supervision and measures such as reducing the dose are recommended. 2. Pregnancy and Lactation The safety of this product in pregnant women has not been established. Therefore, the product should be used in pregnant women, women who may possibly be pregnant only if the expected therapeutic benefits outweigh the possible risks associated with treatment 3. Pediatric Use The safety of this product in children has not been established (insufficient clinical data.)
I	Drug Interactions: (Precautions for concomitant drug use) Type of Drugs: (1) Formulations containing Glycyrrhiza; (2) Formulations containing glycyrrhizinic acid or glycyrrhizinates. Clinical signs/Management: Pseudoaldosteronism is more likely to occur. Myopathy is also more likely to occur as a result of hypokalemia (refer to the section on "Clinically significant adverse reactions".) Mechanism/Risk Factors: Glycyrrhizinic acid has an effect of accelerating potassium excretion from the renal tubules which may lead to decreased serum potassium level
M	Manufactured and distributed by: Tsumura and Co. Address 2-17-11 Akasaka, Minato-ku, Tokyo 107-8521, Japan Tel +81-3-6361-7176 Fax +81-3-5574-6662 Email kudou_kazuho@mail.tsumura.co.jp Web www.tsumura.co.jp

Package	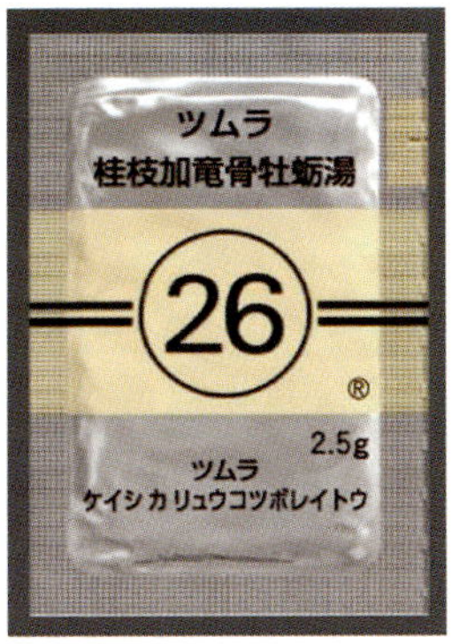
Product	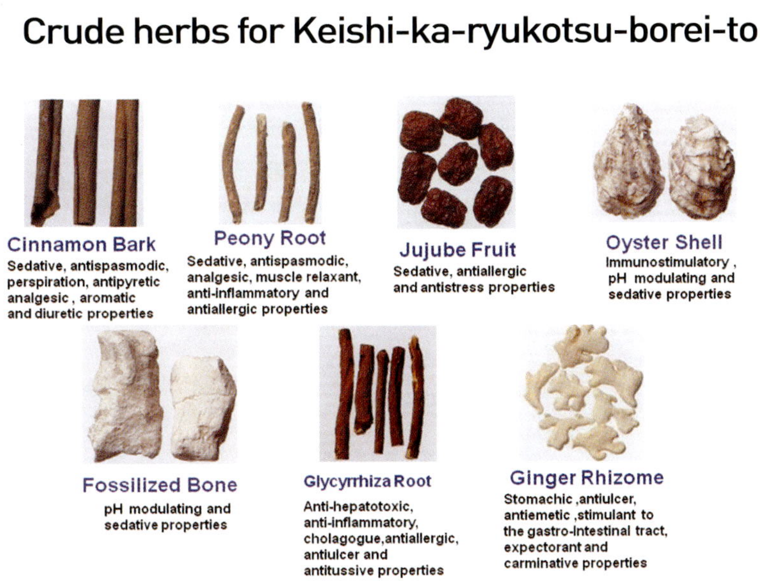

4. Goshajinkigan (TJ-107)

- TSUMURA Goshajinkigan Kampo Extract Formulation for Prescription, Tsumura and Co.

CS	Not stated
AA	Goshajinkigan is indicated for patients with fatigue, cold extremities, decreased urine volume or polyuria, occasional dry mouth presenting the following symptoms or conditions: Leg pain, low back pain, numbness, blurred vision in the elderly, pruritus, dysuria, frequent urination and edema.
T	Extract formulation

S	Goshajinkigan is packaged as 500 g bottles, 5 kg boxes (500 g × 10 bottles), 2.5 g × 42 packets or 2.5 g × 189 packets. 7.5 g of TSUMURA Goshajinkigan contains 4.5 g of dried extract of the following mixture of crude drugs: Rehmannia root .... 5.0 g Achyranthes root .... 3.0 g Cornus fruit .... 3.0 g Dioscorea rhizome .... 3.0 g Plantago seed .... 3.0 g Alisma rhizome .... 3.0 g Poria sclerotium .... 3.0 g Moutan bark .... 3.0 g Cinnamon bark .... 1.0 g Processed Aconite root (powdered).......... 1.0 g
D	The usual adult dose is 7.5 g/day orally in 2 or 3 divided doses before or between meals. The dosage may be adjusted according to the patient' s age, body weight and symptoms.
A	The duration of administration is not specified. Careful Administration (Goshajinkigan should be administered with care to the following patients): (1) Patients with a strong constitution (adverse reactions are more likely to occur, and symptoms may be aggravated.)
	(2) Patients with heat sensitivity, pronounced hot flushes, and red face (palpitation, hot flush, numbness of the tongue, nausea, etc. may occur also.) (3) Patients with an extremely weak gastrointestinal tract (anorexia, gastric distress, nausea, vomiting, abdominal bloating, abdominal pain, diarrhea, constipation, etc. may occur.) (4) Patients with anorexia, nausea or vomiting (these symptoms may be aggravated.)
CP	Important basic precautions (1) When this product is used, the patient' s "SHO" (constitution/symptoms) should be taken into account. The patient' s progress should be carefully monitored, and if no improvement in symptoms/findings is observed, treatment should be discontinued. (2) When this product is concomitantly administered with other Kampo formulations (Japanese traditional herbal medicines), caution should be observed against interactions of duplicating crude drugs. Special care should be exercised when this product is coadministered with formulations containing aconite root to

	prevent toxicity by exceeding the suggested maximum dosage of aconite. SHO: The term "SHO" refers to Kampo diagnosis which matches a particular pathological state with a Kampo prescription. SHO is further categorized according to the patient's constitution, symptoms, abdominal diagnosis, etc. Kampo formulations should be prescribed after the SHO of the patient has been clearly identified.
CI	Not stated
AR	Adverse reactions This product has not been investigated (drug use investigations, etc.) to determine the incidence of adverse reactions. Therefore, the incidence of adverse reactions is not known. (1) Clinically significant adverse reactions a) Interstitial pneumonia: If fever, cough, dyspnea, abnormal pulmonary sound (fine crackle), etc. are observed, discontinue administration of the product, immediately perform examinations such as chest X-ray, and take appropriate measures such as the administration of adrenocortical hormones. The patient should be advised to discontinue the product and to contact the physician immediately if fever, cough, dyspnea, etc. develops. d) Hepatic dysfunction and jaundice: Hepatic dysfunction and/or jaundice with elevation of AST (GOT), ALT (GPT), Al-P and γ-GTP or other symptoms may occur. The patient should be carefully monitored for abnormal findings. Administration should be discontinued and appropriate therapeutic measures should be taken if abnormalities are observed. (2) Other adverse reactions a) Hypersensitivity: rash, redness, pruritus, etc.(If such symptoms are observed, administration should be discontinued.) b) Gastrointestinal: anorexia, gastric distress, nausea, vomiting, abdominal bloating, abdominal pain, diarrhea, constipation, etc. c) Others: palpitation, hot flush, numbness of the tongue, etc.
SC	Precautions 1. Geriatric Use Since elderly patients often have reduced physiological function, careful supervision and measures such as reducing the dose are recommended. 2. Pregnancy and Lactation Use of this product in pregnant women and women who may possibly be pregnant is not recommended. (Achyranthes root and Moutan bark contained in this product may cause premature birth or miscarriage. Adverse reactions due

to Processed Aconite root (powdered) contained in this product are more likely to occur.)

3. Pediatric Use

This product should be administered with care in children (this product contains Powdered Processed Aconite Root.)

Pharmacological effects

[Effects in humans]

1. Effects on numbness of extremities?

Oral administration of Goshajinkigan to patients with diabetic neuropathy reduced the threshold of vibration sensation that had increased[1].

2. Effects on cold sensation

Oral administration of Goshajinkigan to patients with diabetic neuropathy increased forearm skin blood flow[2] and the mean dermal temperature of the dorsal hand[3].

[Effects in animals]

1. Effects on lens opacity

Oral administration of Goshajinkigan to rats with hereditary cataract (ICR/f) delayed the onset of opacity of the nucleus lentis[4].

2. Effects on the velocity of nerve conduction

Oral administration of Goshajinkigan to rats with streptozotocin (STZ)-induced diabetes inhibited the reduction of sciatic nerve conduction velocity[5].

3. Antinociceptive (analgesic) effects

Oral administration of Goshajinkigan to mice with STZ-induced diabetes increased the anti-nociceptive threshold that had decreased[6].

4. Blood flow-increasing actions

Oral administration of Goshajinkigan to rats with STZ-induced diabetes inhibited the decrease in gastrocnemial muscle blood flow[7].

5. Mechanism of actions

Goshajinkigan may exhibit antinociceptive (analgesic) actions via two mechanisms, intravertebral κ opioid receptor stimulation and the promotion of nitric oxide (NO) production at pain-sensing sites. In addition, Goshajinkigan may increase peripheral blood flow by promoting NO production.

(a) Antinociceptive (analgesic) actions

- Treatment with anti-dynorphin antiserum in mice with STZ-induced diabetes reduced the antinociceptive actions of orally administered Goshajinkigan.

Pretreatment with a κ opioid receptor antagonist, norbinal torphimine, also showed a similar effect[6].

- Treatment with an NO synthase inhibitor, NG-nitro-L-arginine methyl ester (L-NAME), in mice with STZ-induced diabetes reduced the antinociceptive actions of orally administered Goshajinkigan. In addition, combination therapy with anti-dynorphin antiserum resulted in the disappearance of the above actions[8].

(b) Blood flow-increasing actions

- Pretreatment with L-NAME in rats with STZ-induced diabetes resulted in the disappearance of the blood flow-increasing actions of intraduodenally administered Goshajinkigan[7].

REFERENCES

1) Tawata, M. et al. Diabetes Res. Clin. Pract. 1994, 26, p.121.
2) Shikano, M. et al. J. Med. Pharm. Soc. WAKAN- YAKU. 1988, 5(3), p.378.
3) Shikano, M. et al. J. Med. Pharm. Soc. WAKAN- YAKU. 1990, 7(3), p.442.
4) Kamei, A. et al. Journal of the Eye. 1994, 11(2), p.270.
5) Nishizawa, M. et al. J. Neurol. Sci. 1995, 132(2), p.177.
6) Suzuki, Y. et al. Jpn. J. Pharmacol. 1999, 79(2), p.169.
7) Suzuki, Y. et al. Meth. Find. Exp. Clin. Pharmacol. 1998, 20(4), p.321.
8) Suzuki, Y. et al. Jpn. J. Pharmacol. 1999, 79(3), p.387.

I	Not Stated.
M	Manufactured and distributed by: Tsumura and Co.
	Address 2-17-11 Akasaka, Minato-ku, Tokyo 107-8521, Japan
	Tel +81-3-6361-7176
	Fax +81-3-5574-6662
	Email kudou_kazuho@mail.tsumura.co.jp
	Web www.tsumura.co.jp

Package

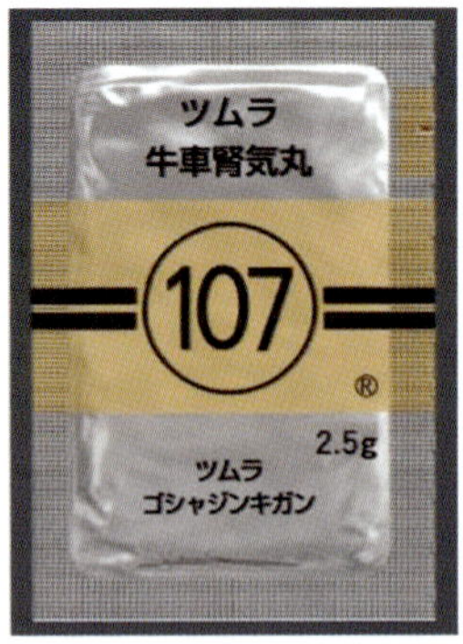

Product

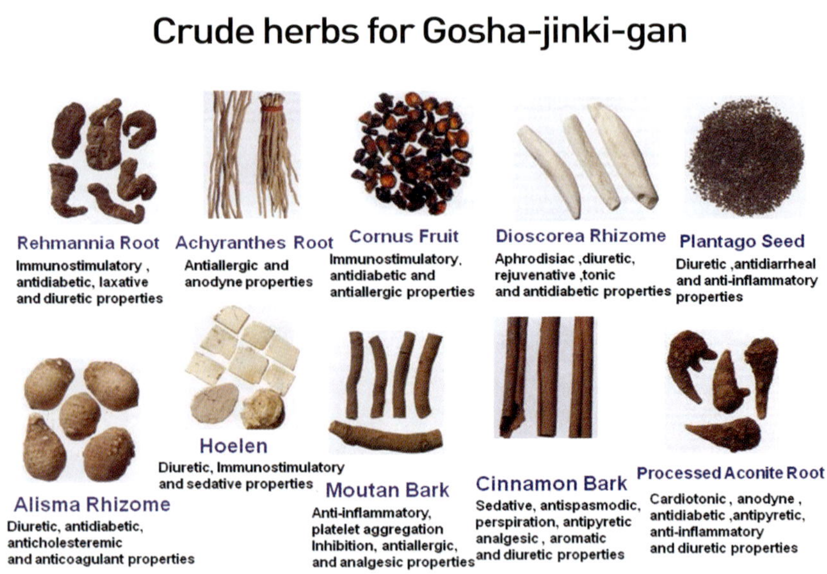

5. Hochuekkito
- TSUMURA Hochuekkito Kampo Extract Formulation for Prescription, Tsumura and Co.

CS	Not Stated
AA	Hochuekkito is indicated for patients who have reduced digestive functions, severe fatigability of the extremities, delicate constitution presenting the following symptoms or conditions: summer emaciation, recuperation from illness, tuberculosis, anorexia, gastroptosis, common cold/influenza, hemorrhoid, anal prolapse, uterine prolapse, impotence, hemiplegia, and hyperidrosis.
T	Extract Formulation

S	Hochuekkito is packaged as 500 g bottles, 5 kg boxes (500 g × 10 bottles), 2.5 g × 42 packets or 2.5 g × 189 packets. 7.5 g of TSUMURA Hochuekkito contains 5.0 g of dried extract of the following mixture of crude drugs. Astragalus root .... 4.0 g Atractylodes Lancea rhizome .... 4.0 g Asian Ginseng root .... 4.0 g Japanese Angelica root .... 3.0 g Bupleurum root .... 2.0 g Jujube fruit .... 2.0 g Citrus Unshiu peel .... 2.0 g Chinese Licorice root .... 1.5 g Cimicifuga rhizome .... 1.0 g Ginger rhizome .... 0.5 g
D	The usual adult dose is 7.5 g/day orally in 2 or 3 divided doses before or between meals. The dosage may be adjusted according to the patient' s age and body weight, and symptoms."
A	The duration of administration is not specified. Careful administration by the clinician is needed.
CP	Important basic precautions (1) When this product is used, the patient' s "SHO" (constitution/symptoms) should be taken into account. The patient' s progress should be carefully monitored, and if no improvement in symptoms/findings is observed, treatment should be discontinued. (2) When this product is concomitantly administered with other Kampo formulations (Japanese traditional herbal medicines), caution should be observed against interactions of duplicating crude drugs. Since this product contains Glycyrrhiza, careful attention should be paid to the serum potassium level, blood pressure, etc., and if any abnormality is observed, administration should be discontinued. SHO: The term "SHO" refers to Kampo diagnosis which matches a particular pathological state with a Kampo prescription. SHO is further categorized according to the patient's constitution, symptoms, abdominal diagnosis, etc. Kampo formulations should be prescribed after the SHO of the patient has been clearly identified.
CI	Not stated
AR	Adverse reactions: This product has not been investigated (drug use investigations, etc.) to determine

the incidence of adverse reactions. Therefore, the incidence of adverse reactions is not known.

(1) Clinically significant adverse reactions

a) Interstitial pneumonia: If fever, cough, dyspnea, abnormal pulmonary sound (fine crackle), etc. develop, discontinue administration of the product immediately perform examinations such as chest X-ray, and take appropriate measures such as the administration of adrenocortical hormones. The patient should be advised to discontinue the product and to contact the physician immediately if fever, cough, dyspnea, etc. develops.

b) Pseudoaldosteronism: Symptoms of pseudoaldosteronism such as hypokalemia, increased blood pressure, retention of sodium and body fluid, edema, increased body weight, etc. may occur. Serum potassium level should be carefully monitored, and if any abnormality is observed, administration should be discontinued and appropriate interventions such as administration of potassium should be employed.

c) Myopathy: Myopathy may occur as a result of hypokalemia. The patient should be carefully monitored, and if any abnormality such as weakness, convulsion or paralysis of limbs, etc. occur, administration should be discontinued and appropriate interventions such as administration of potassium should be employed.

d) Hepatic dysfunction and jaundice: Hepatic dysfunction and/or jaundice with elevation of AST (GOT), ALT (GPT), Al-P and γ-GTP or other symptoms may occur. The patient should be carefully monitored for abnormal findings. Administration should be discontinued and appropriate therapeutic measures should be taken if abnormalities are observed.

(2) Other adverse reactions

a) Hypersensitivity: rash, urticaria, etc. (if these symptoms develop, administration should be discontinued).

b) Gastrointestinal: anorexia, gastric distress, nausea, diarrhea, etc.

SC

Precautions

1. Geriatric Use

Because elderly patients often have reduced physiological function, careful supervision and measures such as reducing the dose are recommended.

2. Pregnancy and Lactation

The safety of this product in pregnant women has not been established. Therefore, the product should be used in pregnant women, women who may possibly be pregnant only if the expected therapeutic benefits outweigh the possible risks associated with treatment.

3. Pediatric Use

The safety of this product in children has not been established (insufficient clinical data.)

Pharmacological effects

1. Effect on reduced physical and mental strength after illness

(a) Effect of improving immunosuppression

Oral administration of Hochuekkito to mice immunosuppressed with MMC inhibited decreases in body weight and thymus weight, and suppressed T and B cell dysfunction[1).

(b) Effect on weakness during infection

- Oral administration of Hochuekkito to rats bearing MRSA in the intestinal tract decreased the fecal viable MRSA count[2)].
- Oral administration of Hochuekkito to C.albicans-infected mice with prednisolone-induced immunosuppression prolonged survival[3)].
- Oral administration of Hochuekkito to a Salmonella infection model using tumor-bearing mice, to which mouse EL-4 lymphoma cells had been implanted, prolonged survival[4)].
- Oral administration of Hochuekkito to herpes simplex virus (HSV) -1-infected mice immunosuppressed with MMC increased the survival rate, and prolonged survival[5)].
- Oral administration of Hochuekkito to MRSA-infected mice immunosuppressed with MMC decreased the liver and blood viable bacterial counts, and increased the survival rate[6)].

(c) Repair of biological defense mechanims in active cancer

- Administration of diet pretreated with Hochuekkito to rats inhibited the growth of tumor[7)].
- Oral administration of Hochuekkito to mice increased anti-tumor immunity as evaluated by immune responses to secondarily implanted Meth-A fibrosarcoma cells. Furthermore, it inhibited the growth of tumor[8)]."

(d) Alleviation of adverse effects from anticancer agents and radiation therapy

- Oral administration of Hochuekkito to mice improved MMC-induced decreases of natural killer (NK) activity and bone marrow function[9)].
- Oral administration of Hochuekkito to mice inhibited an adriamycin-induced decrease in testis weight[10)].
- Oral administration of Hochuekkito in drinking water to X-ray-irradiated mice

prolonged survival[11].

(e) Effect on debility after gastrectomy.

Oral administration of Hochuekkito to rats that underwent total gastrectomy inhibited surgery-induced decreases in the serum calcium level and bone mineral density of the femur, and prevented morphological bone disorder[12].

2. Effect on reduced physical strength in elderly persons

Oral administration of Hochuekkito to elderly mice increased the T and NK cell counts, the CD4/CD8 ratio, and the production of antibody against sheep red blood cell (SRBC) antigen[13], which had decreased in elderly mice compared with juvenile mice.

3. Effect on common cold and influenza

Oral administration of Hochuekkito to mice infected with influenza virus prolonged survival[14].

4. Mechanism of actions

The mechanisms of pharmacological effects of Hochuekkito are the following:

(1) Actions on leukocytes

Oral administration of Hochuekkito to mice inhibited MMC-induced leukocytopenia[6].

(2) Immunomodulating actions

a) Actions on humoral immunity

Oral administration of Hochuekkito to mice increased the production of an antibody against SRBC antigen[13].

b) Actions on cell-mediated immunity

- Administration of diet containing Hochuekkito to rats enhanced the cytotoxic activity of splenic $\gamma\delta$-TCR bearing T cells[15].
- Hochuekkito enhanced the cytotoxic activity of activated T lymphocytes from healthy volunteers and cancer patients (in vitro)[16].

c) Actions on NK activity

- Oral administration of Hochuekkito to mice[8] and rats[7] enhanced the NK activity of splenocytes.
- In a mouse cancer metastasis model prepared by implanting mouse colon cancer cells (Colon 26-L5), removal of NK cells led to a lack of inhibitory effects of Hochuekkito on cancer metastasis[17].

d) Actions on macrophages

- Oral administration of Hochuekkito to mice enhanced the phagocytic activity of peritoneal exudates cells, splenocytes, and bone marrow cells[18].

- Oral administration of Hochuekkito to mice enhanced anti-tumor cytotoxic activity of peritoneal exudates cells[8].

e) Actions on the production of cytokines

- Oral administration of Hochuekkito to mice infected with influenza virus promoted the early production of IFN-α[14].
- Oral administration of Hochuekkito in drinking water to tumor-bearing mice inhibited restraint stress-induced decrease of the serum interleukin (IL)-[12,19].
- Oral administration of Hochuekkito to mice inhibited MMC-induced decrease of the production of IL-1β and IFN-γ[6].

(3) Actions on the testis

- Hochuekkito promoted protein synthesis in hamster ductus epididymidis-derived cells (in vitro)[20].
- Hochuekkito promoted the acrosome reaction in human sperm (in vitro)[21].
- Hochuekkito improved the reduction of sperm motility by anti-sperm antibody in human sperm (in vitro)[22].
- Hochuekkito improved the speed and the direction of sperm motility in sperm from male patients with sterility (in vitro)[25].

I

Drug Interactions: (Precautions for concomitant drug use with Hochuekkito)

Type of Drugs: (1) Formulations containing Glycyrrhiza; (2) Formulations containing glycyrrhizinic acid or glycyrrhizinates.

Clinical signs/Management: Pseudoaldosteronism is more likely to occur. Myopathy is also more likely to occur as a result of hypokalemia (refer to the section on "Clinically significant adverse reactions".)

Mechanism/Risk Factors: Glycyrrhizinic acid has an effect of accelerating potassium excretion from the renal tubules which may lead to decreased serum potassium level

REFERENCES

1) Ri, A. et al. J. Jpn. Assoc. Infectious Disease. 1996, 70(7), p.717.
2) Sumiyama, Y. J. New Remedies and Clinic. 1996, 45(7), p.1266.
3) Abe, S. et al. Immunopharmacol. Immunotoxicol. 1999, 21(2), p.331.
4) Shimizu, S. et al. Jpn. J. Oriental Medicine. 1997, 48(3), p.369.
5) Kido, T. et al. Anticancer Res. 2000, 20(6A), p.4109.
6) Matsui, K. et al. Jpn. J. Oriental Medicine. 1997, 48(3), p.357.
7) Cho, J. et al. in vivo. 1991, 5, p.389.
8) Harada, M. et al. Immunopharmacol. Immunotoxicol. 1995, 17(4), p.687.
9) Maemura, K. et al. Kampo and Immuno-allergy vol.3. Medical Tribune, 1990, p.108.

10) Sudo, K. et al. Folia Pharmacol. Jpn. 1988, 92, p.251.
11) Hosokawa, K. Jpn. J. Cancer Clinics. 1993, 39(14), p.1655.
12) Suzuki, H. et al. Prog. Med. 1999, 19(4), p.965.
13) Utsuyama, M. et al. Mech. Ageing Dev. 2001, 122, p.341.
14) Mori, K. et al. Antiviral Research. 1999, 44(2), p.103.
15) Sato, S. et al. J. New Remedies and Clinic. 1996, 45(7), p.1261.
16) Hong, T. et al. J. Traditional Med. 1999, 16(2), p.58.
17) Saiki I. Biol. Pharm. Bull. 2000, 23(6), p.677.
18) Maruyama, H. et al. Jpn. J. Inflammation. 1988, 8(1), p.65.
19) Li, T. et al. Immunopharmacology. 1999, 43(1), p.11.
20) Noda, Y. et al. Jpn. J. Fertil. Steril. 1993, 38(2), p.262.
21) Mizutani, T. et al. Recent progress of KAMPO MEDI-CINE in obstetrics and gynecology No.5. Shindan to Chiryosha, 1988, p.97.
22) Yamanaka, M. et al. Jpn. J. Urology. 1998, 89(7), p.641.
23) Shibahara, H. et al. Jpn. J. Fertility and Sterility. 1993, 38(4), p.654.

M

Manufactured and Distributed by Tsumura and Co.

Address	2-17-11 Akasaka, Minato-ku, Tokyo 107-8521, Japan
Tel	+81-3-6361-7176
Fax	+81-3-5574-6662
Email	kudou_kazuho@mail.tsumura.co.jp
Web	www.tsumura.co.jp

Package

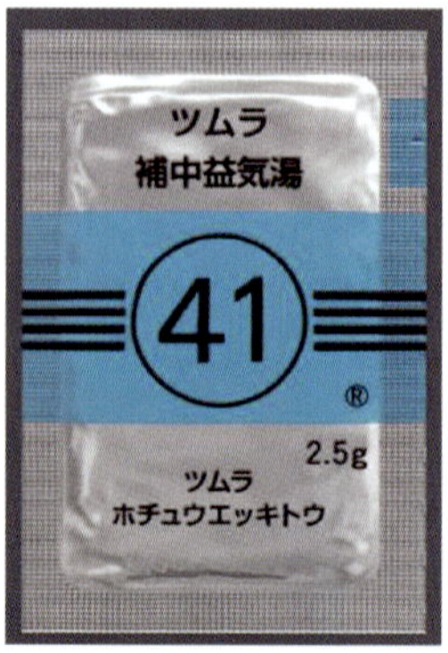

Product

Crude herbs for Hochu-ekki-to

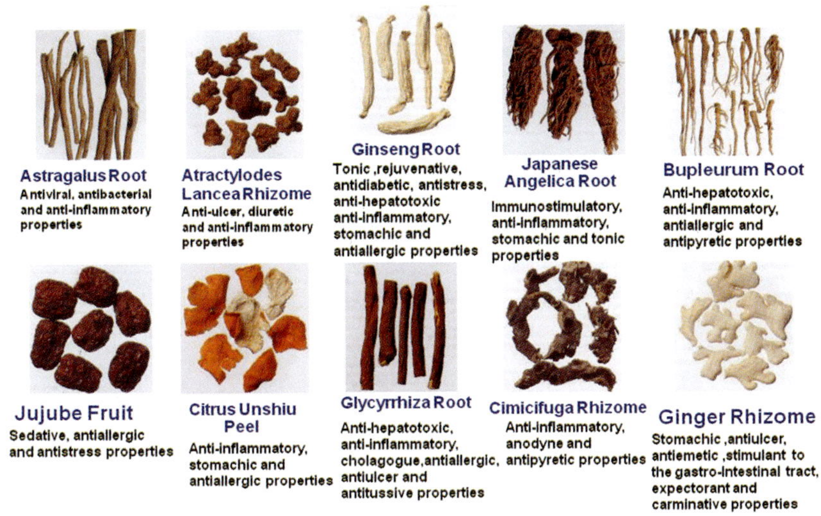

Chapter

5 Korean Products

Jong Kwan Park, Sae Woong Kim,
Sung-Yeoun Hwang, Hyun Jun Park , Nam Cheol Park

1. Cheong-Kwan-Jang Redmax. Korea ginseng corporation

CS	Not stated
AA	Enhancement of general body health for men
T	Tablet
S	Mixing ideally vegetable raw materials (Lycii Fructus, Cuscutae Semen, Rubus coreanus Miq., Torilis japonica fruit, schizandra fruit concentrate) necessary for increase of men' s vital energy and physical strength with six-year-old KRG root concentrate into tablet.
D	Take 3 tablets after meal with water (adult).
A	Duration of application for effectiveness may differ individually.
CP	Ginseng has a history of herbal use going back over 5,000 years. It is one of the most highly regarded of herbal medicines in the Orient, where it has gained an almost magical reputation for being able to promote health, general body vigour and also to prolong life. The root is adaptogen, alterative, carminative, demulcent, emetic, expectorant, stimulant and tonic. It both stimulates and relaxes the nervous system, encourages the secretion of hormones, improves stamina, lowers blood sugar and cholesterol levels and increases resistance to disease. It is used internally in the treatment of debility associated with old age or illness, lack of appetite, insomnia, stress, shock and chronic illness. Ginseng is not normally prescribed for pregnant women, or for patients under the age of 40, or those with depression, acute anxiety or acute inflammatory disease. It is normally only taken for a period of

	3 weeks. Excess can cause headaches, restlessness, raised blood pressure and other side effects, especially if it is taken with caffeine, alcohol, turnips and bitter or spicy foods. The roots are harvested in the autumn, preferably from plants 6 - 7 years old, and can be used fresh or dried. A dose of 10ug/ml of ginseng saponins has been shown to be significantly radio-protective when it is administered prior to gamma-irradiation. The leaf is emetic and expectorant.
CI	Reduce the dosage when symptoms such as fever, skin irritation, indigestion or chest problems occur. Should these symptoms continue in spite of the reduction in dosage, stop taking the ginseng or consult an Oriental doctor before continuing to take the ginseng.
AR	Not stated
SC	Ginseng is one of the most popular herbs in both Eastern and Western countries. It is known as a traditional asian medicine for stimulation of sexual function and studies have shown the effects of ginseng on relaxation of penile corpus cavernous smooth muscle in rabbits.
I	1. Adaptogen 2. Anticholesterolemic 3. Emetic 4. Expectorant 5. Hypoglycemic 6. Nervine 7. Tonic
M	Korea Ginseng Corp.H.Q. Address Kosmo Tower 15F, 1002 Daechi-dong, Gangnam-gu, Seoul, Korea Tel +82-2-2189-6571 Fax +82-2-2189-6530 Email kgcceo1@kgc.or.kr Web www. kgc.or.kr
Package	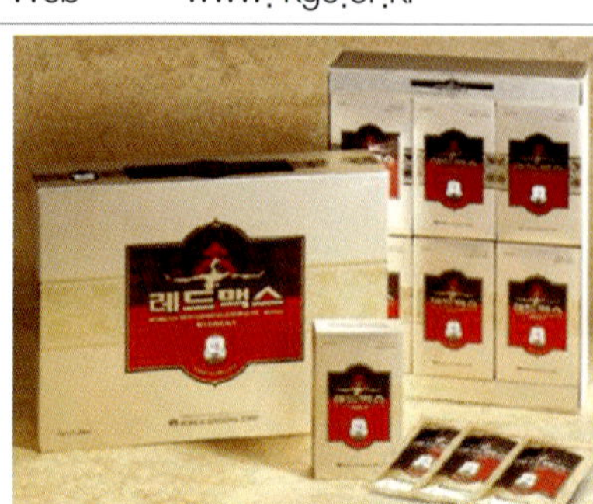

Product	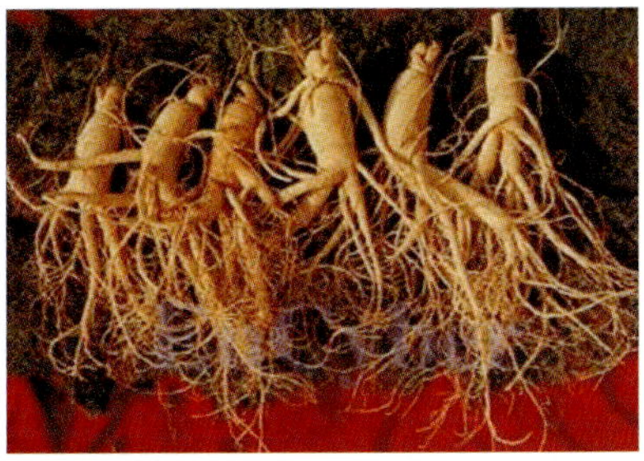

2. Korean Mountain Ginseng Culture Root

CS	Not stated
AA	Enhancement of general body health for men
T	Pack
S	Korean mountain ginseng culture root extract (saponin 140mg/g) 0.024%, Korean red ginseng(red ginseng saponin 70mg/g) 0.15%, Angelica gigas Nakai, Astragalus membrane aceus, fructose
D	One pack per day (180ml x 6 pack/set)
A	Duration of application for effectiveness may differ individually.
CP	A 2002 study by the Southern Illinois University School of Medicine found that in laboratory animals, both Asian and American forms of ginseng enhance libido and copulatory performance. These effects of ginseng may not be due to changes in hormone secretion, but to direct effects of ginseng, or its ginsenoside components, on the central nervous system and gonadal tissues. In males, ginsenosides can facilitate penile erection.
CI, AR	Not stated
SC	Ginseng refers to species within Panax, a genus of 11 species of slow-growing perennial plants with fleshy roots, in the family Araliaceae. They grow in the Northern Hemisphere in eastern Asia (mostly northern China, Korea, and eastern Siberia), typically in cooler climates; Panax vienamensis, discovered in Vietnam, is the southernmost ginseng found. This article focuses on the Series Panax ginsengs, which are the adaptogenic herbs, principally Panax ginseng and P. quinquefolius. Ginseng is characterized by the presence of ginsenoside.
I	1. Increases physical strength after illness 2. Helps recovert from accumulated fatigue 3. Increases the immune system 4. Controls cholesterol

	5. Improves ageing and nutritive conditions in the body
M	Tulip international Inc. Address Room No. 303 Chungsan B/D, 157-19 Samsung-Dong, Kangnam-Gu, Seoul, Korea Tel +82-2-63002580 Fax +82-2-6300-2590 Web http://www.tulipint.com
Package	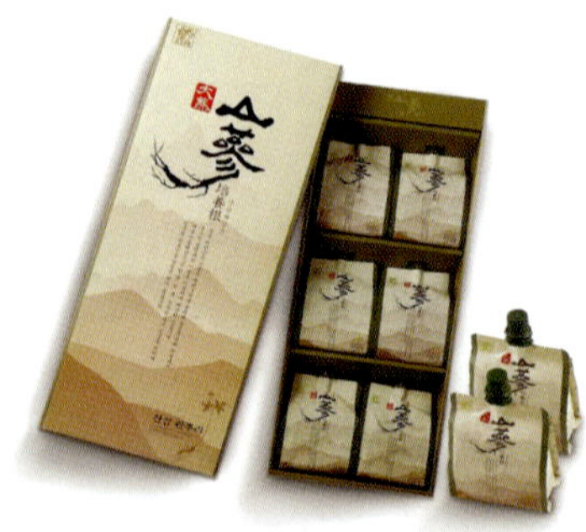
Product	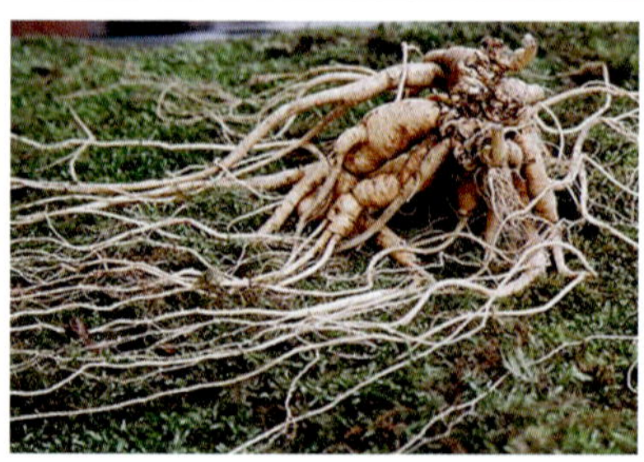

3. Eunhanggaru, Euisung sikpum

CS	Not stated
AA	Sexual dysfunction, enhancement of general body health for men
T	Powder
S	Eunhanggaru is supplied as powder of Ginkgo Biloba 100%. Keep this product in a cool and dry place.
D	Ginkgo supplements are usually taken in the range of 40-200 mg per day.
A	Duration of application for effectiveness may differ individually.
CP	Ginko Biloba is cold in nature and it tastes sweet and has toxicity. Improves lung and stomach function and helps stop breathlessness and coughing. (Dongeuibokam, traditional medical book, Tang section, Fruit-subsection)
CI	1. Ginkgo may have undesirable effects, especially for individuals with blood

	circulation disorders and those taking anticoagulants such as ibuprofen, aspirin, or warfarin, although recent studies have found that ginkgo has little or no effect on the anticoagulant properties or pharmacodynamics of warfarin. 2. Ginkgo should also not be used by people who are taking certain types of antidepressants (monoamine oxidase inhibitors and selective serotonin reuptake inhibitors) or by pregnant women, without first consulting a doctor. 3. Ginkgo side effects and cautions include: possible increased risk of bleeding, gastrointestinal discomfort, nausea, vomiting, diarrhea, headaches, dizziness, heart palpitations, and restlessness. If any side effects are experienced, consumption should be stopped immediately. 4. Ginkgo biloba leaves contain long chain alkylphenols together with the extremely potent allergens, the urushiols (similar to poison ivy)."
AR	Not stated
SC	Ginkgos are very large trees, normally reaching a height of 20-35 m (66-115 feet), with some specimens in China being over 50 m (164 feet). The tree has an angular crown and long, somewhat erratic branches, and is usually deep rooted and resistant to wind and snow damage. Young trees are often tall and slender, and sparsely branched; the crown becomes broader as the tree ages. During autumn, the leaves turn a bright yellow, then fall, sometimes within a short space of time (1-15 days). A combination of resistance to disease, insect-resistant wood and the ability to form aerial roots and sprouts makes ginkgos very long-lived, with some specimens claimed to be more than 2,500 years old: One of the oldest Ginkgo trees is in Shanghai, within the Yuyuan Garden; it is four centuries old. A 3,000 year-old ginkgo has been reported in Shandong province in China. Some old Ginkgos produce aerial roots, known as "chi chi" (Japanese; "nipples") or zhong-ru (Mandarin Chinese), which form on the undersides of large branches and grow downwards. Chi chi growth is very slow, and may take hundreds of years to occur. The function, if any, of these thick aerial roots is unknown.
I	1. Ginkgo is for peripheral vascular disease such as intermittent claudication and, more important, cerebral insufficiency. 2. Ginko extract can improve vascular perfusion, and in German data, it improved chronic cerebrovascular insufficiency. 3. Ginkgo biloba extract contains flavonid glycosides, mainly composed of kaempferol, quercetin isorhamnetin with glucose or rhamnose and characteristic terpenes of ginkgolides, bilobalides. These have a complicated pharmacological action and improve not only damage to the vessel walls but also damage to the tension f blood vessels.

M	Euisung sikpum	
	Address	1) 400-14 Naeduk-dong, Sangdang-gu, Cheongju-sim, Chongbuk Korea 2) 948-1, Daechi 3 dong, Kanagnam-gu, Seoul
	Tel	1) +82-43-293-8005 2) +82-2-2008-2550
	Email	echam@echam.co.kr
Package	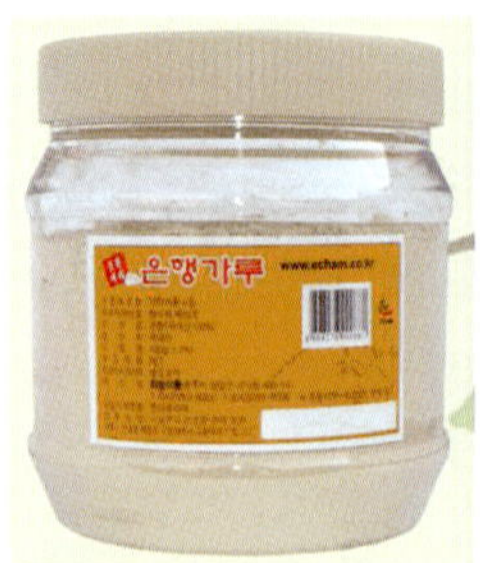 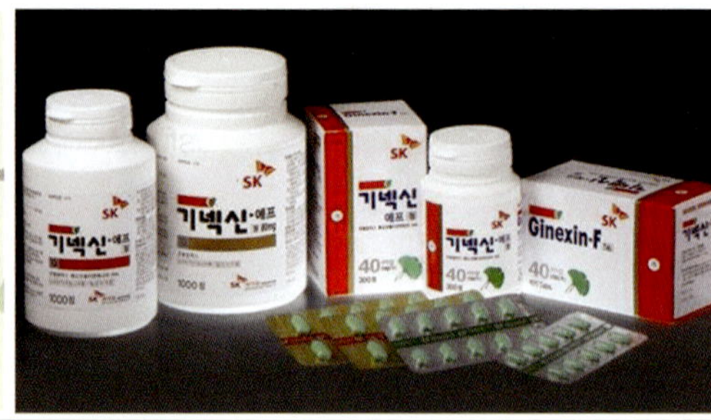	
Product	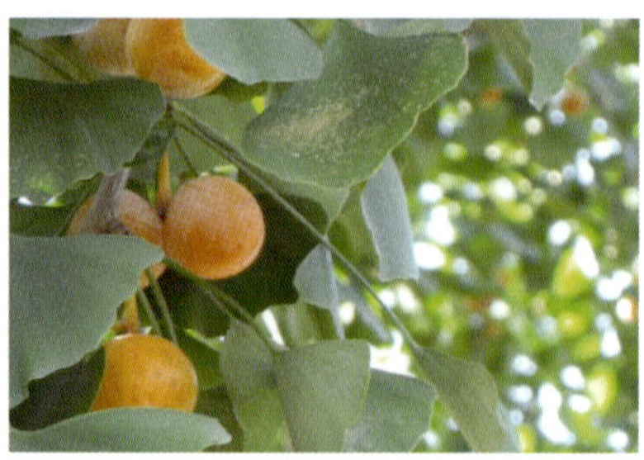	

4. Bokbunja juice, Kochang bokbunja maeul

CS	Not stated
AA	Sexual dysfunction, enhancement of general body health for men
T	Juice
S	Bokbunja juice is supplied as a pack containing 90 ml of Rubus Coreanus 95%, citric acid 3% and honey 2%. Keep this product out of the direct rays of the sun.
D	Take twice (morning and evening) a day.
A	More than 1 year Duration of application for effectiveness may differ individually.
CP	Rubus Coreanus is calming in nature and it tastes sweet and sour and has no toxicity. It cures weak vigor and sexual power in man and sterility in women. It also cures impotence in men, protects liver, improves eyesight and delays graying of hair. (Dong Ui Bo Gam, traditional medical book, Tang section, Fruit-subsection)
CI, AR	Not stated

SC	A decidious Shrub growing to 3meter by 3meter. It is hardy to zone 6. It is in flower from July to August, and the seeds ripen from August to October. The flowers are hermaphrodite (have both male and female organs) and are pollinated by insects. The plant prefers light (sandy), medium (loamy) and heavy (clay) soils and requires well-drained soil. The plant prefers acid, neutral and basic (alkaline) soils. It can grow in semi-shade (light woodland) or no shade. It requires moist soil.
I	The fruit is an aphrodisiac, an astringent, a restorative and a tonic. It is taken internally in the treatment of complaints associated with disturbed liver and kidney functions, back pain, urinary dysfunction, premature greying, blurred vision, infertility, impotence and premature ejaculation. The fruit is harvested when fully ripe and can be used fresh or dried. The juice of the bruised leaves or a decoction of the root are used in the treatment of ophthalmia. The seed is astringent and tonic.
M	Kochang bokbunja maeul Address 300, Jugok-ri , Kochang-eub, Kochang-gun Jeonbuk Korea Tel +82-63-564-4928 Email yys1581@yahoo.co.kr Web www.mybokbunha.co.kr
Package	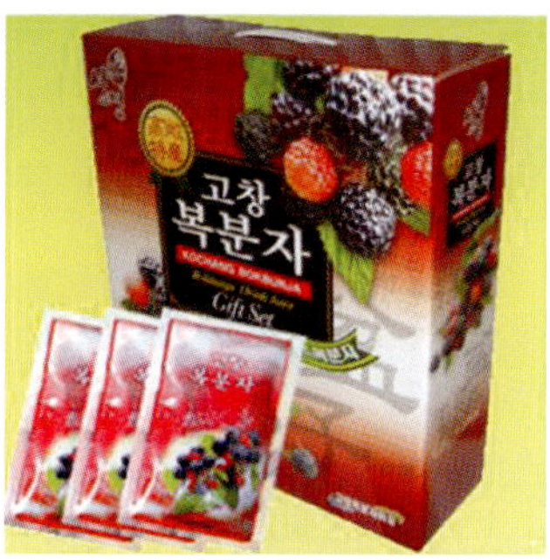
Product	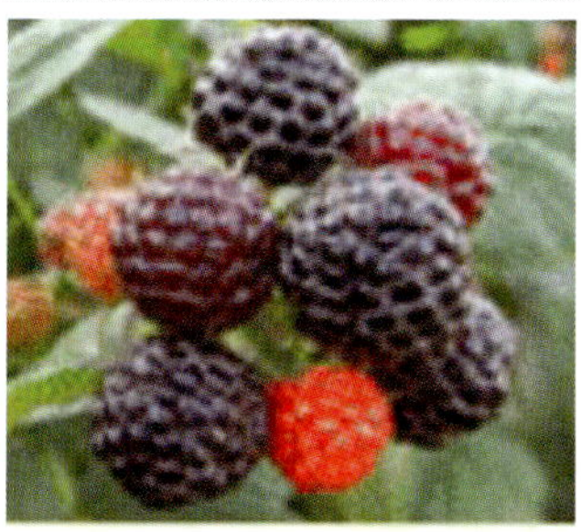

5. Sansuyu 1000

CS	Not stated
AA	Sexual dysfunction, enhancement of general body health for men
T	Pill
S	Sansuyu 1000 is supplied as a plastic container containing 90 g pills of Cornus officinalis 49%, Chinese matrimony vine, Rubus coreanus and Arginine 1000 mg. Keep this product out of the direct rays of the sun and keep in cool place or store under refrigeration.
D	Take 1-2 times anytime in a day (40 pills for adult).
A	More than 1 month Duration of application for effectiveness may differ individually.
CP	*Cornus Officinalis* is little bit warm in nature and it tastes sour and puckery and has no toxicity. It makes the negatives dynamic and reinforces sexual power, vigor and raises sexual function and makes the penis strong and large. Also it reinforces marrow, warms waist and kneel and helps vigor. It cures frequent urination and it assists with incontinence in elderly men. It cures head palsy, nose stuffiness and deafened ear (Donguibogam, traditional medical book, Tang section, Mok-subsection)
CI	1. Persons who have high body temperature, sweating and priapism should not take this product. 2. There is low toxicity but avoid long term application.
AR	Not stated
SC	Sansuyu is deciduous tree that is cultivated around the mountains in the south central part of Korea. The height is 7m, bark of the tree is divided lengthwise irregularly. It' s grey brown and symmetry and ovoid, and it's long and sharp on the tip of its leaves. The edge of the leaves are plain, back side is yellowish green, front side is deep green and has long brown hair. Its flower is androgynous, yellow and the diameter is 4 to 5 mm. The flower blooms before the leaves in early spring and usually 20~30 floweres bloom. The bract is 4 yellowish green, oval and sharp on its tip. The peduncle is 10mm long and its ovary has hair.
	The fruit is drupe oval and red has gloss, organic acid, gallic acid, mallic acid, racemic acid. Skin of the fruit has morroniside, loganin which is iridoide glycoside. 60% of Sansuyu in Korea is from Gurye, Jeonnam, and only this kind is being exported to Japan, Taiwan, Hongkong.
I	1. It warms liver and kidney and stops sweat and involuntary emission of semen.

Therefore it is effective on involuntary emission of semen, too much urine, constant sweat, hypermenorrhea caused by weak kidney.

It strengthens bones and sinews, is good when loins and knees are cold and sore, and when it feels powerless in arms and legs.

2. It gives effect to obscurity of eyes and vertigo caused by weak liver.

3. Pharmacology

Through pharmacologic experiments, it has been proven that it has strong diuretic effects, reduction of blood pressure, anticarcinogenic effects, and anti-biotic effects. Also, helps digest proteins and shows strong diuretic effects which temporally reduces the blood pressure.

M

Chunho Food Industry Co., Ltd.

Address	Chunho B/D, 389-2, Deokpo-2dong, Sasang-gu, Busan 617-814 Korea
Tel	+82-51-3031005
Fax	+82-51-3031586
Email	chunho@chunho.net
Web	www.chunho.net

Package

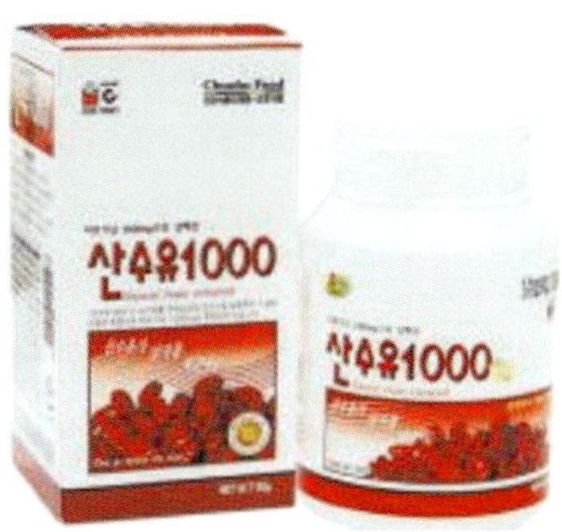

Product

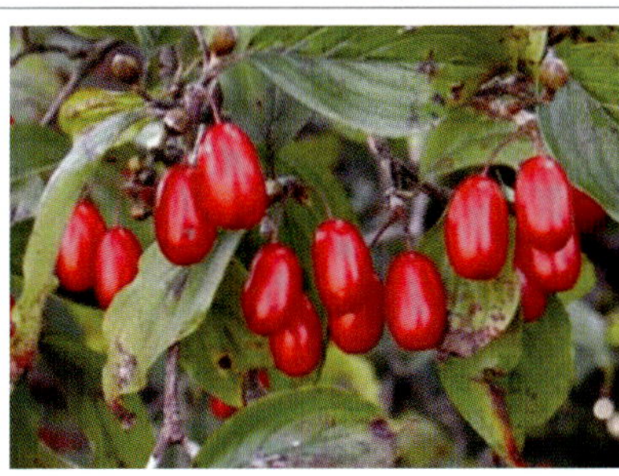

6. Lycium chinense Mill Pill

CS	Not stated
AA	Sexual dysfunction, enhancement of general body health for men
T	Pill
S	Lycium chinense Mill Pill is supplied as a plastic container containing 180 g pills of Lycium chinense Mill 80%, Rubus coreanus and Arginine.
D	Take 2-3 times anytime in a day (30-40 pills for adult).
A	Duration of application for effectiveness may differ individually.
CP	Chinese boxthorn is a major Chinese tonic herb with a history of almost 2,000 years of medicinal use. Both the berries and the root are used and traditionally the plant is believed to promote long life. The fruit is one of the most popular tonics used in Chinese herbal medicine. A decoction is used to clear the vision, strengthen the kidneys, restore semen and nourish the liver. The fruit protects the liver from damage caused by exposure to toxins. It is also used in the treatment of diabetes mellitus, vertigo, nocturnal emissions and aching back and legs. The fruit of many members of this genus is a very rich source of vitamins and minerals, especially in vitamins A, C and E, flavonoids and other bio-active compounds. It is also a fairly good source of essential fatty acids, which is fairly unusual for a fruit. It is being investigated as a food that is capable of reducing the incidence of cancer and also as a means of halting or reversing the growth of cancers. The seed is used as a hemostat for the control of bleeding, with a special action on the kidneys and sex organs. The root bark is antibacterial, antipyretic, hepatic, hypoglycemic and vasodilator. It stimulates the parasympathetic nervous system, which controls involuntary bodily functions such as digestive secretions. The root is used in the treatment of pulmonary tuberculosis and pneumonia in small children, chronic febrile disease, night sweats, cough and asthma, tuberculosis, hypertension and diabetes mellitus. The root can be harvested at any time of the year but traditionally it is harvested in the spring and can be dried for later use. The root bark contains betaine. This can increase the rate of growth of farm animals and increase the weight and amount of eggs. It is used in the treatment of achlorhydria, atherosclerosis and hepatic diseases. Hemostatic.
CI, AR	Not stated
SC	Lycium barbarum (goji) is in the family Solanaceae and its ripe fruit has been used in Asian countries, such as China, Korea, and Japan, for more than 2500 years a traditional herbal medicine and functional food for its benefits to anti-aging, vision, kidney, and liver functions. In his Compendium of Medica, Li Shi-zen named L.

barbarum as a top-grade medicinal material that can nourish the liver and kidney, supplement energy, and improve eyesight. Shennong' s Classic of Materia Medica (Shennong Bencaojing) also mentioned that "long term use of goji can contribute to agility and longevity." Ni Zhu-Mo, the renowned Chinese herbalist, also said in his Ben Cao Hui Yan (Convergent Speech on the Materia Medica) that "Goji can supplement energy, blood, adjust yin and yang, reduce internal heat and resist wind and humidity, and enjoys ten magic functions." 1 In support of these traditional properties assigned to L.barbarum, recent studies indicate that extracts from L.barbarum fruit possess a range of biological activities, including effects on aging, neuroprotection, antifatigue/ endurance, increased metabolism, glucose control in diabetics, glaucoma, antioxidant properties, immunomodulation, antitumor, activity, and cytoprotection.

I

1. Antibacterial
2. Antipyretic
3. Cancer
4. Haemostatic
5. Hepatic;
6. Hypoglycemic
7. Infertility
8. Kidney
9. Ophthalmic
10. Tonic
11. Vasodilator

M

Chunho Food Co., Ltd

Address	Chunho building, #389-2, Deokpo2-dong, Sasang-ku, Busan City, Korea
Tel	+82-51-303-1005
Fax	+82-51-303-1586
Email	chunho@chunho.net
Web	www.chunho.net

Package

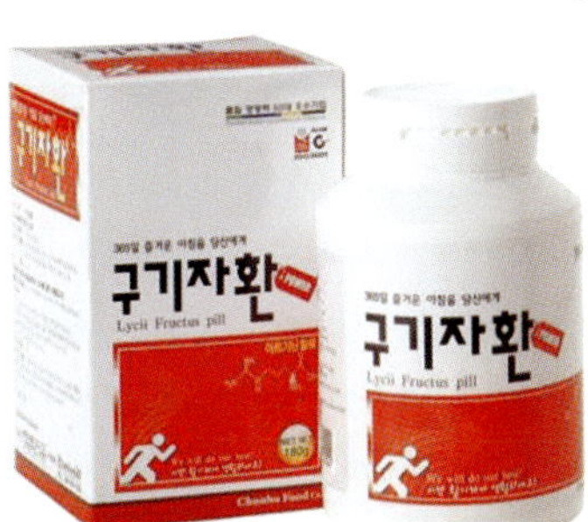

Product	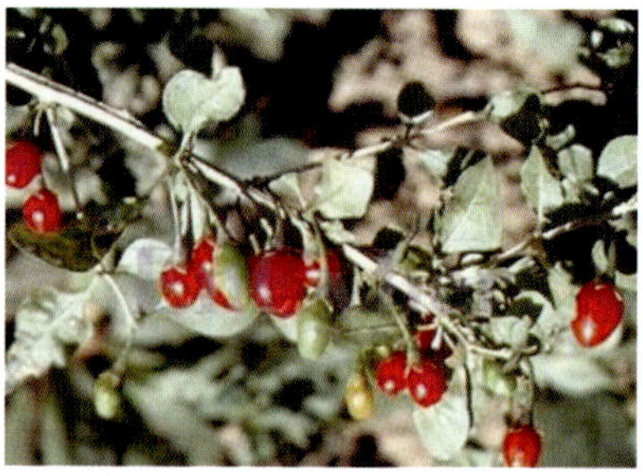

7. MACA Power, MORIGANA

CS	Not stated
AA	Has been used for energy, stamina, athletic performance, impotence, fertility enhancement, aphrodisiac qualities, erectile dysfunction, hormone balancing and increased testosterone levels
T	Pill
S	MACA Power is supplied as abottle of 360 g pills of MACA powder 49.9%, bean powder 6.0%, Adlay powder 6.0%, Polygonum multiflorum powder 5.0% excl. Keep this product out of the direct rays of the sun and keep in cool place or store under refrigeration.
D	Take 3 times anytime in a day (1 pills for one time).
A	More than 1 month according to the directions Duration of application for effectiveness may differ individually.
CP	Lab studies have shown that MACA can increase sperm production, sex hormone levels and sexual activity in male and female rodents. The few clinical trials that have investigated MACA' s effectiveness have resulted in increase sperm count and motility as well as sexual desire. Human studies are also necessary to confirm the supplement's effects.
CI	MACA supplement use hasn' t been extensively studied in humans, so there' s little information about the safety of long term use or high doses.
AR	Not stated
SC	Lepidium meyenii or MACA is an herbaceous biennial plan or annual plan native to the high Andes of Bolivia and Peru. It is grown for its fleshy hypocotyl (actually a fused hypocotyls and raproot), which is used as a root vegetable and a medicinal herb. Its Spanish and Quechua names include *maca-maca*, *maino*, *ayak chichira*, and *ayak willku*. For approximately 2,000 years, MACA has been an important traditional food and

	medicinal plant in its limited growing region, where it is well-known and celebrated. It is regarded as a highly nutritious, energy-imbuing food, and as a medicine that enhances strength, endurance and also acts as an aphrodisiac. During Spanish colonization MACA was used as currency.
I	12-week double blind, placebo-controlled, randomized, parallel trial in which active treatment with different doses of Gelatinized MACA was compared with Placebo. Logistic regression analysis showed that MACA has an independent effect on sexual desire at 8 and 12 weeks of treatment, and this effect is not because of changes in either Hamilton scores for depression or anxiety or serum testosterone and estradiol levels. In conclusion, treatment with MACA improved sexual desire.
M	Morigana Address A-1603, Shangjaerijae Center, Daechi-dong, Gangnam-gu, Seoul 889-5, Korea Tel +82-2-5665790 Fax +82-2-5390063 Web www.morigana.co.kr
Package	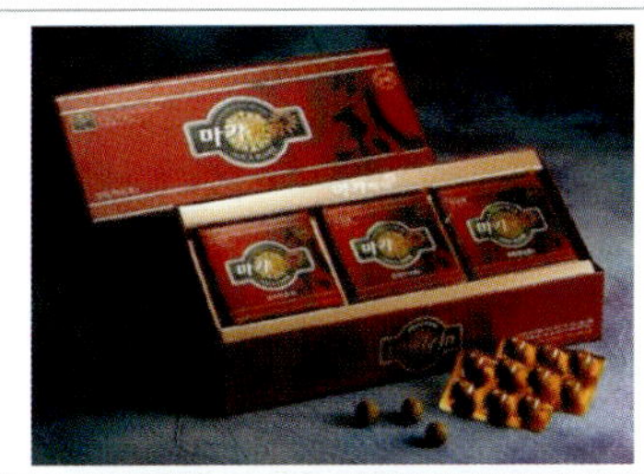
Product	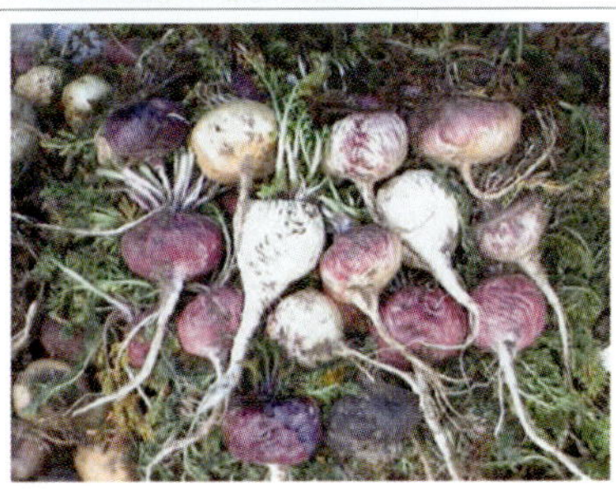

8. Nuegra

CS	Not stated
AA	Effective not only in boosting men' s vigor, but also in helping one to recover from physical exhaustion. Young and old men with reduced physical function or strength, weak urinary function, or complaints off fatigue.

T	Pill
S	*Nuegra* is supplied as a plastic container of 99 g pills of Royal gelly 20%, *Silkworm and cocoon* 18.2%, *Acanthopanax senticosus* 5.6%, *Rubus coreanus*, *Schisandra chnensis* Baillon. Keep this product out of the direct rays of the sun and keep in cool place or store under refrigeration
D	Take 3 times anytime in a day (2 pills for one time).
A	More than 10 days according to the direction Duration of application for effectiveness may differ individually.
CP	*Nuegra* is made from male silkworm pupae and is expected to make great contributions to the silkworm industry, as well as people's health. Korean ancient medical records, including 'Dong ui bo gam', the bible of oriental medicine say the male silkworm moth is effective in strengthening men's vitality.
CI	1. Nuegra produces mild adverse effects such as digestive difficulty, sputum production, temporary chest palpitation, drowsiness and increased stool frequency. 2. There is low toxicity but avoid long term application.
AR	Not stated
SC	The silkworm is the larva or caterpillar of Bombyx mori, the domesticated silkworm moth. A moth in the family Bombycidae, it is very important economically as the producer of silk. It is entirely dependent on humans for its reproduction and no longer occurs naturally in the wild. Sericulture has been practiced for at least 5,000 years in China. A silkworm's preferred food is white mulberry leaves, but it may also eat the leaves of the Osage Orange or the Tree of Heaven. It is native to northern China.
I	1. Nuegra is effective in improving general conditions especially insomnia, muscular weakness and fatigue. 2. Pharmacology To prove it, RDA scientists let animals feed on the extraction of male silkworms for three weeks, in a series of experiments. The results showed that the animals (rat)' male hormone levels increased by 33 percent and their sperm count jumped by 33 percent, while their athletic endurance rose by 60 percent. Conducted field tests on 30 men to evaluate the efficacy of Nuegra with the first batch of production. It was revealed that the medicine is effective not only in boosting men's vigor, but also in helping one to recover from physical exhaustion.
M	KunWha Pharmaceutical Co., Ltd. Address KunWha B/D, 94, Garak-dong, Songpa-gu, Seoul 138-160, Korea

	Tel	+82-2-4313100
	Fax	+82-2-4435757
	Email	webmaster@kunwha.com
	Web	http://www.Kunwha.com
Package	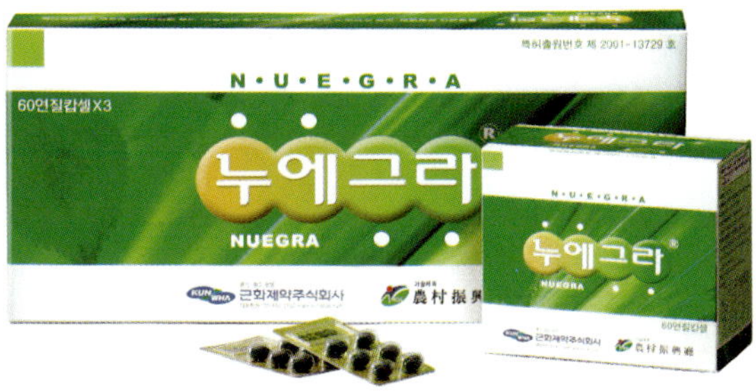	
Product	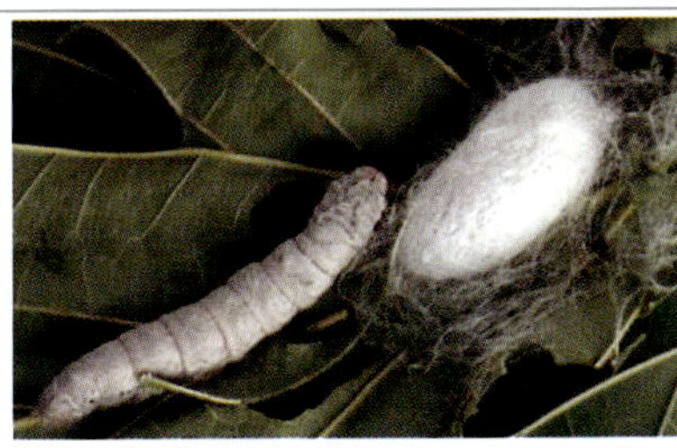	

9. Cheon Bo Gong Shin Dan

CS	Not stated
AA	Hepatic hypofunction caused by stress and overdrinking and Chronic fatigue
T	Pill
S	Easily portable due to individual packaging by pills
D	Chew it slowly with warm water, 2(two) pills a day (one in the morning and the other in the evening), 6g per pill
A	Duration of application for effectiveness may differ individually Child to be recommended 1/2 quantity of adult
CP	Gong Shin Dan(拱辰丹) which had been treated only to Emperors is developed by Mr. Wei Yi Lin, a famous doctor of Yuan Dynasty of China. It is described in Shi Yi De Xiao Fang (世醫得效方) which was an oriental medicine book. It was widely used for weakness at the convalescent stage and hepatic hypofunction caused by excessive stress and overdrinking.
CI, AR	Not stated
SC	Title of invention: Composition for immune enhancement comprising the extract of

	Young antler, Cornus officinalis, Ligusticum acutilobum, Chinese matrimony vine, Yam, Aurantill nobilis pericarpium, Gastrodia elata blume, Agastache rugosa, Cinamomum loueirii, Ginseng steamed red and Schizandra chinensis, as an active ingredient
I	Not stated
M	Korea Bio Medical Science Institute Co., Ltd. Address 7th Floor, Shinhan Bldg, 80-1, Nonhyun-Dong, Gangnam-Gu, Seoul, Korea Tel +82-2-3443-9252 Fax +82-2-3444-9252 Email admin@kbmsi.com Web http://www.kbmsi.com
Package	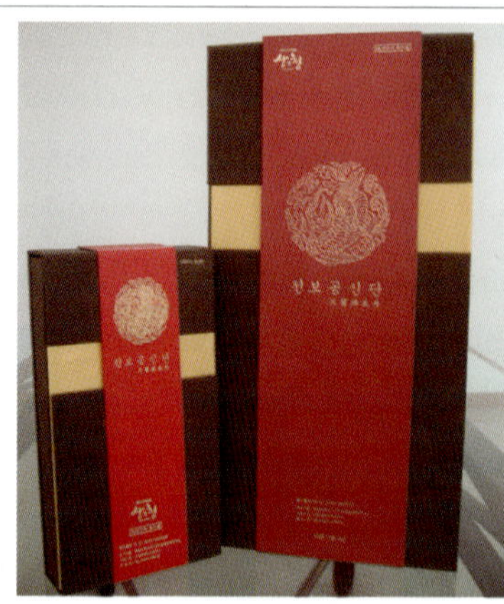
Product	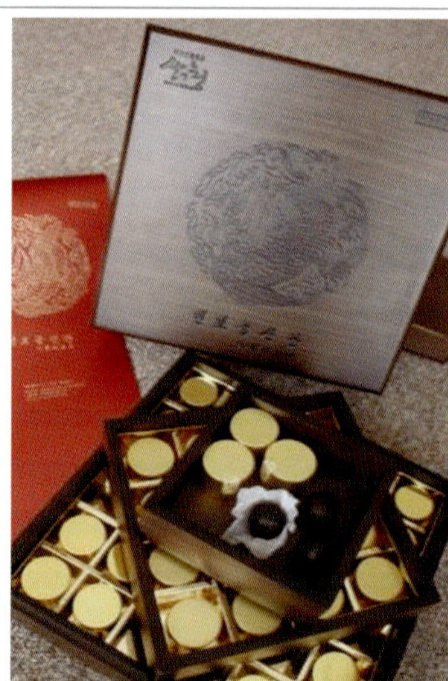

10. SS Cream

CS	Not stated
AA	Treatment of premature ejaculation (PE)
T	Cream
S	SS-cream is a topical agent derived from the extracts of nine natural products (Ginseng Radix Alba, Angelicae Gigantic Radix, Cistanchis Herba, Zanthoxylli Fructus, Torilidis Fructus, Asiasari Radix, Caryophylli Flos, Cinnamomi Cortex, and Bufonis Venenum).
D	Rub cream over the use region (1 pack , 0.2g) before 1 hour After 0.5~1 hours washes with water
A	Duration of application for effectiveness may differ individually
CP	SS cream is a topical agent for treatment of PE which was made with carefully selected extracts of nine natural products, which is based on the traditional herb remedy and the action mechanisms of SS cream are believed to have local desensitizing effects and enhancing capabilities of the local blood flow and was effective in the treatment of PE in the pilot, clinical studies.
CI	Some patients complained of its unpleasant small and color. It has also been reported that a local anesthetic desensitizing the glans, but it may cause numbness of the glans and prolong the waiting time.
AR	Not stated
SC	SS cream is a mixture of nine traditional medicines, including Korean ginseng, Bufonis Venenum, cinnamon, etc. which have been shown to possess a local desensitizing effect and proved to be safe and effective for PE treatment upon local application on the glans penis. Animal studies showed that SS cream inhibited a pin-prick induced corneal reflex dose dependently and prolonged latency and reduced amplitude of SEP of rabbits in a dose-dependent fashion.
I	1. Treatment of premature ejaculation 2. Satisfaction for both male and female partner 3. Excellent Safety 4. Proven High Efficacy
M	CJ Address CJ Bldg. 500, Namdaemunro 5-ga, Jung-gu, Seoul, Korea Tel +82-2-726-8114 Fax +82-2-726-8179 Email webmaster@CJ.net Web www.cj.co.kr / www.ssclinic.com

Package

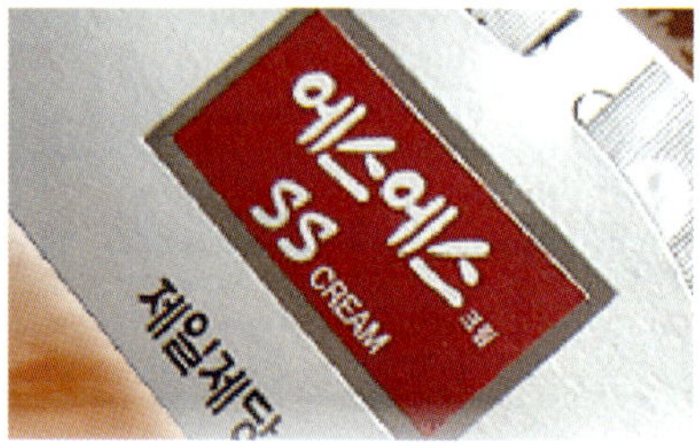

Crude herbs for SS Cream

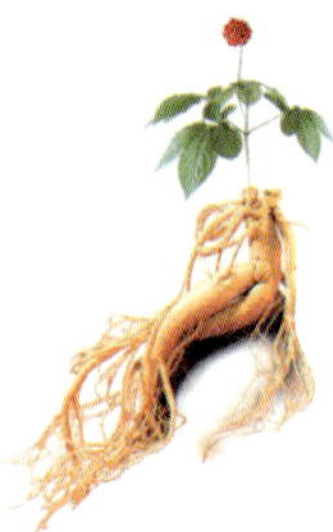
Ginseng Radix Alba

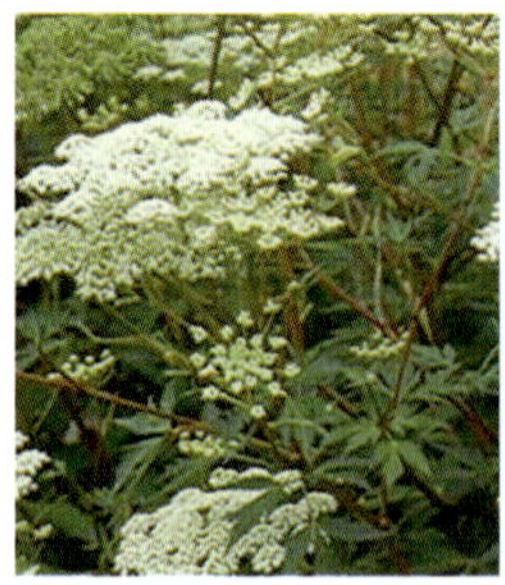
Angelicae Gigantis Radix

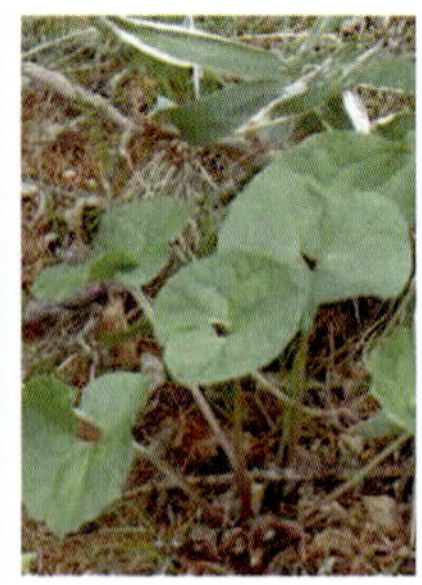
Asiasari Radix

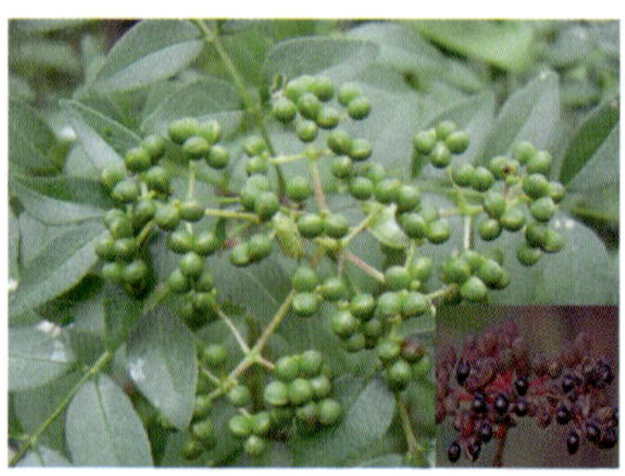
Zanthoxyli Fructus

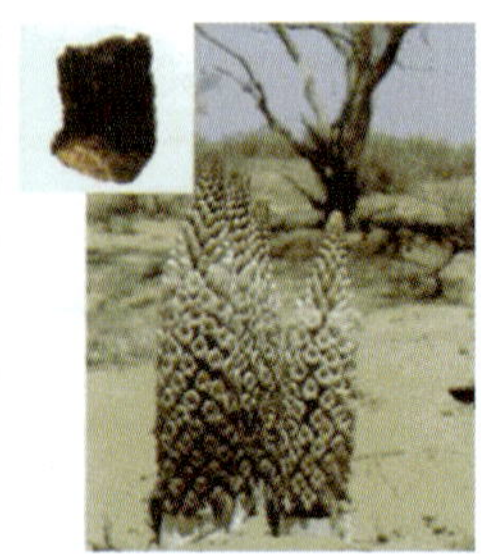
Cistanchis Herba

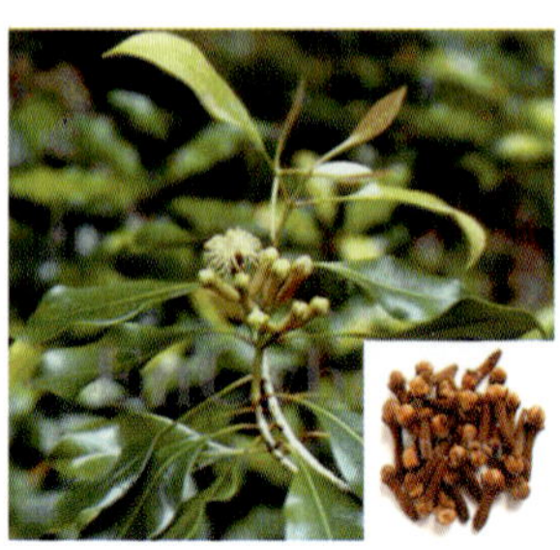
Caryophylli Flos

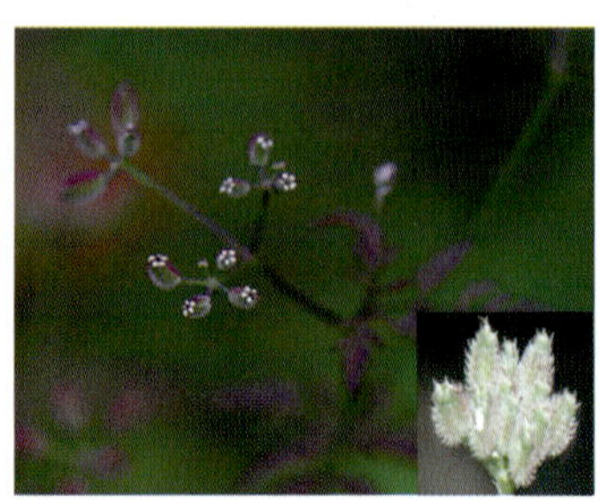
Torilidis Fructus

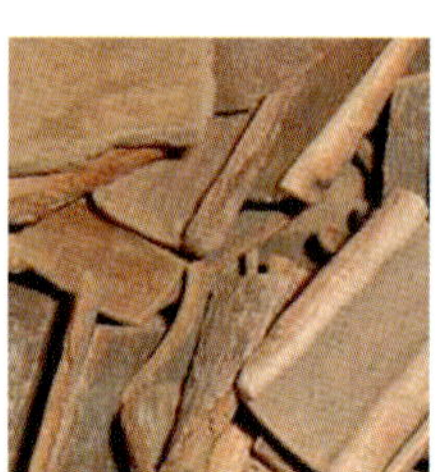
Cinnamomi Cortex

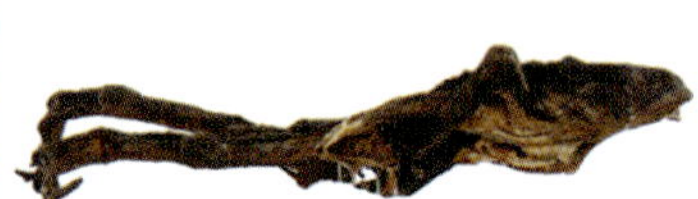
Bufonis Venenum

Chapter 6

Taiwanese Products

Han-Sun Chiang, Chun-Hou Liao

I. Single Prescription

1. Horny Goat Weed(Yin yang huo)

CS	Not stated
AA	kidney-yang deficiency: impotence, spermatorrhoea, premature ejaculation, lumbago, cold hands and feet, fear of cold; rheumatic discomforts of "wind-damp" excess; spasms; numbness
T	Tablet
S	Leaves of Epimedium Sagittatum(Berberidaceae)
D	10-15g per day
A, CP	Not stated
CI	Deficiency of "Yin", high sexual desire
AR	Not stated
SC	The drug dilates the capillaries and larger blood vessels; lowers blood pressure; common ingredient in "Spring Wine"; remedies absent mindedness by flooding the brain with blood
I	Not stated
M	KO DA PHARMACEUTICAL CO. LTD Address No.20-1, Gongye 3rd Rd., Pingjhen City, Taoyuan County 324, Taiwan Tel 886-3-4696105 Fax 886-3-4690546

	Email	koda@koda.com.tw
Web	http://www.koda.com.tw	
Product	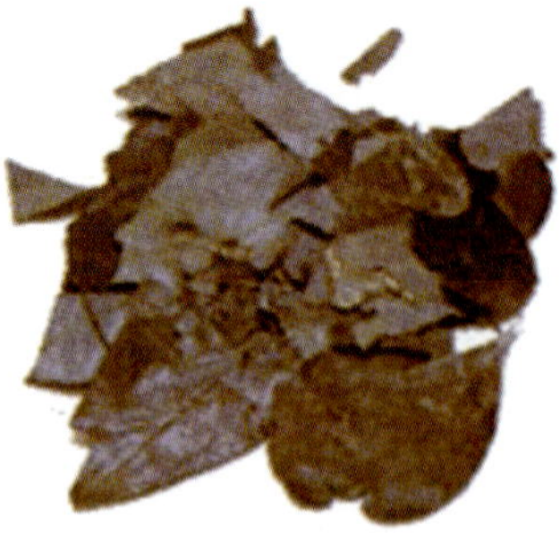	

2. She chuang zi

CS	Not stated
AA	kidney-yang deficiency: especially impotence and female sterility
T	Tablet
S	Fruits of Cnidium Monnieri (Umbelliferae)
D	5-10g
A, CP	Not stated
CI	Deficiency of "Yin", high sexual desire
AR	Not stated
SC	A decoction of this herb is a highly effective antiseptic wash for vaginal itching, yeast infection, parasites, etc
I	Not stated
M	Sun Ten Phmarmaceutical Co., Ltd Address 3F., No.11, Sec. 2, Roosevelt Rd., Jhongjheng District, Taipei City 100, Taiwan Tel +886-2-23957070 Fax +886-2-23213707 Email sunten@sunten.com.tw Web w3.sunten.com.tw

3. Broomrape(Rou cong rong)

CS	Not stated
AA	kidney-yang deficiency: impotence, spermatorrhoea, premature ejaculation, lumbago, weak bones and sinews; constipation due to dry intestines
T	Tablet
S	Fleshy stems of Cistanche Salsa (Orobanchaceae)
D	10-15g
A, CP	Not stated
CI	Deficiency of "Yin", high sexual desire
AR	Not stated
SC	Tonifies yin as well as yang; lower blood pressure
I	Not stated
M	KO DA PHARMACEUTICAL CO. LTD Address No.20-1, Gongye 3rd Rd., Pingjhen City, Taoyuan County 324, Taiwan Tel +886-3-4696105 Fax +886-3-4690546 Email koda@koda.com.tw Web http://www.koda.com.tw
Product	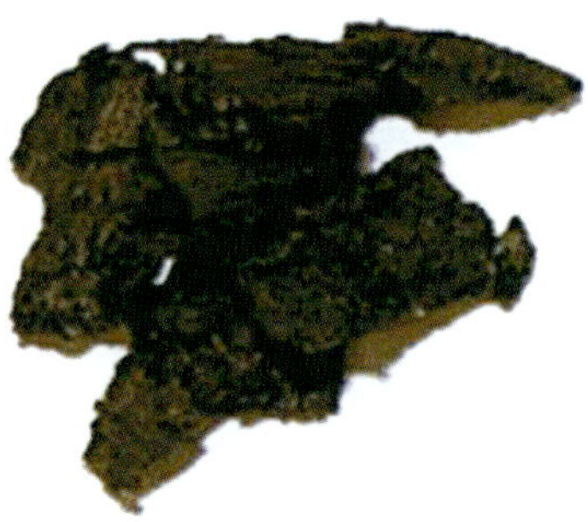

4. Spotted Deer (Lu rong)

CS	Not stated
AA	kidney-yang deficiency (insufficient secretions of sexual hormones): impotence, watery semen, cold extremities, lumbago, clear and profuse urine, anemia, weight loss, slow growth in children, weak bone and sinews, dysmenorrhoea, leucorrhoea; 13th and 14th meridian deficiencies
T	Tablet

S	Horn and velvet antler of Cervus Nippon (Cervidae)
D	3-5g
A, CP, CI, AR	Not stated
SC	This is one of the most renowned and popular sexual tonics in the ben cao; the best is tender new horn still in velvet with the dried blood still visible in the cartilage; the most potent essence is obtained by drinking the fresh blood and secretions directly from the freshly cut horn
I	Not stated
M	Hong Shing Phmarmaceutical Co., Ltd Address No.1-1, Nanyuan Rd., Jhongli City, Taoyuan County 320, Taiwan Tel +886-3-4623628 Web http://hongshing.com.tw

5. Blackberry (Fu pen zi)

CS	Not stated
AA	Kidney deficiency; impotence, spermatorrhoea, premature ejaculation, urinal incontinence, bed-wetting
T	Tablet
S	Unripe berries of Rubus Coreanus(Rosaceae)
D	5-10g
A, CP	Not stated
CI	Deficiency of "Yin", high sexual desire, void difficult
AR	Not stated
SC	The drug improves vision in liver and kidney deficient symptoms
I	Not stated
M	Sun Ten Phmarmaceutical Co., Ltd Address 3F., No.11, Sec. 2, Roosevelt Rd., Jhongjheng District, Taipei City 100, Taiwan Tel +886-2-23957070 Fax +886-2-23213707 Email sunten@sunten.com.tw Web w3.sunten.com.tw

6. Black cardamom(Yi zhi ren)

CS	Not stated	
AA	Kidney-yang deficiency: impotence, premature ejaculation, frequency and profuse urine, urinal incontinence; "cold" spleen symptoms: diarrhea, profuse salivation, cold and pain in abdomen	
T	Tablet	
S	Seeds of Alpinia oxyphylla (zingiberaceae)	
D	3-10g	
A, CP	Not stated	
CI	Deficiency of "Yin", high sexual desire	
AR, SC, I	Not stated	
M	Sun Ten Phmarmaceutical Co., Ltd	
	Address	3F., No.11, Sec. 2, Roosevelt Rd., Jhongjheng District, Taipei City 100, Taiwan
	Tel	+886-2-23957070
	Fax	+886-2-23213707
	Email	sunten@sunten.com.tw
	Web	w3.sunten.com.tw

7. Caltrop (Ci ji li)

CS	Not stated	
AA	Kidney-yang deficiency: impotence, premature ejaculation, frequency and profuse urine, ringing in the ears, lumbago, leukorrhowa; blurry vision due to liver deficiency	
T	Tablet	
S	Mature fruits of Tribulus Terrestris (zygophylaceae)	
D	10-15g	
A, CP, CI, AR	Not stated	
SC	The drug facilitates labour contractions during difficult childbirths	
I	Not stated	
M	Sun Ten Phmarmaceutical Co., Ltd	
	Address	3F., No.11, Sec. 2, Roosevelt Rd., Jhongjheng District, Taipei City 100, Taiwan
	Tel	+886-2-23957070
	Fax	+886-2-23213707
	Email	sunten@sunten.com.tw
	Web	w3.sunten.com.tw

8. Dodder (Tu si zi)

CS	Not stated	
AA	Kidney-yang deficiency: impotence, premature ejaculation, frequency and profuse urine, ringing in the ears, lumbago, leukorrhowa; blurry vision due to liver deficiency	
T	Dried Seeds	
S	Seeds of Cuscuta japonica (convulvulaceae)	
D	10-15g	
A, CP, CI, AR	Not stated	
SC	Be aware for blood deficiency	
I	Not stated	
M	KO DA PHARMACEUTICAL CO. LTD	
	Address	No.20-1, Gongye 3rd Rd., Pingjhen City, Taoyuan County 324, Taiwan
	Tel	+886-3-4696105
	Fax	+886-3-4690546
	Email	koda@koda.com.tw
	Web	http://www.koda.com.tw/main.aspx

9. Songaria Cynomorium Herb

CS	Not stated	
AA	Impotence, constipation, weak extremities	
T	Dried stem	
S	Stem of Cynomorium songaricum Rupr.	
D	10-15g	
A, CP	Not stated	
CI	High kidney-yang	
AR, SC, I	Not stated	
M	Sun Ten Phmarmaceutical Co., Ltd	
	Address	3F., No.11, Sec. 2, Roosevelt Rd., Jhongjheng District, Taipei City 100, Taiwan
	Tel	+886-2-23957070
	Fax	+886-2-23213707
	Email	sunten@sunten.com.tw
	Web	w3.sunten.com.tw/index.php

II. Combination Prescription

1. You Gui Wan "C.A." ; Yow Guei Pill "L.L." ; You-Kuei-Wan "Sun-Ten"

CS	Not stated
AA	kidney-yang deficiency, cold extremities, impotence, edema, residual urine
T	Tablet
S	Shu di huang 68 mg; Cassia(Chinese Cinnamon)(rou gui) 17 mg; Fu tzyy 17 mg; Corni Fructus 34 mg; Chinese yam(shan yao) 34 mg; Dodder(tu si zi) 34 mg; Eucommia(du zhong) 34 mg; Chinese Wolfberry(gou qi zi) 34 mg; Luh Jeau Jiau 26.1 mg; Dang gui 26.1 mg; Honey(feng mi) 275.8 mg
D	Twice daily or directed by doctor of traditional Chinese medicine
A, CP, CI, AR, SC, I	Not stated
M	Sun Ten Phmarmaceutical Co., Ltd Address 3F., No.11, Sec. 2, Roosevelt Rd., Jhongjheng District, Taipei City 100, Taiwan Tel +886-2-23957070 Fax +886-2-23213707 Email sunten@sunten.com.tw Web w3.sunten.com.tw/index.php
Package	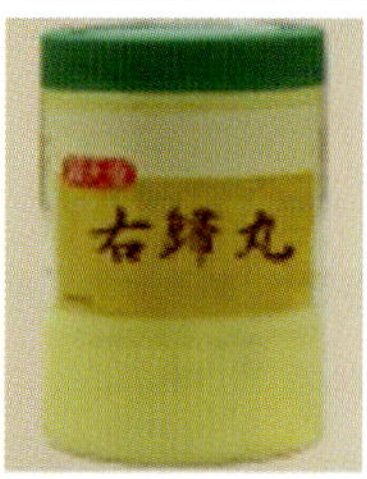

2. Jin Suoo Guh Jing Pill

CS	Not stated
AA	kidney-yang deficiency ; semen leak; cold sweating; tinnitus; extremities weakness
T	Tablet
S	Seeds of Astragalus complanatus R. (shayuanzi) 66.6 mg; Foxnut (qian shi) 66.6 mg; Nelumbinis Stamen 66.6 mg; Dragon bones(long gu) 33.3 mg; Oyster Shells(mu li) 33.3 mg; Lotus seed 66.6 mg; Honey(feng mi) 167 mg
D	Three times a day
A, CP, CI, AR, SC, I	Not stated
M	Fung Song Pharm. Biotechnology Co., Ltd Address No.60, Chenggong St., Guantian Township, Tainan County 720, Taiwan Tel +886-6-6987396 Email fung.song@msa.hinet.net Web http://www.pharmed.com.tw/index.asp

3. Hwan Shaw Dan Wan

CS	Not stated
AA	Kidney and spleen deficiency, cold sweating, semen leak, turbid urine
T	Tablet
S	Chinese yam(shan yao) 37.5 mg; Achyranthes bidentata(niu xi) 37.5 mg; Subterranean fungus(Tuckahoe, Indian bread, virgina truffle)(fu ling) 25 mg; Dogwood Tree(shan zhu yu) 25 mg; Papermulberry Fruit 25 mg; Eucommia(du zhong) 25 mg; Schisandra(we wei zi) 25 mg; Radix Morindae Officinalis 25 mg; Broomrape(rou cong rong) 25 mg; Polygalaceae)(Yuan zhi) 25 mg; Fennel (hui xiang) 25 mg; Rock Sweet-Flag(shi chang pu) 12.5 mg; Shu di huang 12.5 mg; Chinese Wolfberry(gou qi zi) 12.5 mg; Chinese Jujube (cultivated variety)(da zao) 12.5 mg; Honey(feng mi) 150 mg
D, A, CP, CI, AR, SC, I	Not stated
M	Jin-An Phmarmaceutical Co., Ltd Address No.9, Ln. 260, Sec. 3, Jianguo Rd., Minsyong Township, Chiayi County 621, Taiwan Tel +886-5-2213018

Fax	+886-5-2218833
Email	changmp@ch-angmp.com.tw
Web	http://www.ch-angmp.com.tw/

4. Shuenn-An Huanglong Medicated Wine

CS	Not stated
AA	kidney deficiency, impotence, lumbago
T	Drink
S	Poria cocos 1.870mg; Longan fruit (long yan rou) 15.025mg; Polygalaceae(Yuan zhi) 2.560mg; Blackberry (fu pen zi) 1.870mg; Teasel (xu duan) 0.510mg; Safflower(hong hua) 1.280mg; Codonopsis pilosula 2.560mg; Broomrape(rou cong rong) 3.744mg; She chuang zi 1.870mg; Shu di huang 3.744mg; Rosa laevigata Michx 0.380mg; Eleutheros(wu jia pi) 0.890mg; Umbelliferae(Dang gui) 1.870mg; Leguminosae(huang qi) 1.690mg; Psoraleae Ftuctus 1.870mg; Chinese Wolfberry(gou qi zi) 3.744; Polygonatum sibiricum Red. 0.890mg; Scrophulariaceae(gan di huang) 1.280; Chinese Licorice(gan cao) 1.080; Horny Goat Weed(yin yang huo) 3.744mg; Dodder(tu si zi) 2.560mg; Songaria Cynomorium Herb 0.770mg; Ligusticum chuanxiong Hort 0.770mg
D, A, CP, CI, AR, SC, I	Not stated
M	Taiwan Shuenn-An Biotechnology Phmarmaceutical Co., Ltd Address No.876, Fonglin 2nd Rd., Daliao Township, Kaohsiung County 831, Taiwan Tel +886-7-7870228 Fax +886-7-7889118 Web http://www.shunan.com.tw/

5. Da Xiong Wan Film Coating Tablet

CS	Not stated
AA	Kidney-yang deficiency, general weakness, low back pain"
T	Tablet
S	Spotted Deer (lu rong); 30.0 mgDodder(tu si zi) 30.0 mg; Eucommia(du zhong) 30.0 mg; Radix Morindae Officinalis 30.0 mg; Broomrape(rou cong rong) 30.0 mg; Shu di

	huang 68.4 mg; Poria cocos 43.2 mg Ginseng 59.4 mg; Cinnamomum cassia 43.2 mg; Chinese Wolfberry(gou qi zi) 30.0 mg; Umbelliferae(Dang gui) 30.0 mg; Root of Paeonia lactiflora Pall 30.0 mg; Dogwood Tree (shan zhu yu) 43.2 mg; Bai zhu 43.2 mg; Achyranthes bidentata(niu xi) 43.2 mg; Chinese Licorice(gan cao) 16.2 mg
D, A, CP, CI, AR, SC, I	Not stated
M	Hong Shing Phmarmaceutical Co., Ltd Address No.1-1, Nanyuan Rd., Jhongli City, Taoyuan County 320, Taiwan Tel +886-3-4623628 Web http://hongshing.com.tw
Package	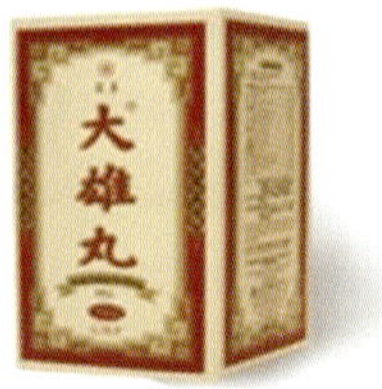

6. Zhuang Chunren Nan Po Jian Li Wan Tablet

CS	Not stated
AA	Kidney-yang deficiency; low back pain, extremities cold
T	Tablet
S	Spotted Deer (lu rong) 15 mg; Shu di huang 62 mg; Schisandra(we wei zi) 8 mg; Eucommia(du zhong) 31 mg Corni Fructus山 31 mg; Chinese Wolfberry(gou qi zi) 31 mg; Achyranthes bidentata(niu xi) 31 mg; Subterranean fungus (Tuckahoe, Indian bread, virgina truffle)(fu ling) 31 mg; Chinese yam(shan yao) 31 mg; Ophiopogonis Radix 31 mg Dodder(tu si zi) 31 mg; Honey(feng mi) 167 mg
D, A, CP, CI, AR, SC, I	Not stated
M	Zhuang Chunren Pharmaceutical Co. Ltd Address No.252, Sec. 3, Jhongjheng Rd., Rende Township, Tainan County 717, Taiwan Tel +886-06-2236191

7. Shuenn-An Ren Shen Lu Rong Pellet

CS	Not stated
AA	Deficiency of kidney and spleen, weak energy, low back pain, dizziness
T	Tablet
S	Spotted Deer (lu rong) 18 mg; Ginseng 36 mg; Chinese Wolfberry(gou qi zi) 18 mg; Radix Morindae Officinalis 18 mg; Broomrape(rou cong rong) 18 mg; Dodder(tu si zi) 18 mg; Dang gui 18 mg; Cassia(Chinese Cinnamon)(rou gui)27 mg; Eucommia(du zhong) 18 mg; Root of Paeonia lactiflora Pall 18 mg; Shu di huang 45 mg; Corni Fructus 27 mg; Bai zhu 27 mg; Subterraneanfungus(tuckahoe, Indian bread, virgina truffle)(fu ling) 27 mg; Achyranthes bidentata Blumb 27 mg Chinese Licorice(gan cao) 9 mg; Honey(feng mi) 131 mg
D	Twice daily or directed by doctor of traditional Chinese medicine
A, CP, CI, AR, SC, I	Not stated
M	Sun Ten Phmarmaceutical Co., Ltd Address 3F., No.11, Sec. 2, Roosevelt Rd., Jhongjheng District, Taipei City 100, Taiwan Tel +886-2-23957070 Fax +886-2-23213707 Email sunten@sunten.com.tw Web hongshing.com.tw

III. Combination with Chinese and Western Medicine

1. Yuan Shu Lon Capsules Aifuhao

CS	Not stated
AA	Androgen deficiency
T	Tablet
S	Thiamine nitrate Tocopherol acetate alpha dl Pantothenate calcium Bezoar orientale Pyridoxine HCL Methyltestosterone

	Cyanocobalamin (Vitamin B12) Riboflavin (Vitamin B12)	
D	1-2 tablet daily	
A, CP, CI, AR, SC, I	Not stated	
M	Chenho Pharmaceutical Co., Ltd	
	Address	No.23, Singong Rd., Sinying City, Tainan County 730, Taiwan
	Tel	+886-6-6529311
	Fax	+886-6-6528563
	Email	Not stated
	Web	www.chenho.com.tw
Tablet	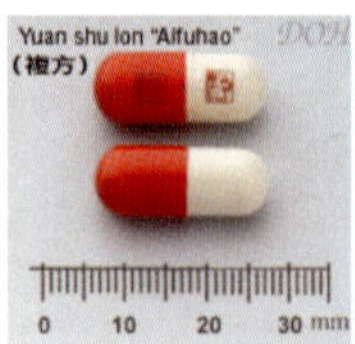 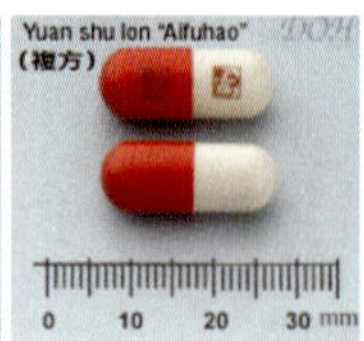 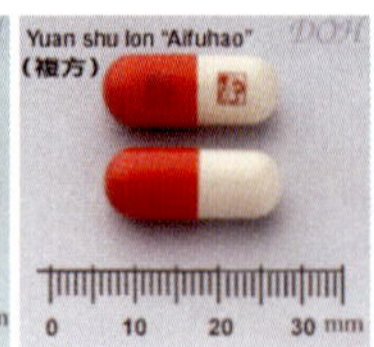 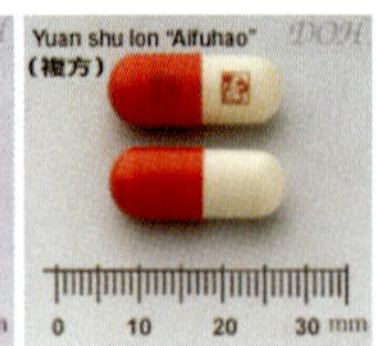	

2. Pu Ri Su Capsule Sinphar

CS	Not stated	
AA	Androgen deficiency	
T	Tablet	
S	Calcium Glycerophosphate Methyltestosterone Thiamine HCL (Thiamine chloride hydrochloride) Taurine	
D, A, CP, CI, AR, SC, I	Not stated	
M	Sinphar Pharmaceutical Co., Ltd	
	Address	5F., No.69, Dongsing Rd., Sinyi District, Taipei City 110, Taiwan
	Tel	+886-2-27603688
	Fax	+886-2-27699918
	Web	http://www.sinphar.com.tw/

3. Bouseng-P S.C. Tablets

CS	Not stated	
AA	Androgen deficiency	
T	Tablet	
S	Epimedii herba Methyltestosterone Bezoar orientale Riboflavin (Vitamin B2) Thiamine mononitrate Ginseng	
D, A, CP, CI, AR, SC, I	Not stated	
M	Shou Chan Industrial Co., Ltd	
	Address	No.27, Renhe Rd., Nantou City, Nantou County 540, Taiwan
	Tel	+886-49-2254221
	Web	http://www.shou-chan.com/

4. Honsamin

CS	Not stated	
AA	Androgen deficiency	
T	Tablet	
S	Glinseng Methyltestosterone Thiamine HCL (Thiamine chloride hydrochloride) Riboflavin (Vitamin B2) Pyridoxine HCL Caffeine anhydrous	
D, A, CP, CI, AR, SC, I	Not stated	
M	Long Shin Biopharma Co,Ltd	
	Address	No.115-1, Jiafu Village, Jiali Township, Tainan County 722, Taiwan
	Tel	+886-2-8773-0792
	Fax	+886-2-8773-3431
	Email	service@lsbiopharma.com.tw
	Web	http://www.lsbiopharma.com.tw/indromain.htm

5. Wang Lih Grnaules Shiteh

CS	Not stated	
AA	Androgen deficiency	
T	Tablet	
S	Fluoxymesterone Thiamine HCL (Thiamine chloride hydrochloride) Rutin Niacinamide (Nicotinamide) Pantothenate calcium	
D, A, CP, CI, AR, SC, I	Not stated	
M	Shiteh Organic Pharmaceutical Co., Ltd	
	Address	No.36, Ln. 560, Jhongjheng N. Rd., Sanchong City, Taipei County 241, Taiwan
	Web	http://www.shiteh.com.tw/

6. Lilipo Capsules T.L.B

CS	Not stated
AA	Decreased enegry, weak sexual finction, androgen deficiency
T	Tablet
S	Methionine dl Calcium Glycerophosphate Taurine Methyltestosterone Pyridoxine HCL Niacinamide (Nicotinamide) Riboflavin (Vitamin B2) Thiamine HCL (Thiamine chloride hydrochloride) Cyanocobalamin (Vitamin B12)
D	Once daily
A, CP	Not stated
CI	Prostate cancer, pregnancy, hepatic failure
AR	Hepatotoxicity, GI upset
SC, I	Not stated

M	Hor Chen Chem. and Pharm. Co.,Ltd.	
	Address	No.15, Gongye 10th Rd., Pingjhen City, Taoyuan County 324, Taiwan
	Tel	+886-3-4696792
	Fax	+886-3-4696964

Chapter 7 Thailand Products

Apichat Kongkanand, Kavirach Tantiwongse, Narisa Nakpairat

1. Compound Butea Superba Capsule

CS	Not stated
AA	Oral Agent for Sexual Dysfunction
T	Capsule
S, D, A, CP	Not stated
CI	Malaise Leg pain Vasodilatation flushing, skin thickening but not effective or strong enough for blood pressure change
AR, SC, I	Not stated
M	Herbal One Co., Ltd. Web www.herbalone.co.th
Package and Capsule	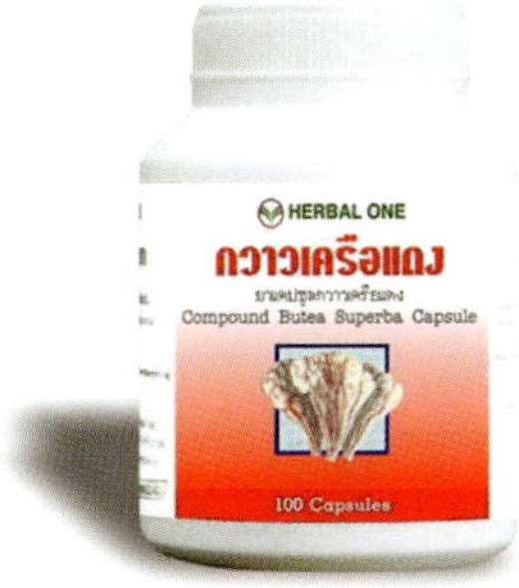 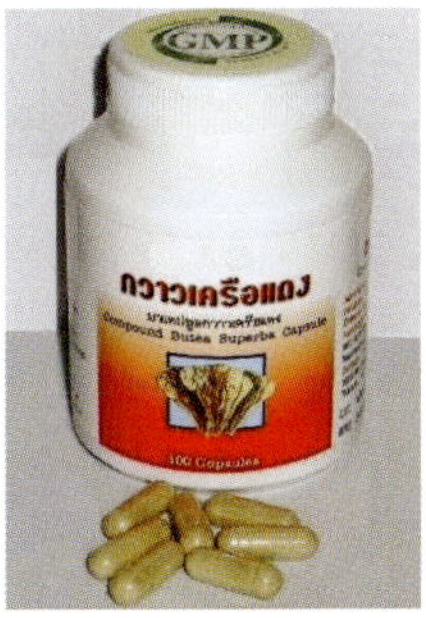

2. Joyce Tonic Capsule Formula 2

CS	Not stated	
AA	Oral Agent for Sexual Dysfunction	
T	Capsule	
S, D, A, CP, CI, AR, SC, I	Not stated	
M	JOYCE Cosmetic	
	Address	119/4 M., Soi. CHARANSANITHWONG 4 , CHARANSANITHWONG Rd., , TAIWA-CHO , ,BANGKOKYAI , Bangkok 10700
	Tel	+662-4576568
	Web	www.joycecosmetics.com
Package	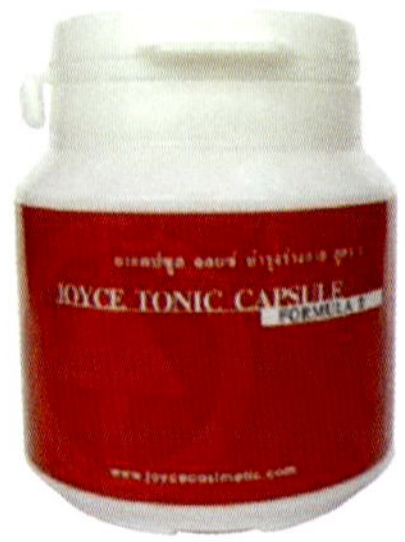	

3. Natural Plus

CS, AA	Not stated	
T	Bar soap	
S, D, A, CP, CI, AR, SC, I	Not stated	
M	TRIO INTELGATE CO.,LTD.	
	Address	Information not supplied
	Tel	+038-948770-1
	Fax	+038-865100
	Email	Information not supplied
	Web	www.triobiz.net

Package	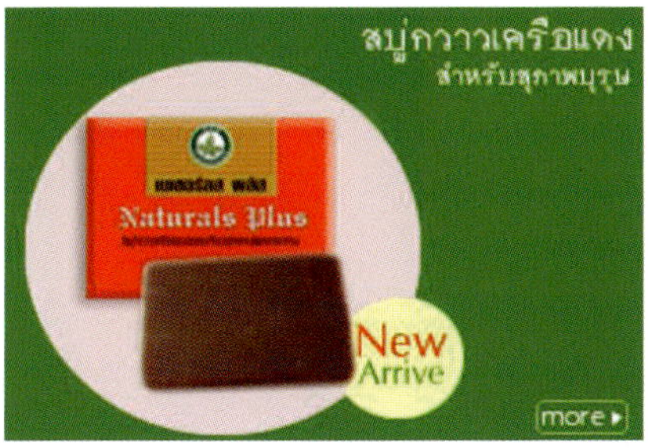

4. Compound Kaempferia parviflora Capsule

CS	Not stated
AA	For tonic, promotes vitality and stamina and reduce fatique
T	Capsule
S	100 capsules
D	Take two capsules three times a day with main meals, should be taken regularity for consistent results.
A	Not stated
CP	Always read the label, use only as directed.
CI	Not stated
AR	None noted in the literature at the recommended usage
SC, I	Not stated
M	Herbal One Co., Ltd. Web www.herbalone.co.th
Package	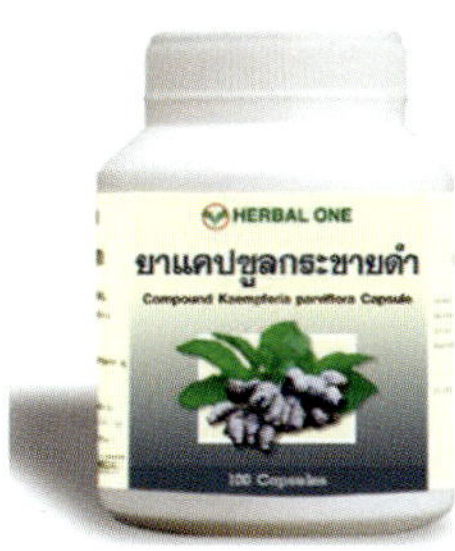

5. Khao-La-Or

CS	Not stated	
AA	Oral agent for sexual dysfunction	
T	Capsule	
S	100 capsules, 30 capsules	
D, A	Not stated	
CP	Sometimes USED for antiflatulence	
CI	Not stated	
AR	Very rare	
SC, I	Not stated	
M	Khao-La-Or Laboratories Ltd,Part	
	Address	146/22 Suksawad Rd, Samutprakarn 10290, Thailand
	Tel	+662-819-7991~5
	Fax	+662-425-8332
	Email	info@khaolaor.com
	Web	www.khaolaor.com
Package and Capsules	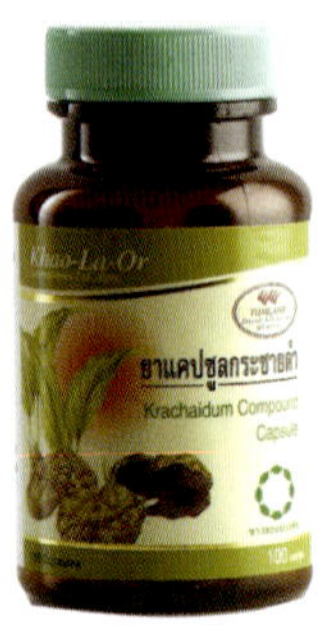 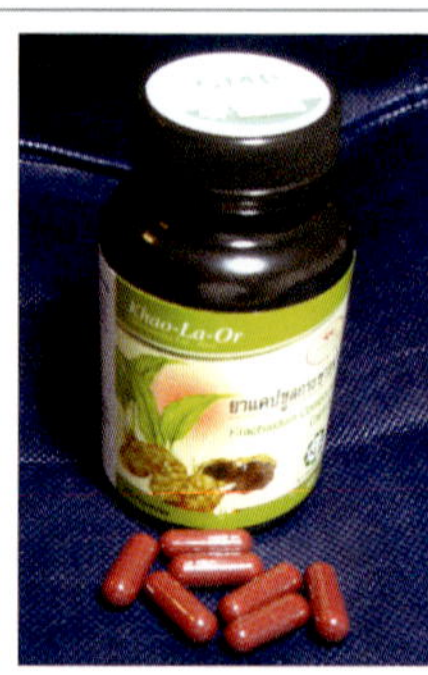	

6. Nature Zone

CS	Not stated
AA	Good Health Promotio, Sexual Health
T	roast & grind
S	150 gm.
D, A, CP, CI, AR, SC, I	Not stated
M	Nature Zone Address Bangkok 10800 Thailand Tel +662-9121115 Fax +662- -9121116 Web www.naturezoneathome.com
Package	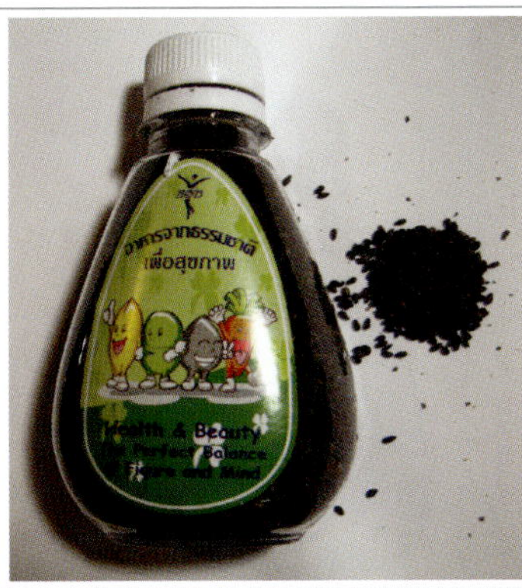

Part III

The Atlas of Medicinal Herb

Photographs and Descriptions by Jong Hee Park
Illustrations by Seung Ho Moon

Modern Oriental Phytotherapy in Sexual Medicine

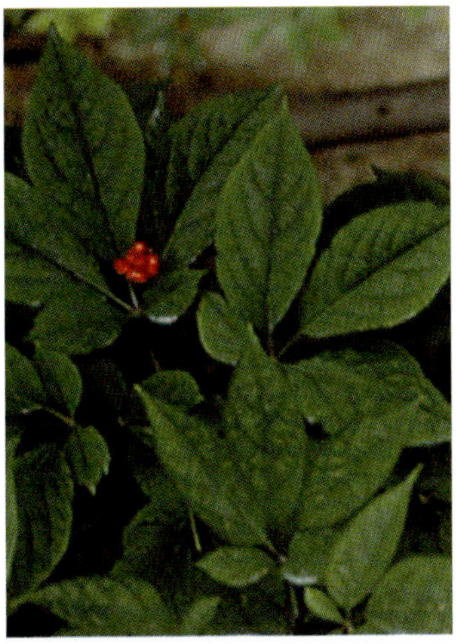

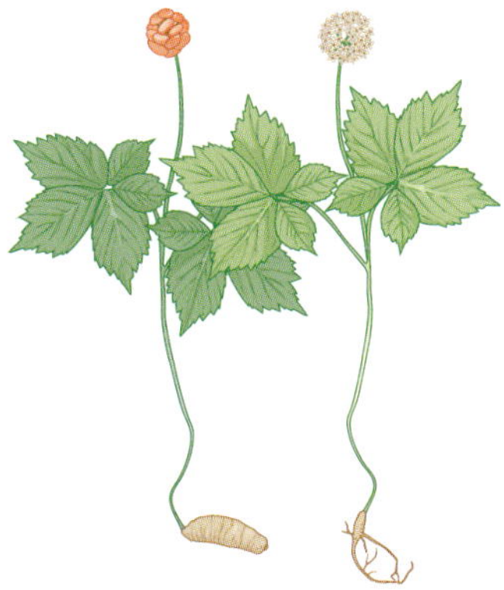

American Ginseng

- Common Names: American ginseng, Xi yang shen
- Latin Name: *Panax quinquefolius*
- Family: Araliaceae
- Parts Used: Roots
- Habitat: Eastern part of North America in the U.S.A and Canada

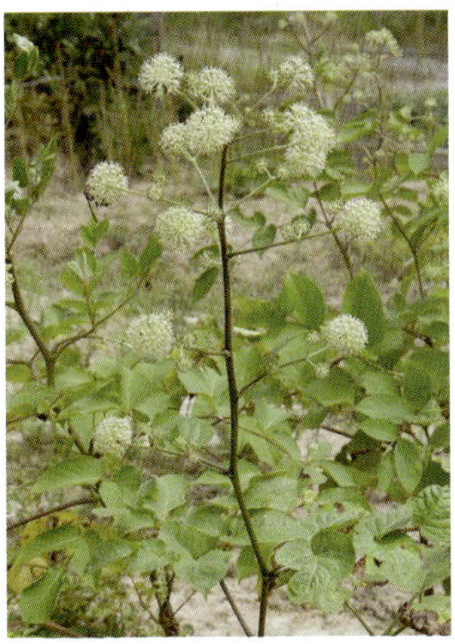

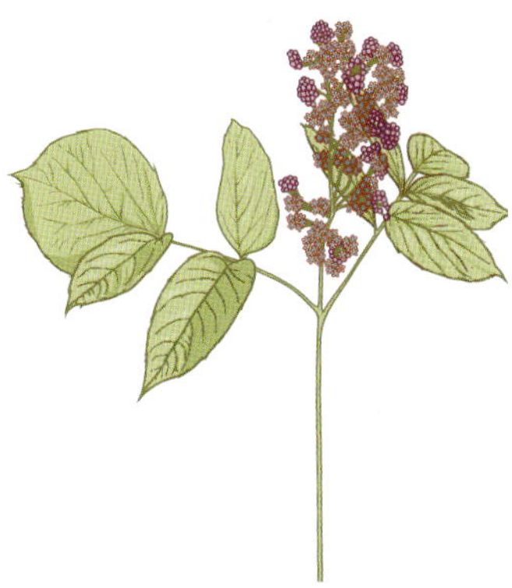

Angelica Root

- Common Names: Angelica root
- Latin Name: *Aralia continentalis*
- Family: Araliaceae
- Parts Used: Roots, Leaves and Seeds
- Habitat: Korea and China

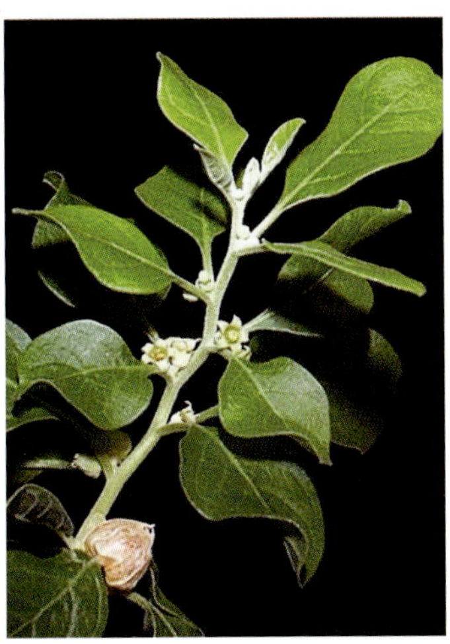

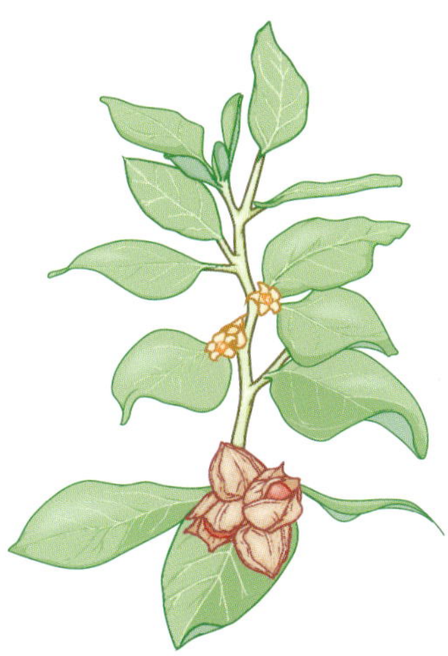

Ashwagandha

- Common Names: Ashwagandha, Winter cherry
- Latin Name: *Withania somnifera*
- Family: Solanaceae
- Parts Used: Roots, Seeds and Leaves
- Habitat: India, Africa, Mediterranean, Middle East, and around the world

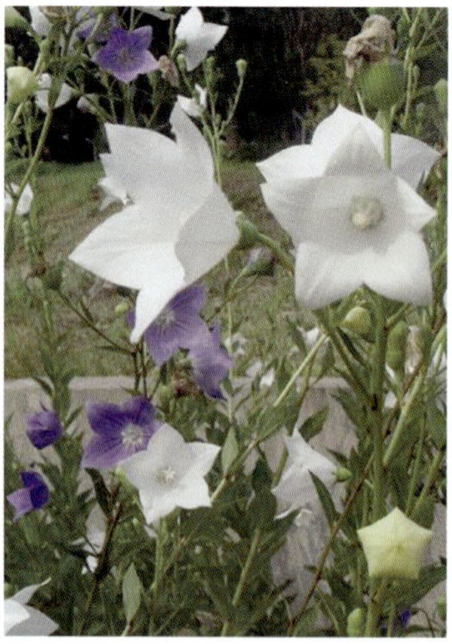
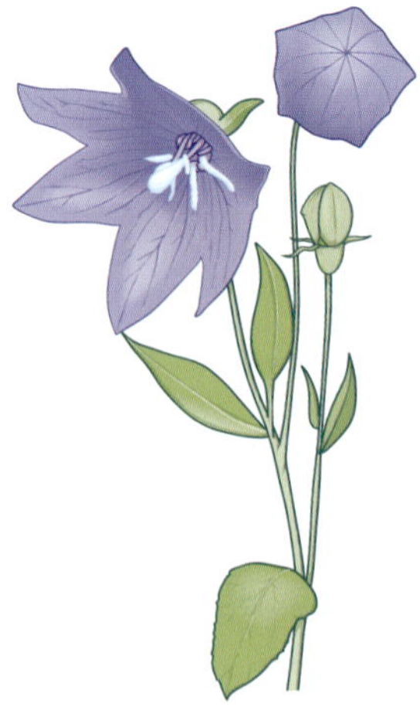

Balloon Flower

- Common Names: Balloon flower, Chinese bellflower
- Latin Name: *Platycodon glandiflorum*
- Family: Campanulaceae
- Parts Used: Roots
- Habitat: Korea, China and Japan

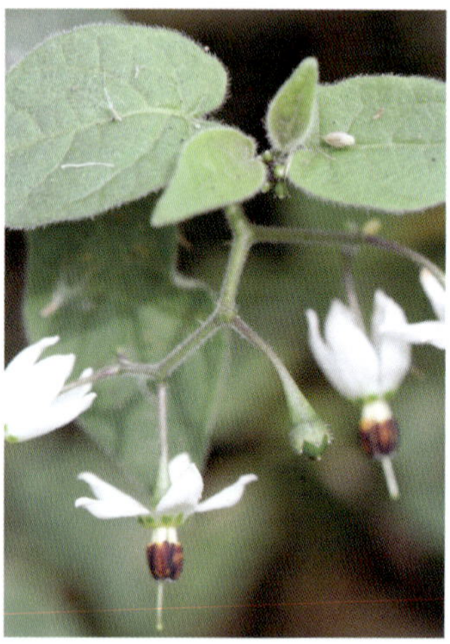
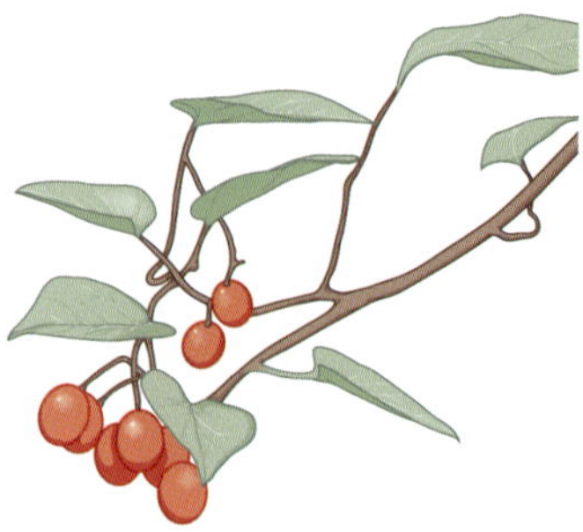

Bittersweet

- Common Names: Bittersweet
- Latin Name: *Solanum lyratum*
- Family: Solanaceae
- Parts Used: Roots and Leaves
- Habitat: Europe and Asia

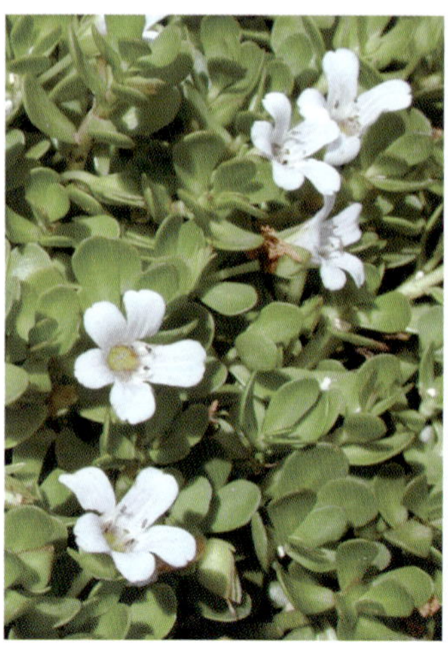
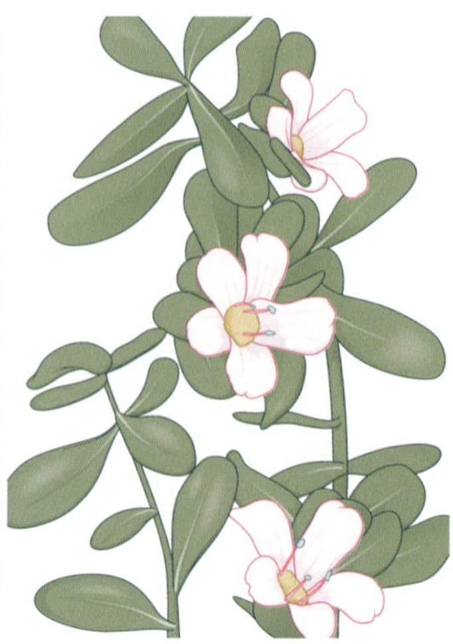

Brahmi

- Common Names: Brahmi
- Latin Name: *Bacopa monniera*
- Family: Scrophulariaceae
- Parts Used: Plants, Roots, Leaves and Stalks
- Habitat: South India

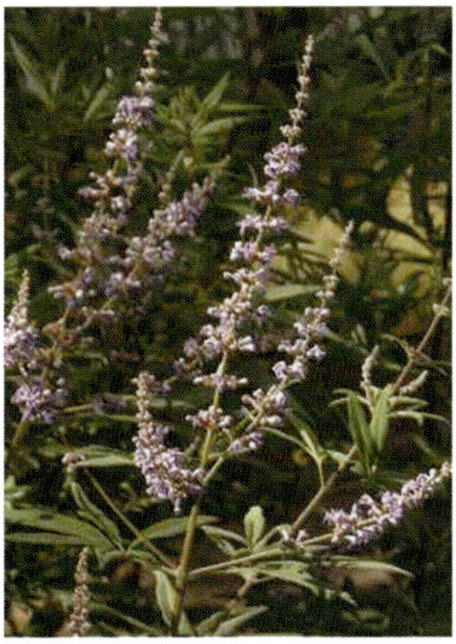

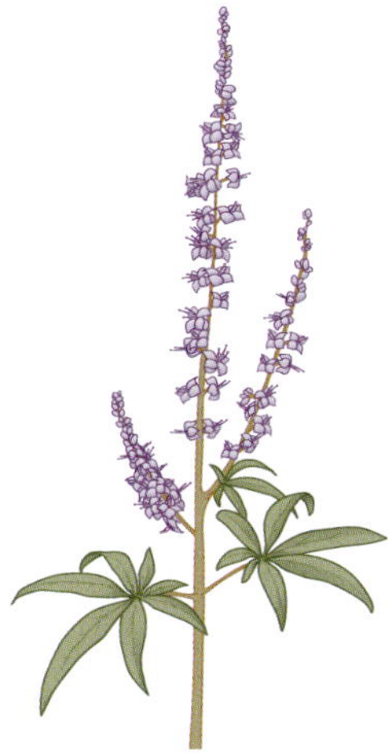

Chaste Tree

- Common Names: Chaste tree, Chaste berry, Monk' s pepper, Agnus castus
- Latin Name: *Vitex agnus-castus*
- Family: Verbenaceae
- Parts Used: Fruits
- Habitat: Native to the Mediterranean region of southern Europe and western Asia

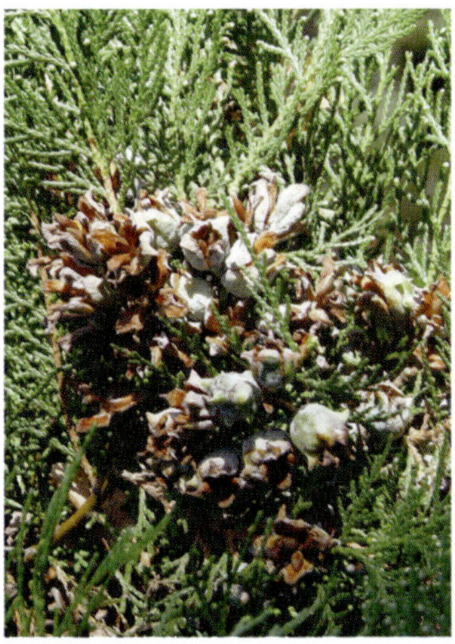

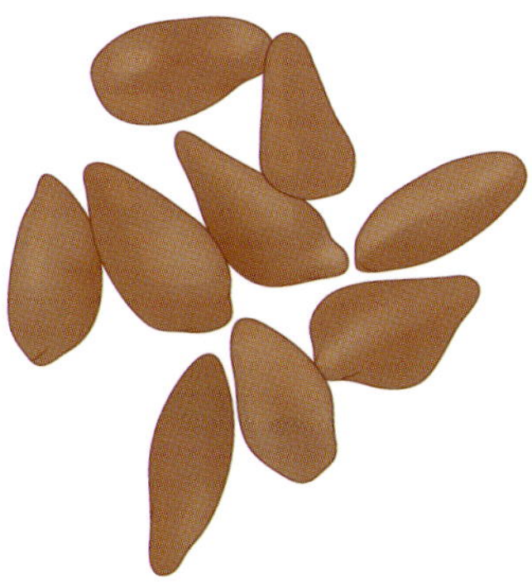

Chinese Arborvitae Kernel

- Common name: Chinese Arborvitae, Platycladus orientalis
- Latin name: *Thuja orientalis*
- Family: Cupressaceae
- Part Used: Seeds
- Habitat: China

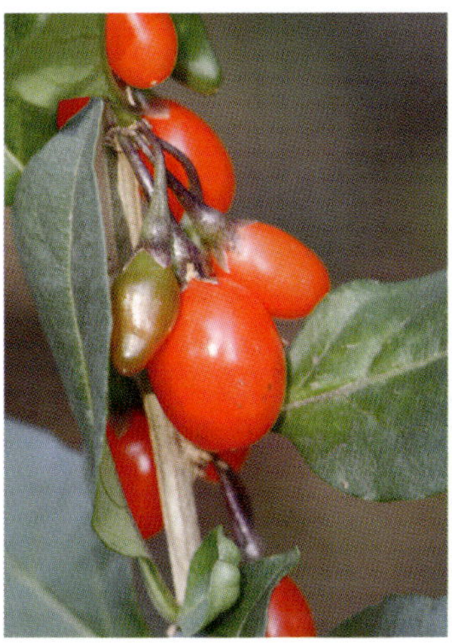

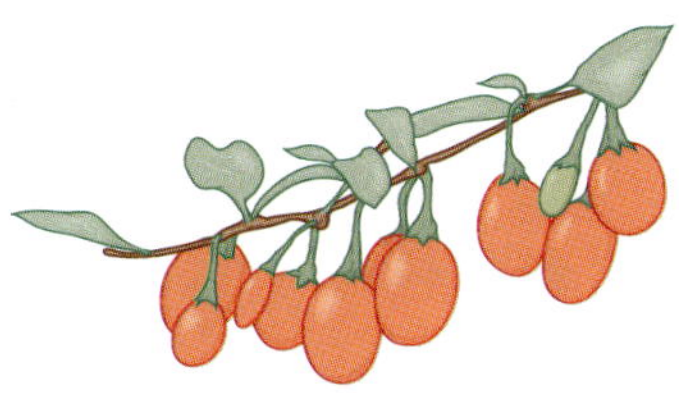

Chinese Boxthorn

- Common Names: Chinese boxthorn, Chinese desert-thorn
- Latin Name: *Lycium chinense*
- Family: Solanaceae
- Parts Used: Fruits
- Habitat: Korea, Japan, China, naturalized in Europe and United States

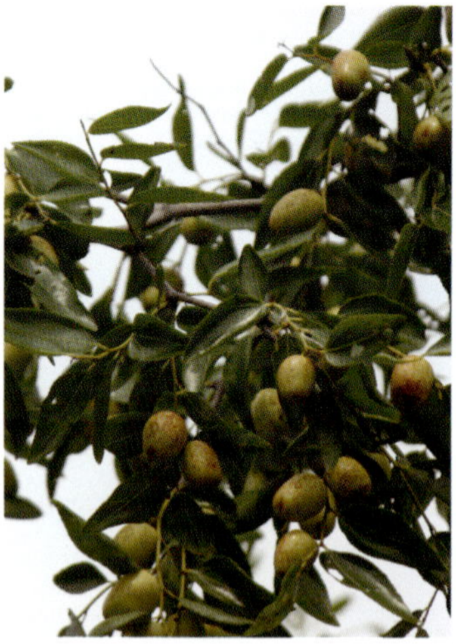

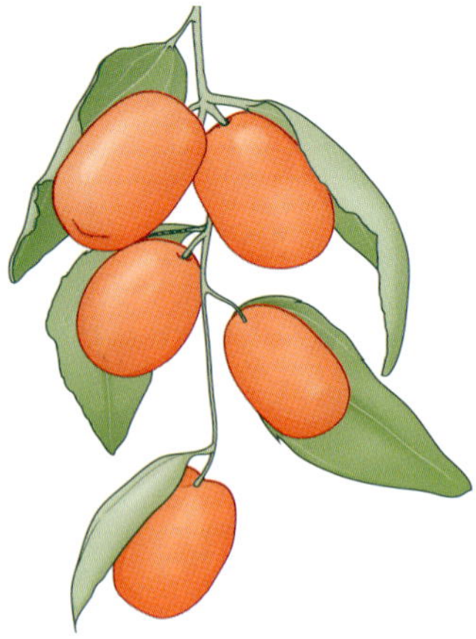

Chinese Date

- Common name: Chinese Date, Jujube
- Latin name: *Zizyphus jujuba* var. *inermis*
- Family: Rhamnaceae
- Part Used: Fruits
- Habitat: Korea, China, Japan, India, Afghanistan and Malaysia

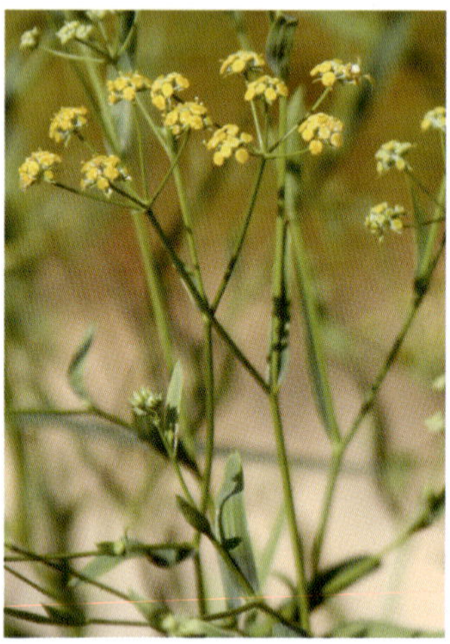

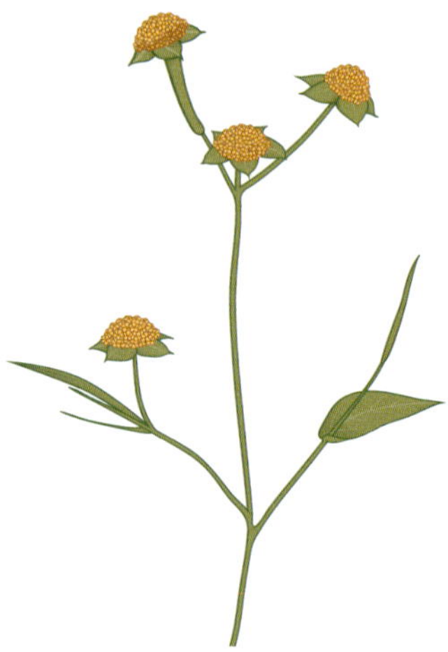

Chinese Thorowax

- Common name: Chinese Thorowax
- Latin name: *Bupleurum falcatum*
- Family: Umbelliferae
- Part Used: Roots
- Habitat: Korea, China and Japan

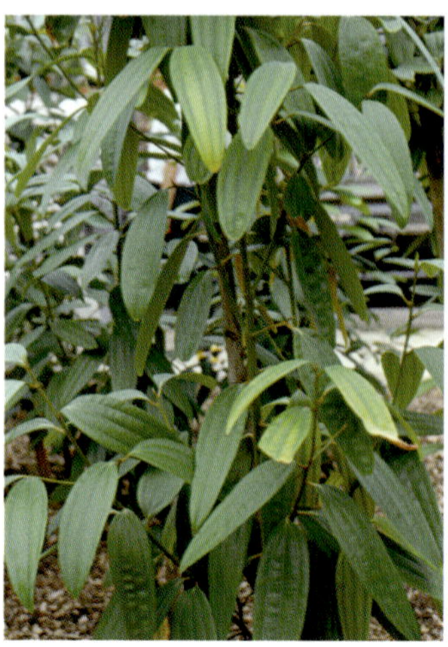

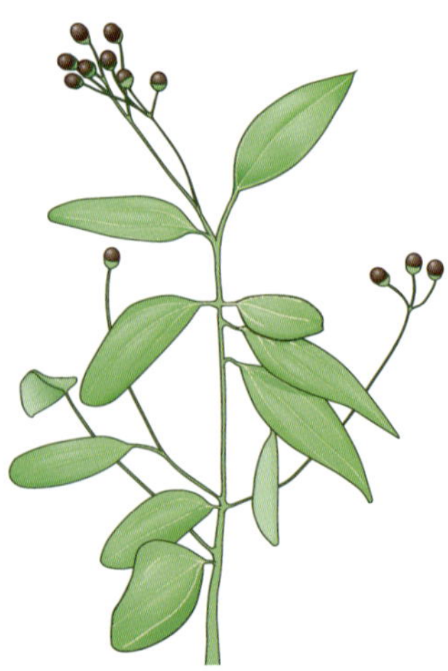

Cinnamon Tree

- Common name: Cinnamon Tree, Cassia Bark
- Latin name: *Cinnamomum cassia*
- Family: Lauraceae
- Part Used: Barks and Leaves
- Habitat: Burma, India, South China and Sri Lanka

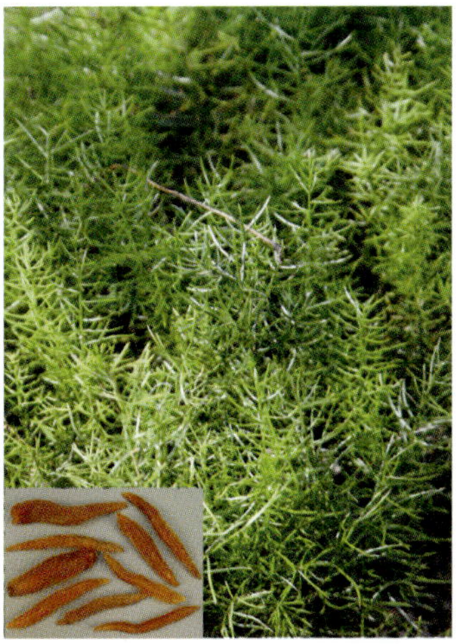

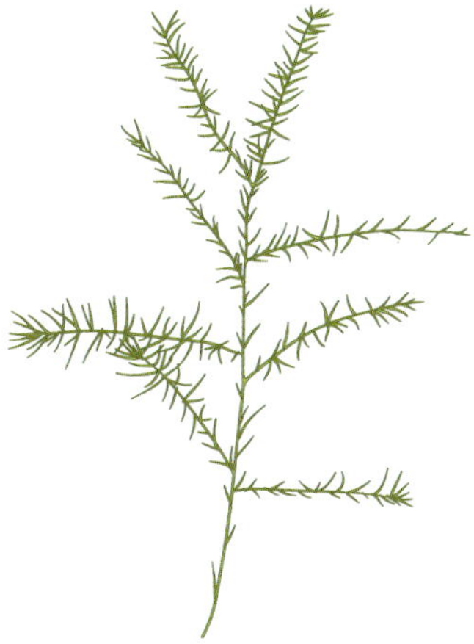

Cochinchinese Aspargus Root

- Common name: Cochinchinese Aspargus Root
- Latin name: *Asparagus lucidus*
- Family: Liliaceae
- Part Used: Roots
- Habitat: Korea, China, Japan, Laos and Viet Nam

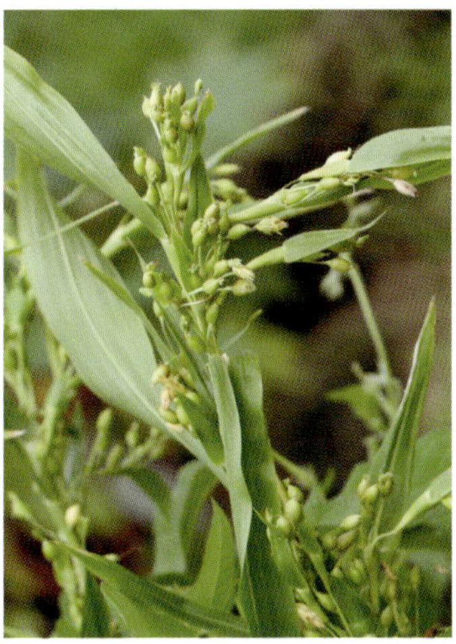

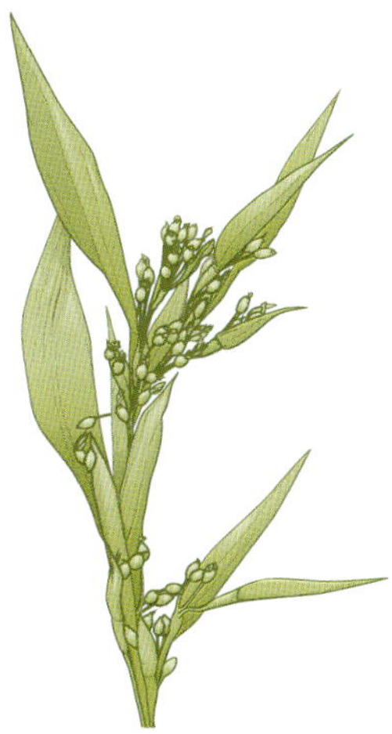

Coix Seed

- Common name: Coix Seed
- Latin name: *Coix lachyma-jobi var. mayuen*
- Family: Gramineae
- Part Used: Dried Seeds
- Habitat: South east Asia, Taiwan and Mainland China

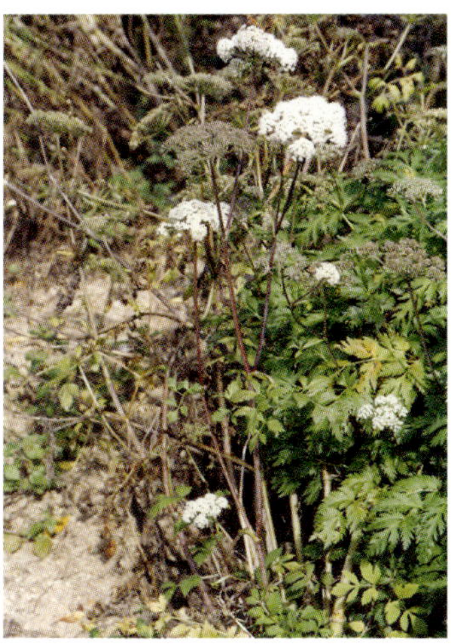

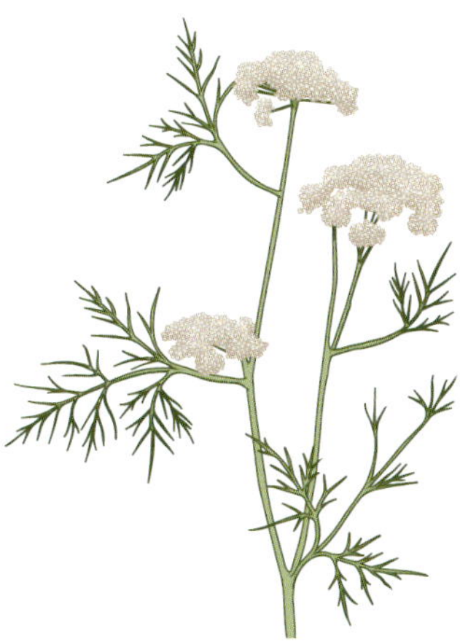

Common Cnidium Fruit

- Common name: Common Cnidium Fruit
- Latin name: *Torilidis japonica(Korea, Japan), Cindium monnieri(China)*
- Family: Umbelliferae
- Part Used: Fruits
- Habitat: Korea, China and Japan

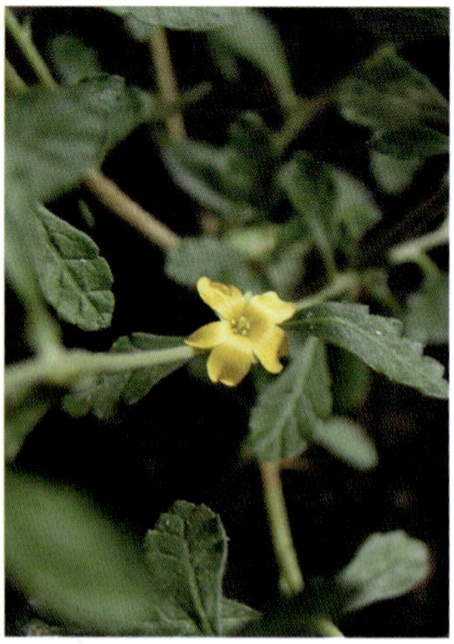

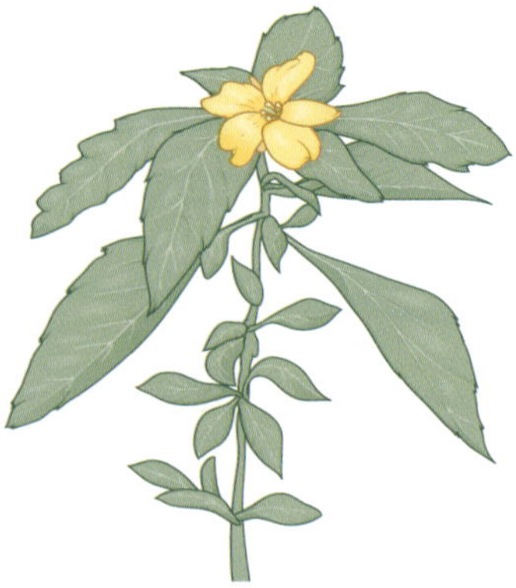

Damiana

- Common Names: Damiana
- Latin Name: *Turnera diffusa var. aphrodisiaca*
- Family: Turneraceae
- Parts Used: Dried leaves and Stems
- Habitat: Southern USA, Mexico and parts of sub-tropical America and Africa

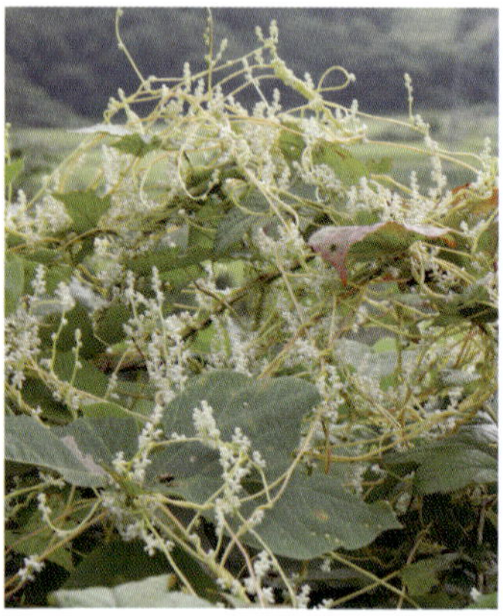

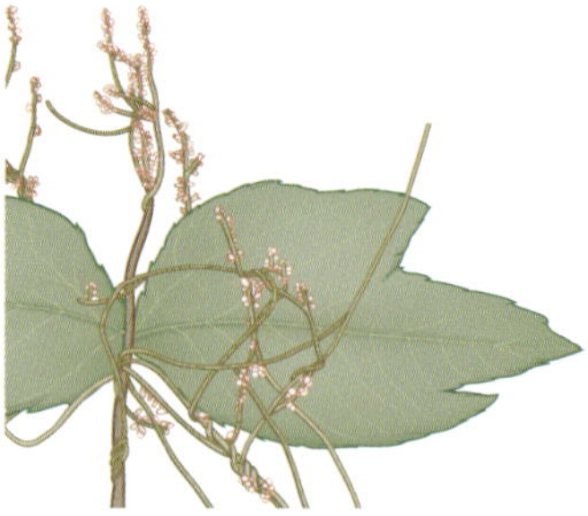

Dodder Seed

- Common name: Cuscuta seed, Chinese dodder seed
- Latin name: *Cuscuta chinensis*
- Family: Convolvulaceae
- Part Used: Seeds
- Habitat: Asia, Europe and Southern Africa

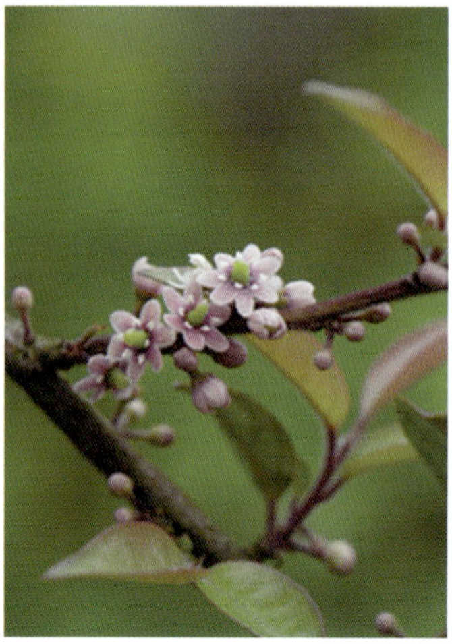

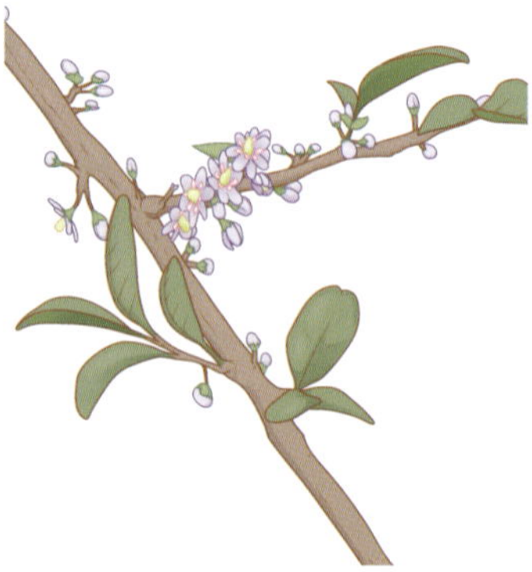

Downy Holly

- Common Names: Downy Holly
- Latin Name: *Ilex pubescens*
- Family: Aquifoliaceae
- Parts Used: Roots
- Habitat: Southern China

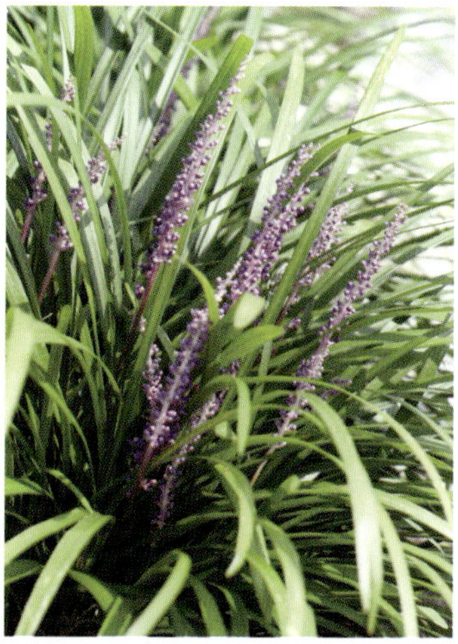

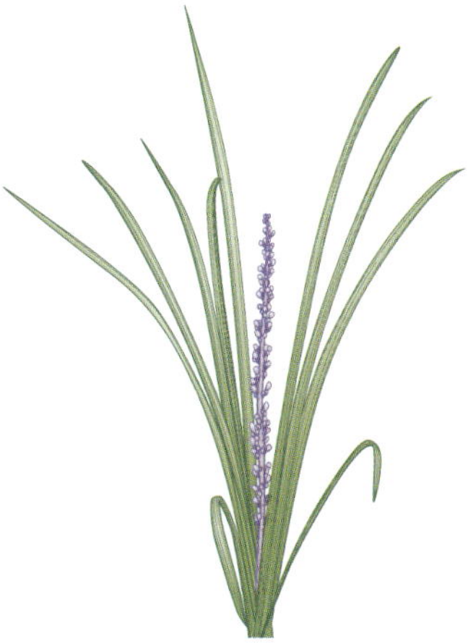

Dwarf Lilyturf Tuber

- Common name: Ophiopogon root(China, Japan), Liliepe(Korea), Lilyturf root, Dwarf Mondo Grass, Dwarf Monkey Grass, Dwarf Lilyturf, Ophiopogon Root, Ophiopogonis Radix
- Latin name: *Liriope platyphylla (Korea), Ophiopogon japonicus (Japan, China)*
- Family: Liliaceae
- Part Used: Tubers
- Habitat: Korea, China and Japan

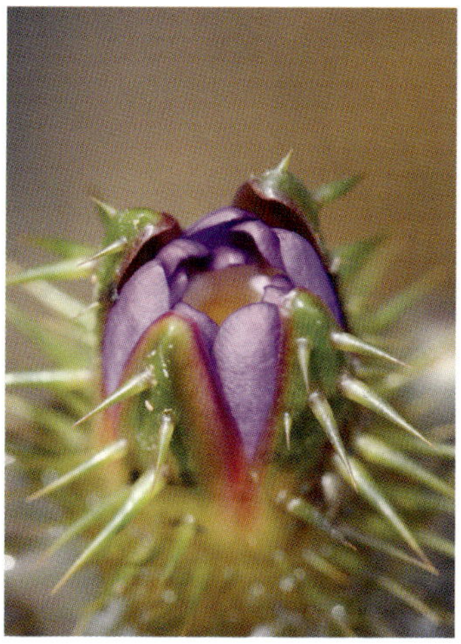

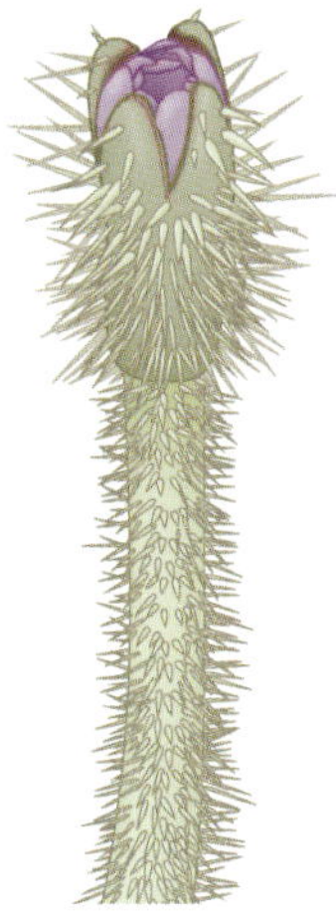

Euryale Seeds

- Common name: Prickly lily seed, Euryale seeds, Foxnut
- Latin name: *Euryale ferox*
- Family: Euryalaceae
- Part Used: Seeds
- Habitat: Korea, China, Japan and India

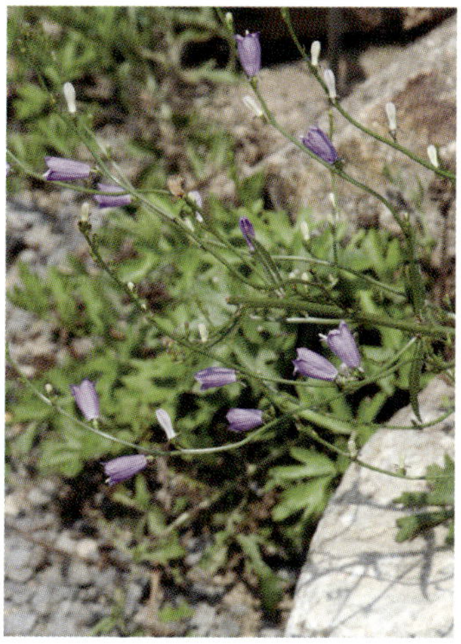

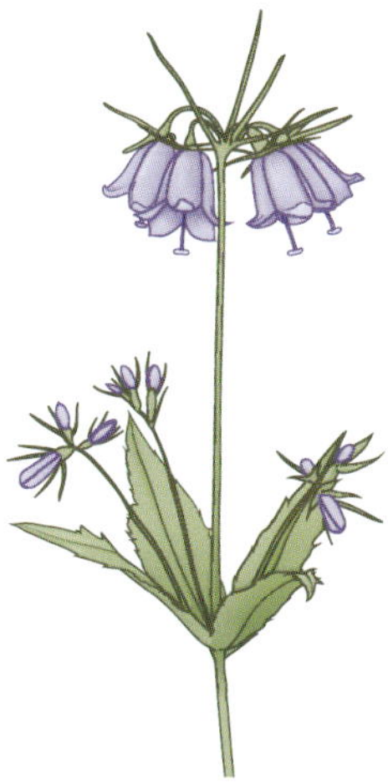

Fourleaf Ladybell

- Common name: Fourleaf Ladybell
- Latin name: *Adenophora triphylla*
- Family: Campanulaceae
- Part Used: Dried Roots
- Habitat: Korea and China

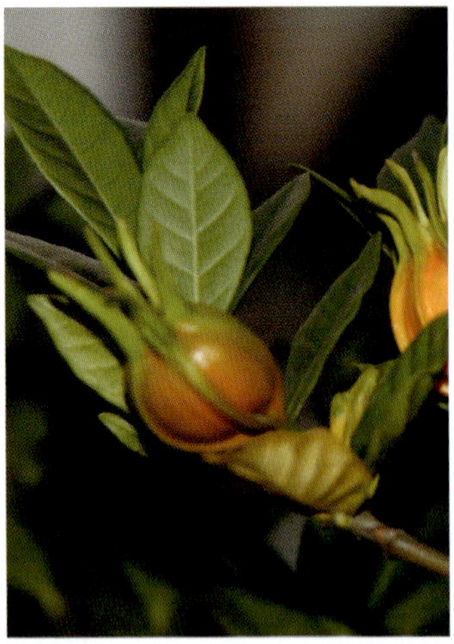

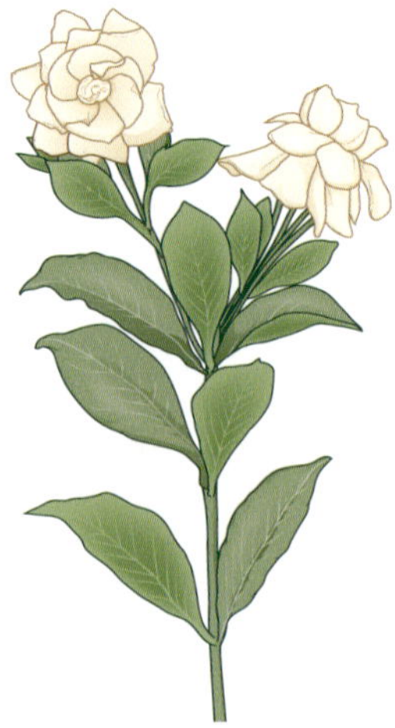

Gardenia

- Common Names: Gardenia
- Latin Name: *Gardenia jasminoides*
- Family: Rubiaceae
- Parts Used: Fruits
- Habitat: Korea, China, Northern India and Persia

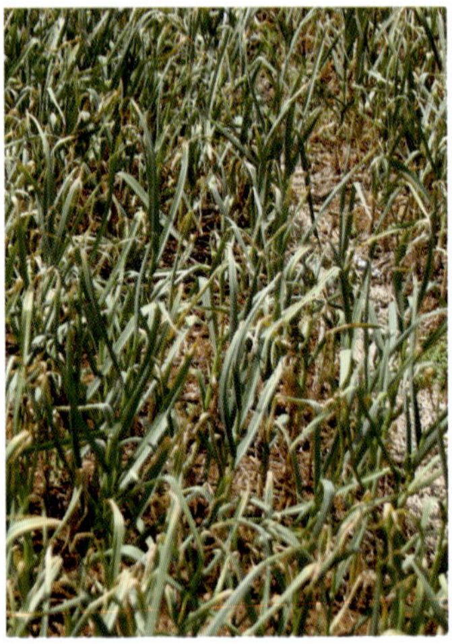

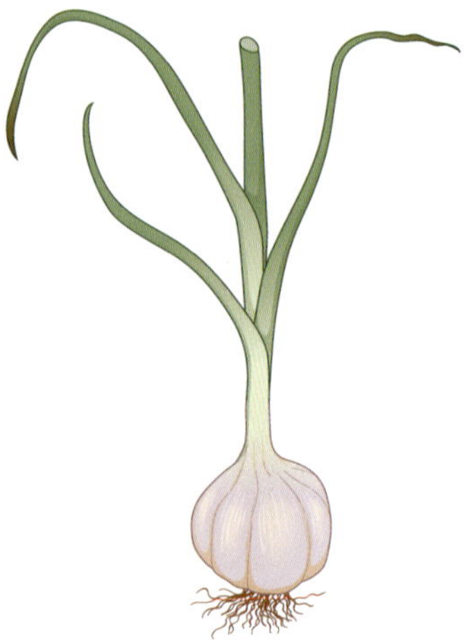

Garlic

- Common Names: Garlic
- Latin Name: *Allium sativum var. pekinense*
- Family: Alliaceae
- Parts Used: Bulbs
- Habitat: Asia and Southern Europe

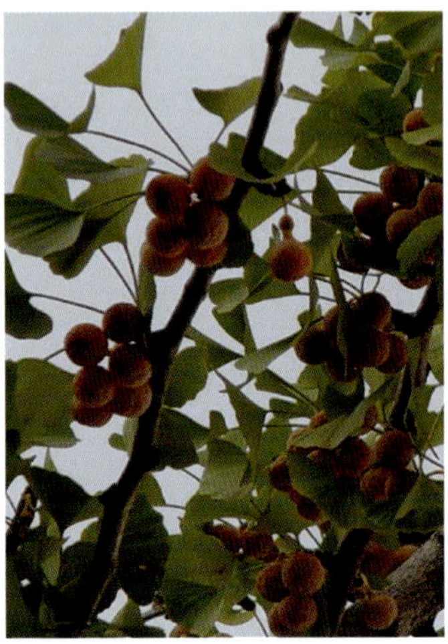

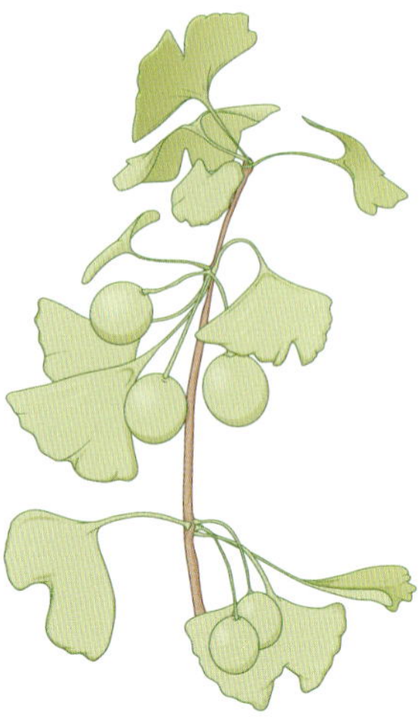

Ginko

- Common Names: Ginko, maidenhair tree, *yin-hsing*, *bao gou*(female seeds)
- Latin Name: *Ginko biloba*
- Family: Ginkgoaceae
- Parts Used: Leaves and Seeds
- Habitat: Korea, China, Japan, France and Southeastern United States

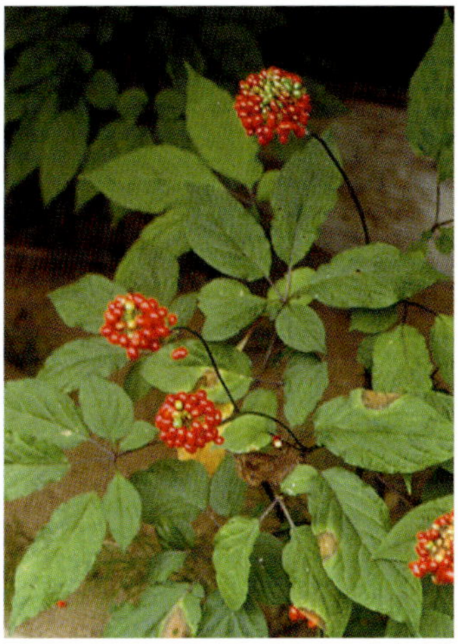

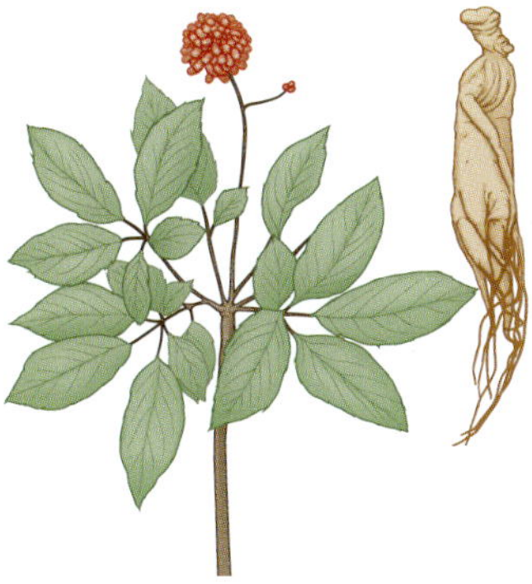

Ginseng

- Common name: Ginseng, Korean Ginseng, Asian Ginseng
- Latin name: *Panax ginseng*
- Family: Araliaceae
- Part Used: Roots, Leaves
- Habitat: Korea, China and Japan

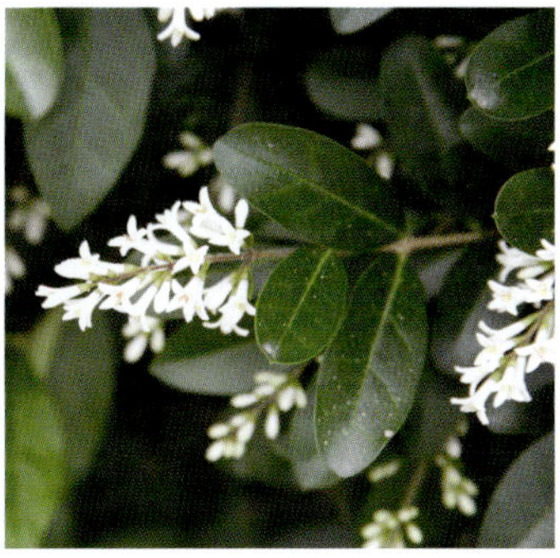

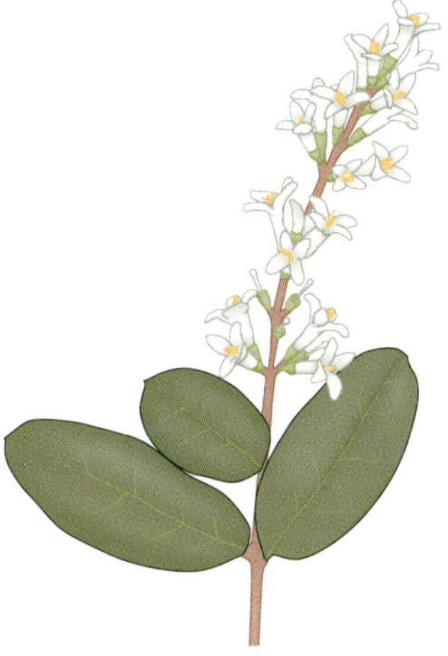

Glossy Privet Fruit

- Common name: Glossy Privet Fruit
- Latin name: *Ligustrum lucidum*
- Family: Oleaceae
- Part Used: Fruits
- Habitat: Korea, China and Japan

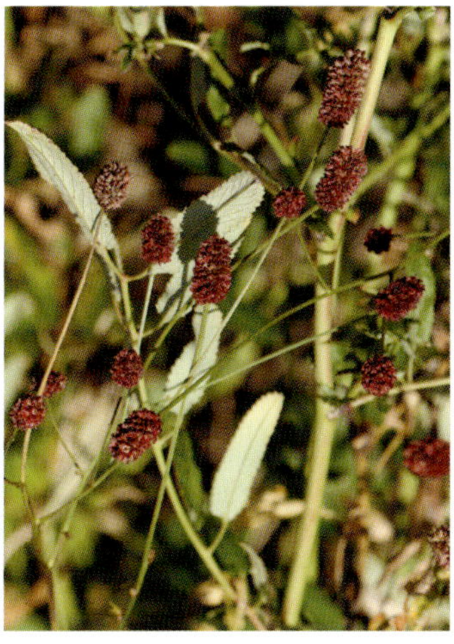

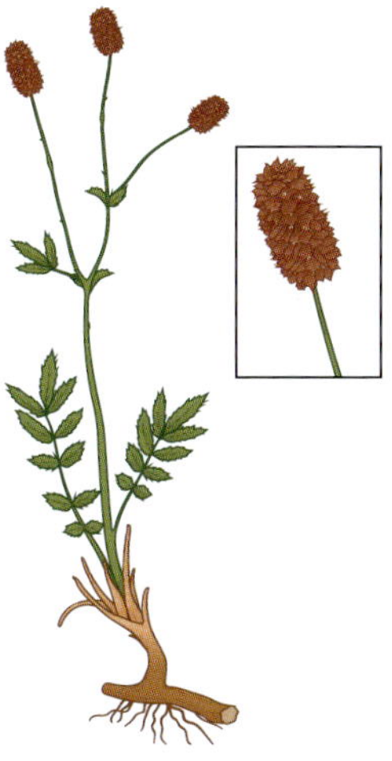

Great Burnet

- Common Names: Great Burnet
- Latin Name: *Sanguisorba officinalis*
- Family: Rosaceae
- Parts Used: Roots
- Habitat: Korea, China and Japan

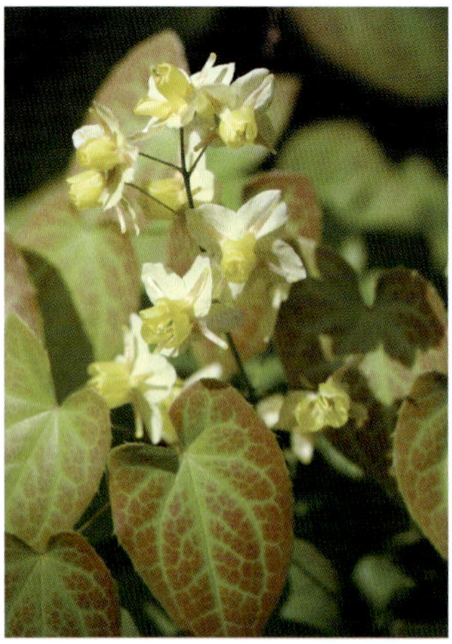

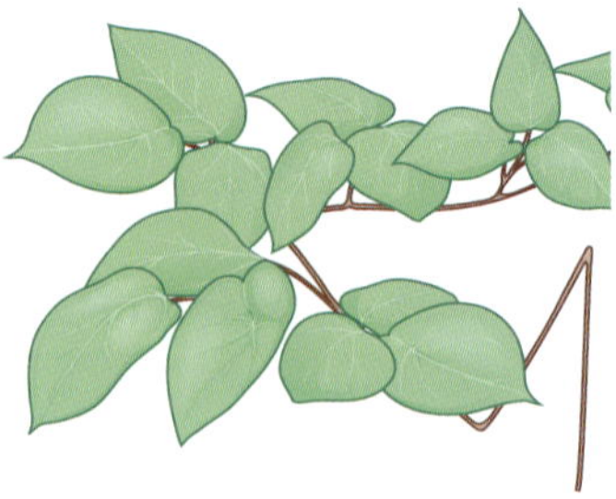

Horny Goat Weed

- Common Names: Horny Goat Weed
- Latin Name: *Epimedium Koreanum, Epimedium sagittatum*
- Family: Berberidaceae
- Parts Used: Whole plants
- Habitat: Korea, China and Japan

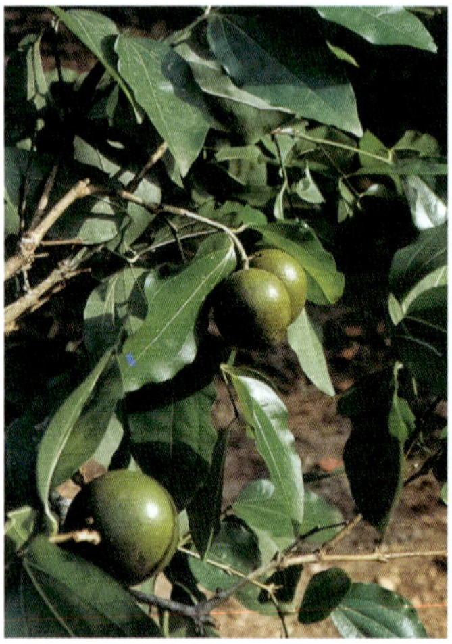

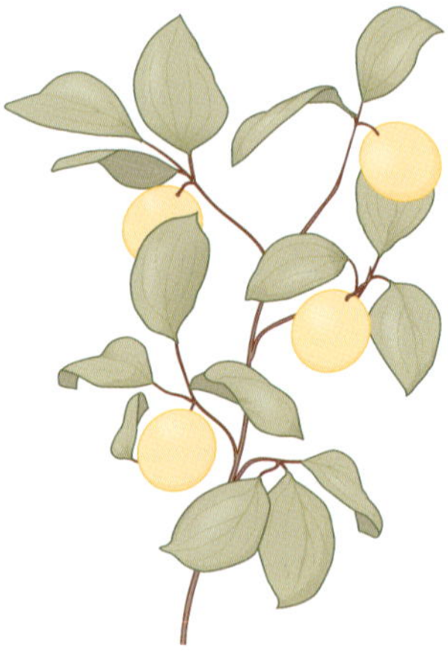

Ignatius Bean

- Common Names: Ignatius bean, St. Ignatius bean, *Kkatbalonga, Ffaba ignatii*, Poison nut
- Latin Name: *Strychnos nux-vomica*
- Family: Loganiaceae
- Parts Used: Seeds
- Habitat: Southeast Asia, Philippines and Vietnam.

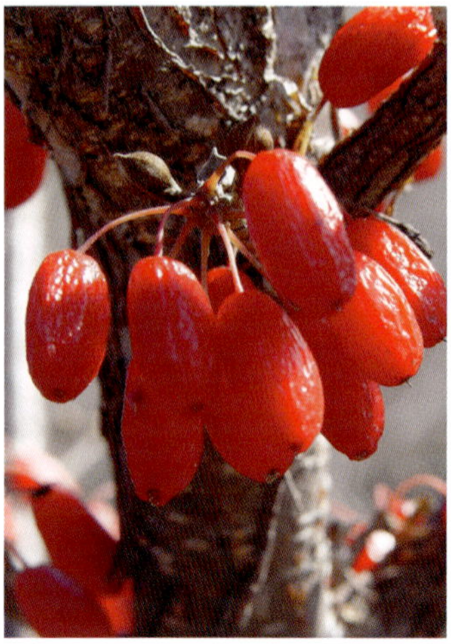

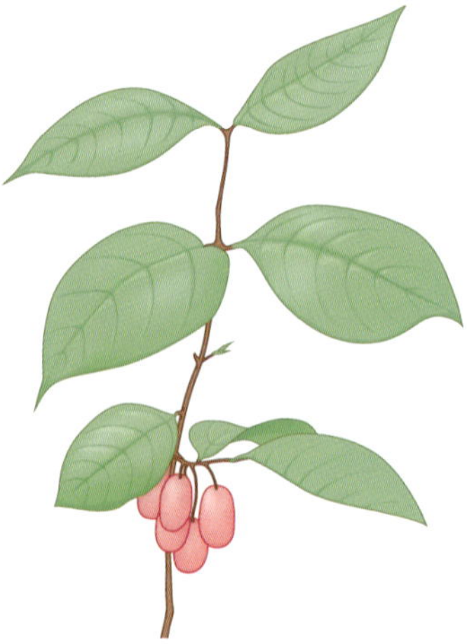

Japanese Cornel Dogwood

- Common Names: Japanese Cornel Dogwood
- Latin Name: *Cornus officinalis*
- Family: Cornaceae
- Parts Used: Fruits
- Habitat: Korea, China and Japan

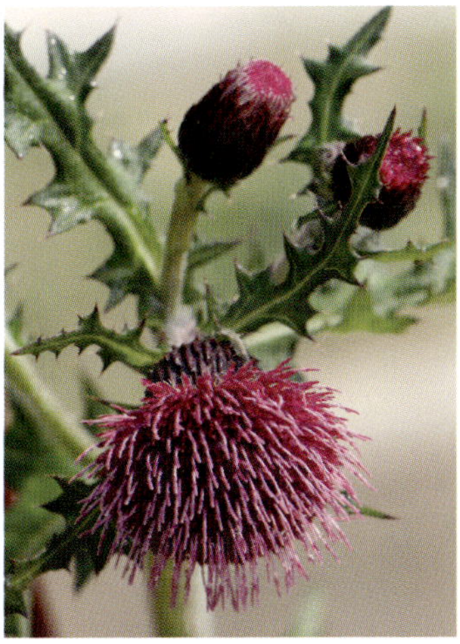

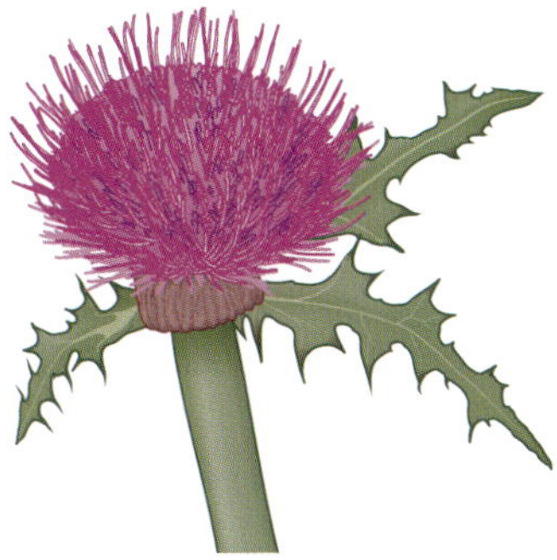

Japanese Thistle

- Common name: Japanese Thistle
- Latin name: *Cirsium japonicum*
- Family: Compositae
- Part Used: Dried roots
- Habitat: Korea, China and Japan

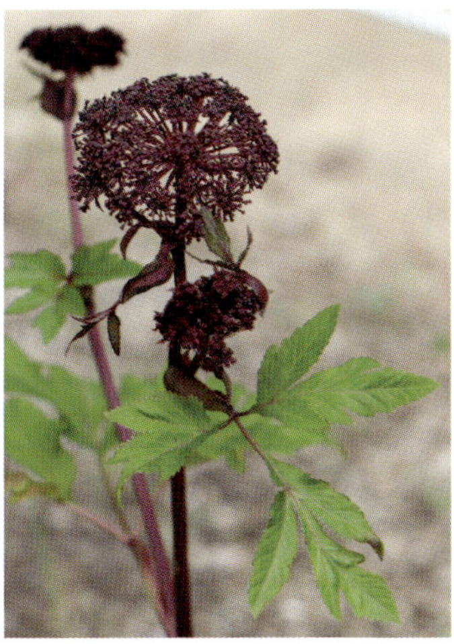

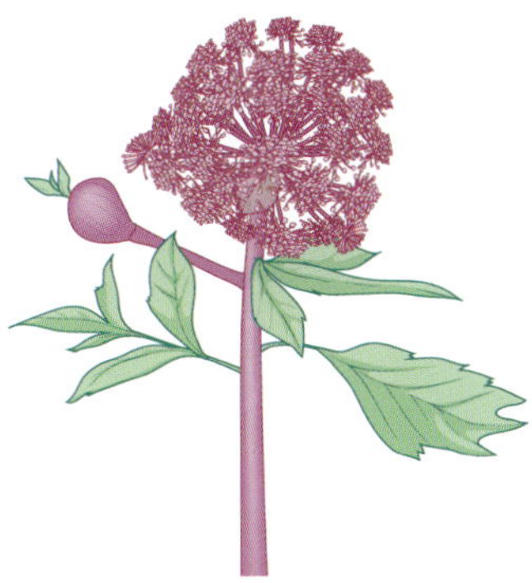

Korean Angelica

- Common name: Korean angelica
- Latin name: *Angelica gigas*
- Family: Umbelliferae
- Part Used: Dried roots
- Habitat: Korea and northern China

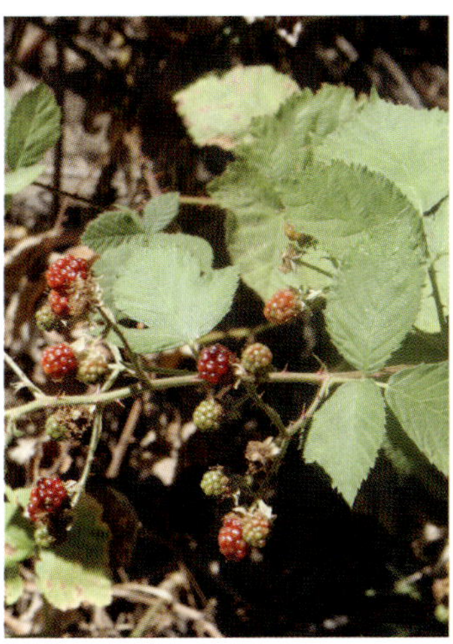

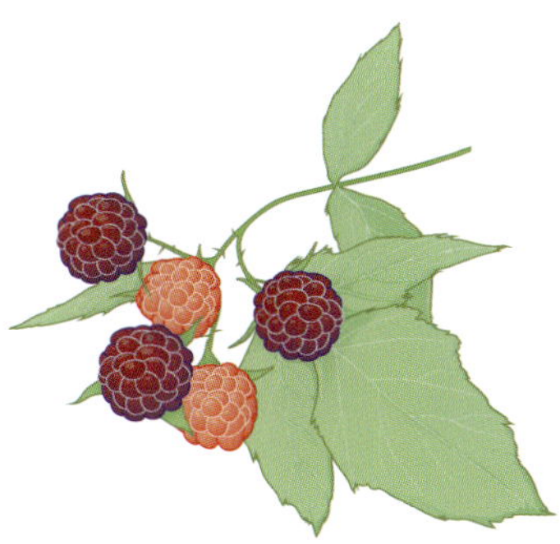

Korean Black Raspberry

- Common Names: Korean Black raspberry, Korean bramble
- Latin Name: *Rubus coreanus*
- Family: Rosaceae
- Parts Used: Fruits
- Habitat: Korea

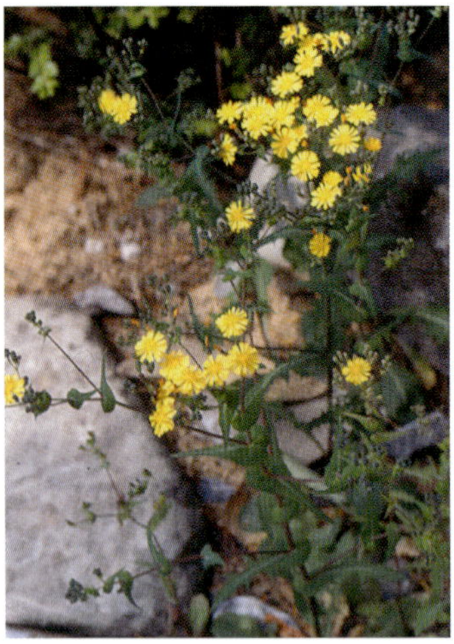
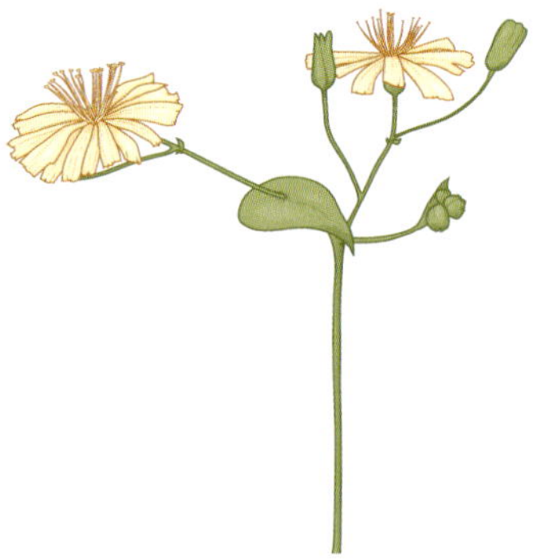

Korean Lettuce

- Common Names: Korean lettuce
- Latin Name: *Ixeris sonchifolia*
- Family: Compositae
- Parts Used: Leaves
- Habitat: Korea, China and Japan

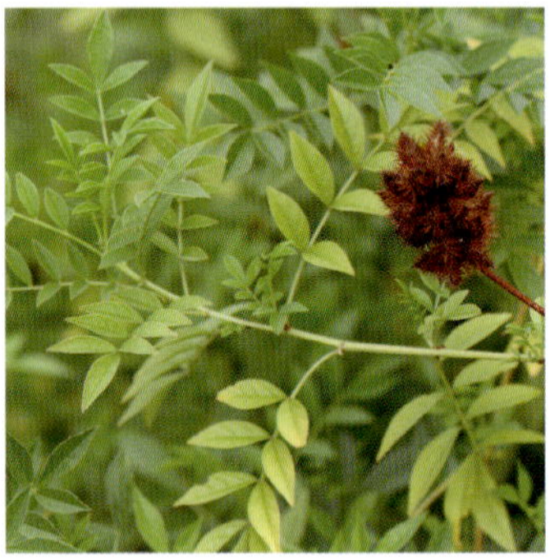
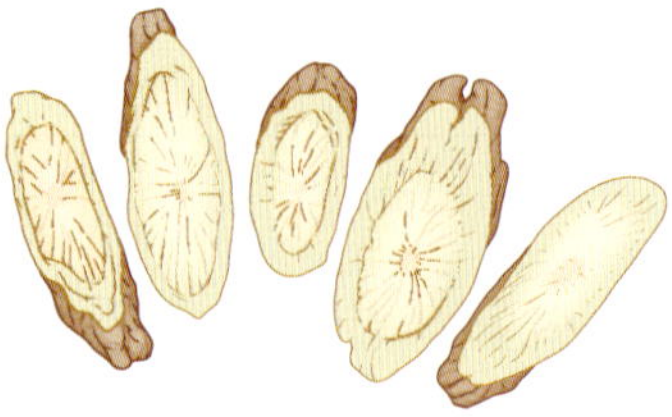

Liquorice Root

- Common name: Liquorice Root
- Latin name: *Glycyrrhiza glabra* var. *glandulifera*
- Family: Leguminosae
- Part Used: Dried roots and Stolons
- Habitat: China, Mongolia and Afghanistan

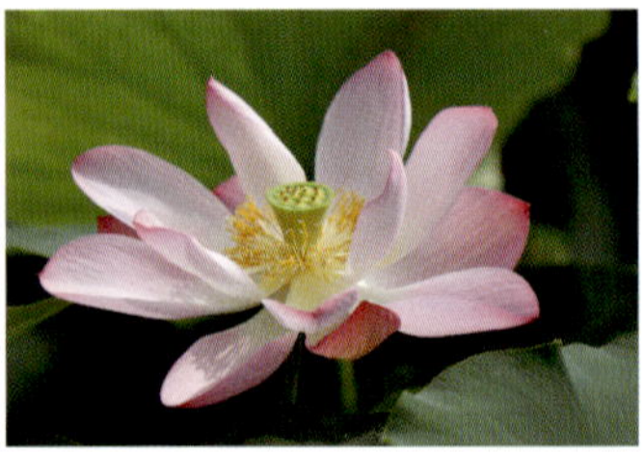
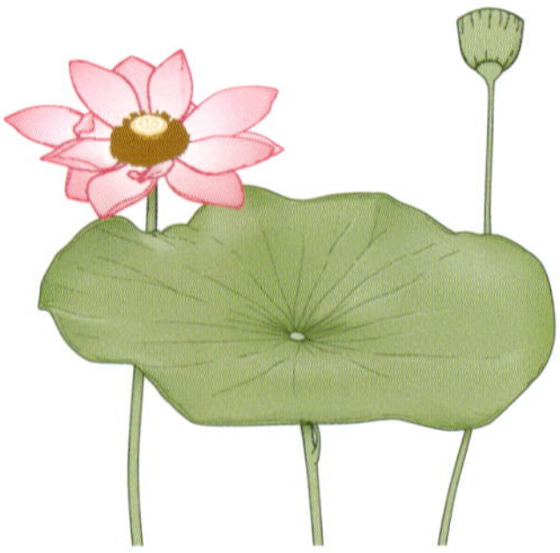

Lotus

- Common name: Lotus, Sacred lotus, East Indian Lotus
- Latin name: *Nelumbo nucifera*
- Family: Nelumbonaceae
- Part Used: Flower Petals, Seeds, Leaves and Roots
- Habitat: Korea, China, Japan and India

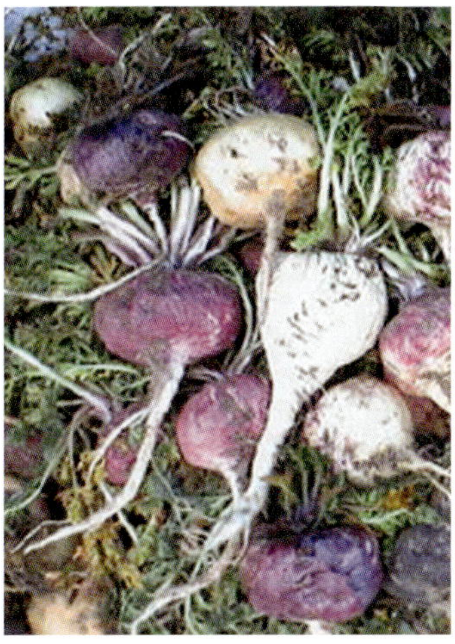

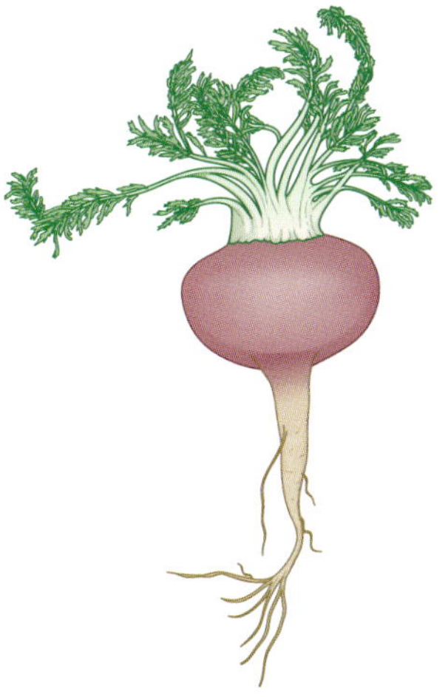

Maca

- Common Names: Maca, Peruvian ginseng, maka, Mace, Maca-maca, Maino, Ayak chichira, Ayuk willku, Pepperweed
- Latin Name: *Lepidium meyenii*
- Family: Brassicaceae
- Part Used: Roots
- Habitat: High Andes of Peru

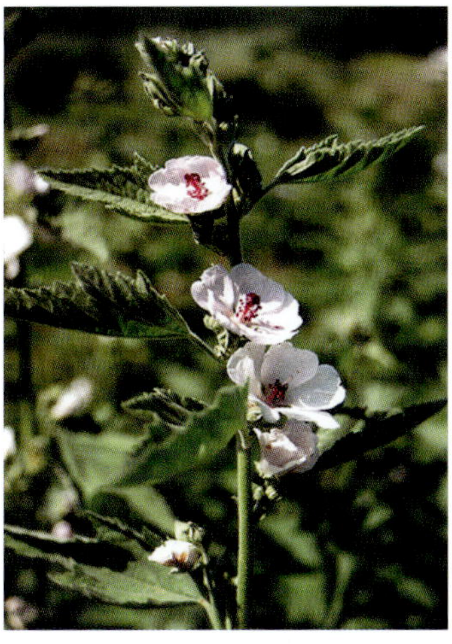

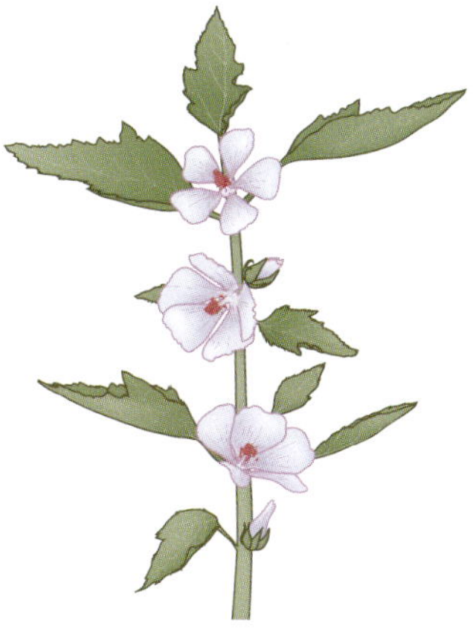

Marshmallow

- Common Names: Marshmallow, White mallow, Althaea, Althea
- Latin Name: *Althaea officinalis*
- Family: Malvaceae
- Parts Used: Roots, Leaves and Flowers
- Habitat: Europe and western Asia

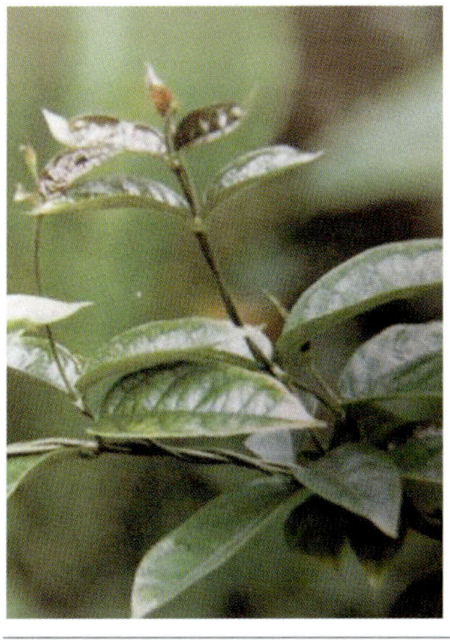

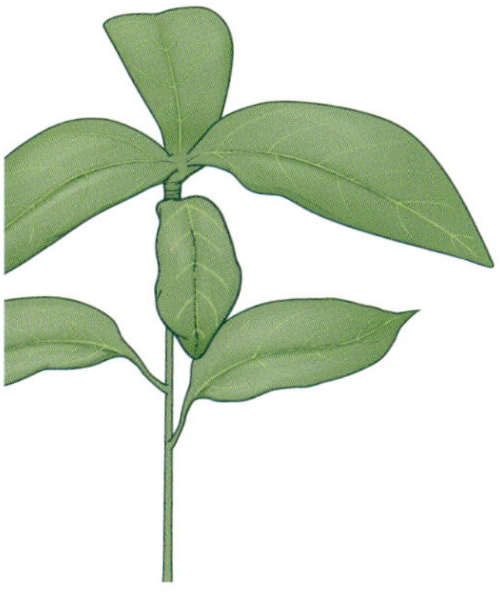

Morinda

- Common Names: Morinda, Morinda Root
- Latin Name: *Morinda officinalis*
- Family: Rubiaceae
- Parts Used: Roots
- Habitat: North Viet Nam

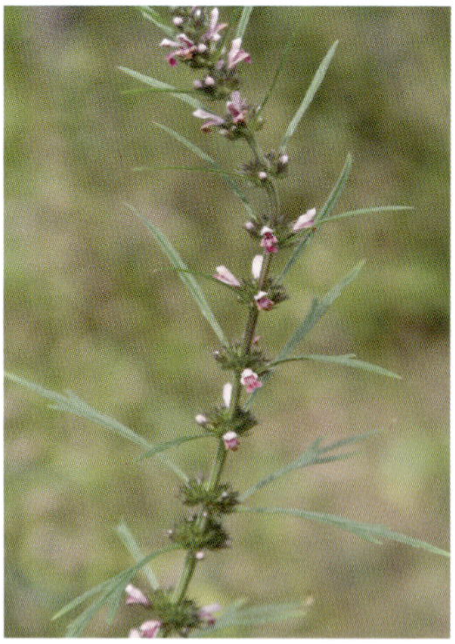

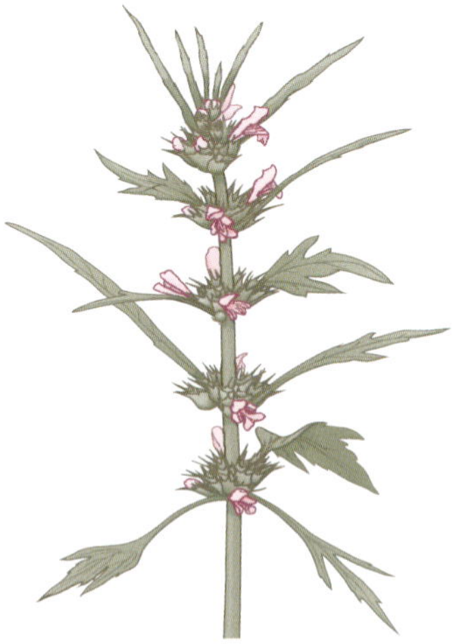

Motherwort Herb

- Common name: Motherwort, Common motherwort, Lion's tail, Lion's tart, Lion's ear, Throwwort, Roman motherwort, Throw-wort, Agripalma, Aslankuyrugu, Hartgespan
- Latin name: *Leonurus japonicus*
- Family: Labiatae
- Part Used: Aerial parts
- Habitat: Korea, China, Japan and northeast Asia

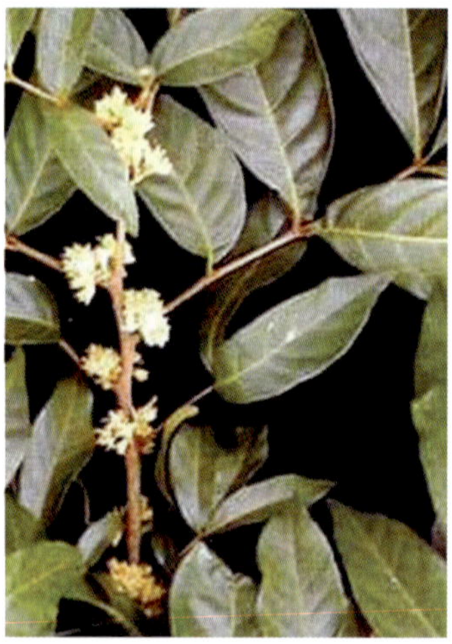

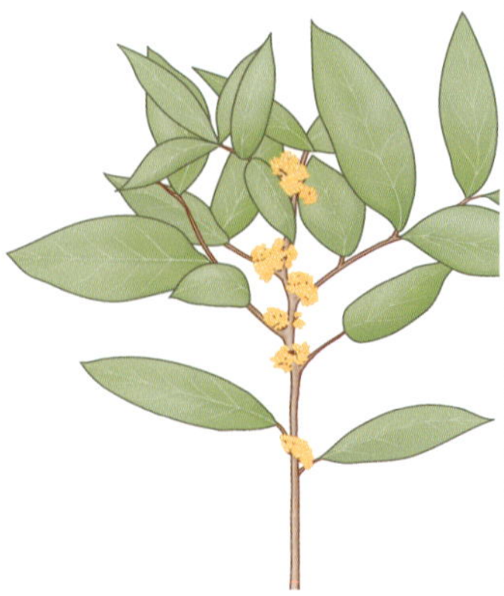

Muira Puama

- Common Names: Muira Puama, Marapuama, Marapama, Potency Wood, Potenzholz
- Latin Name: *Liriosma ovata*
- Family: Olacaceae
- Parts Used: Roots and Barks
- Habitat: Amazon region of Brazil

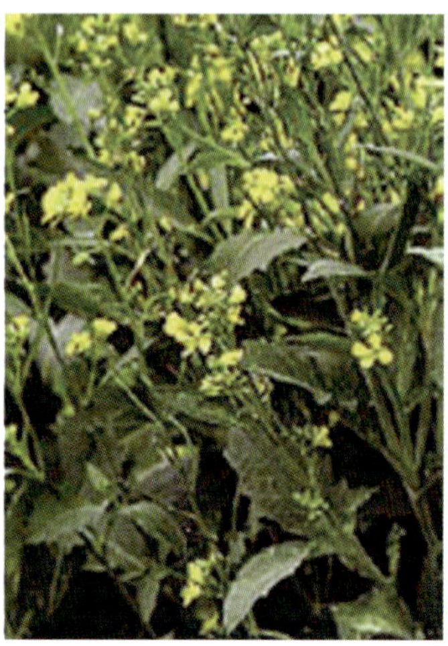

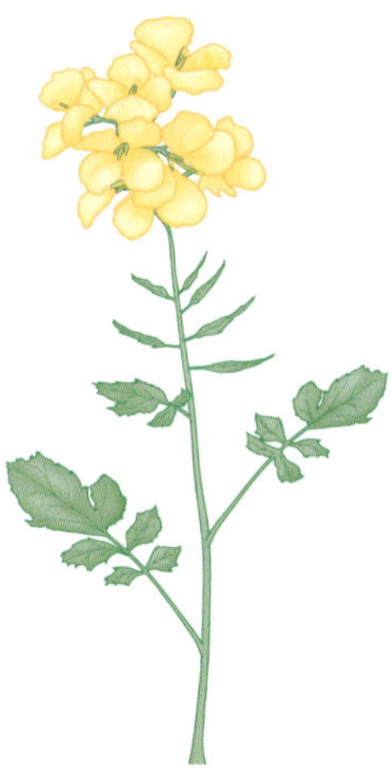

Mustard

- Common Names: Mustard
- Latin Name: *Brassica juncea*
- Family: Brassicaceae
- Parts Used: Leaves and Seeds
- Habitat: Korea and China

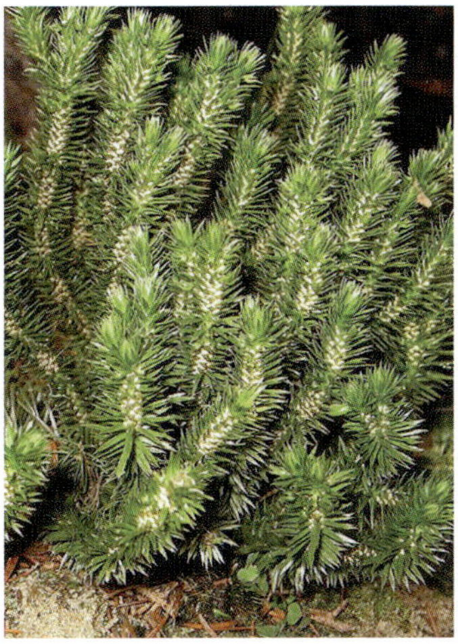
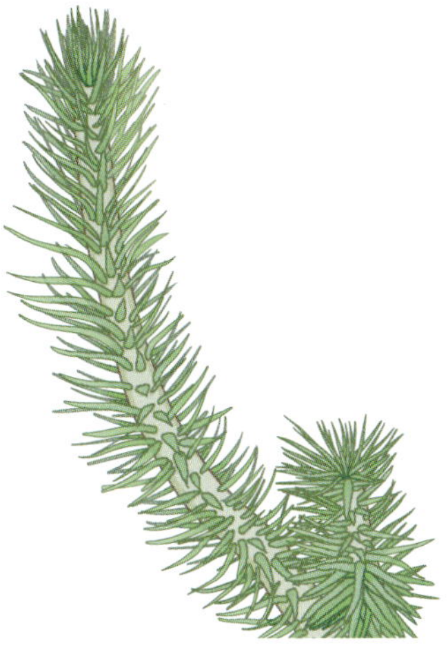

Northern Firmoss

- Common Names: Northern Firmoss
- Latin Name: *Hyperzia serrata*
- Family: Huperziaceae
- Parts Used: Stalks and Leaves
- Habitat: China

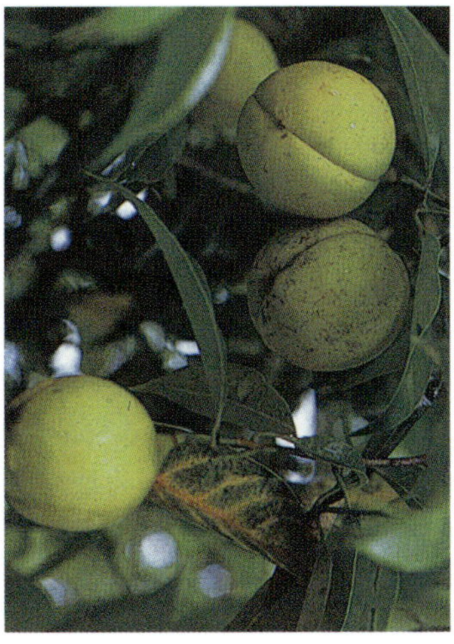
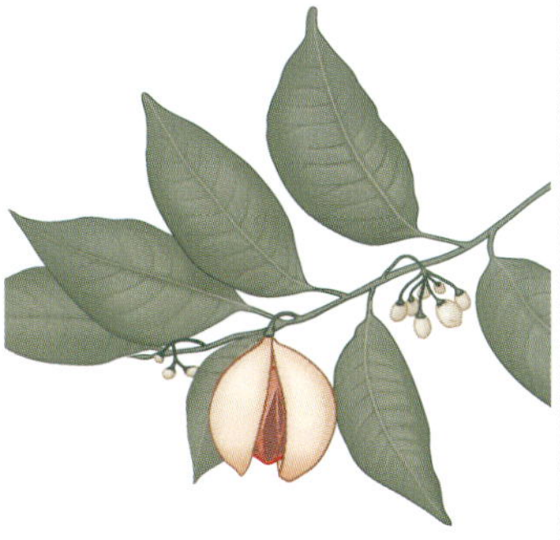

Nutmeg

- Common Names: Mace
- Latin Name: *Myristica fragrans*
- Family: Myristicaceae
- Parts Used: Seeds
- Habitat: Indonesia and India

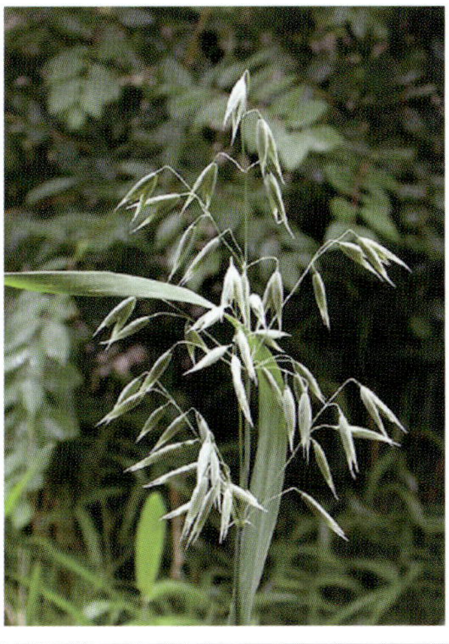
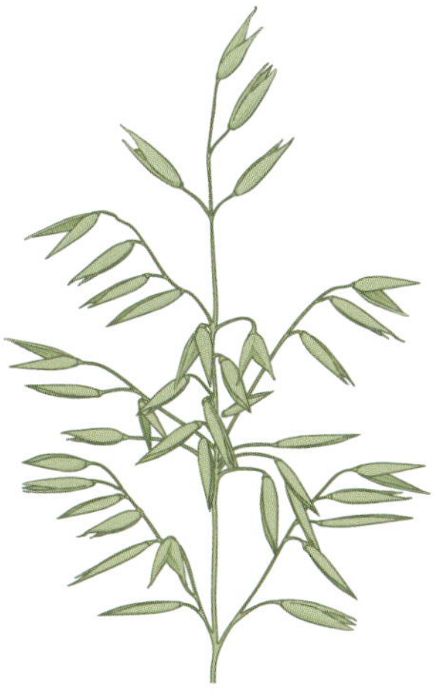

Oats

- Common Names: Wild Oats, Wild Grass, Oat Straw, Wild Oats Milk seed
- Latin Name: *Avena sativa*
- Family: Poaceae
- Parts Used: Seeds
- Habitat: Northern Europe

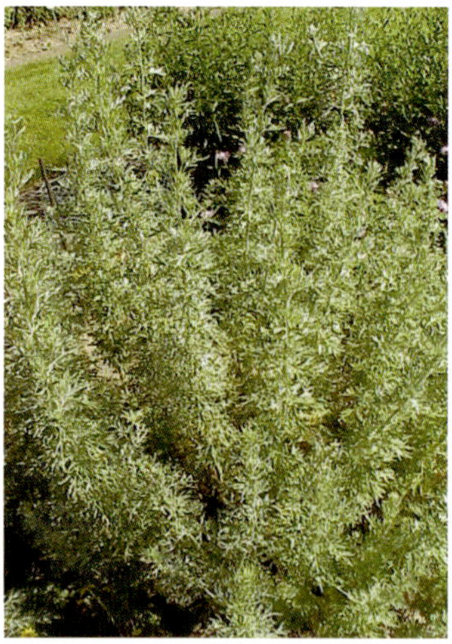

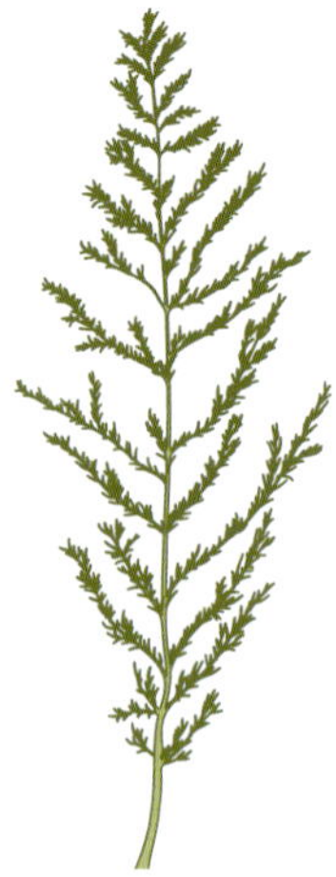

Oriental Wormwood

- Common Names: Oriental wormwood
- Latin Name: *Artemisia absinthium*
- Family: Compositae
- Parts Used: Whole plants
- Habitat: Central Asia, Asia Minor, Western and Eastern Siberia, in the Maritime Territory, Manchuria, Mongolia, part of the USSR and European

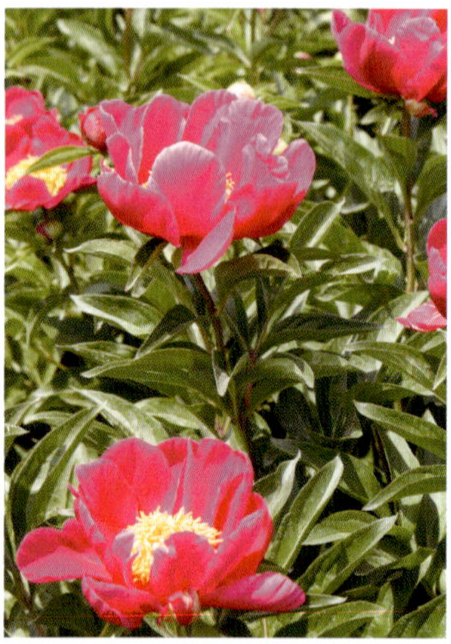

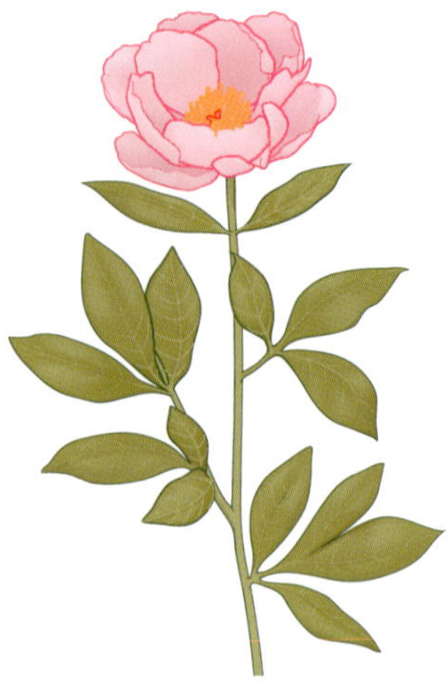

Peony

- Common Names: Peony
- Latin Name: *Paeonia lactiflora*
- Family: Paeoniaceae
- Parts Used: Roots
- Habitat: Korea, China, Japan, Tibet and Siberia

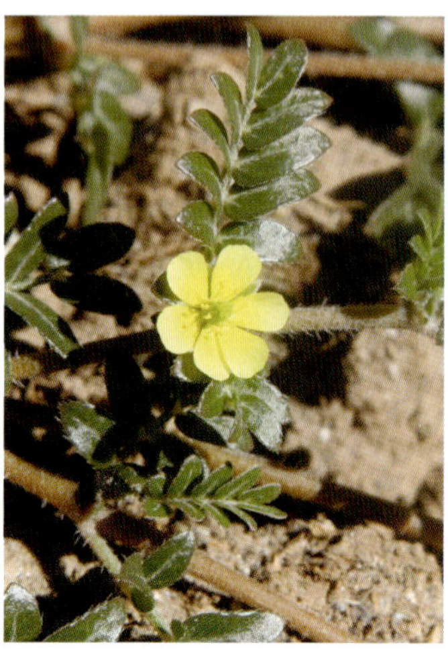

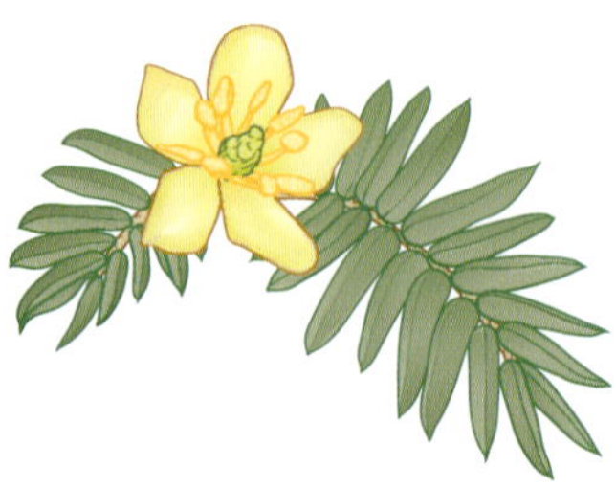

Puncture Vine

- Common Names: Puncture Vine, Land Caltrops, Gokhru
- Latin Name: *Tribulus terrestris L.*
- Family: Zygophyllaceae
- Parts Used: Fruits and Seeds
- Habitat: Europe and United States

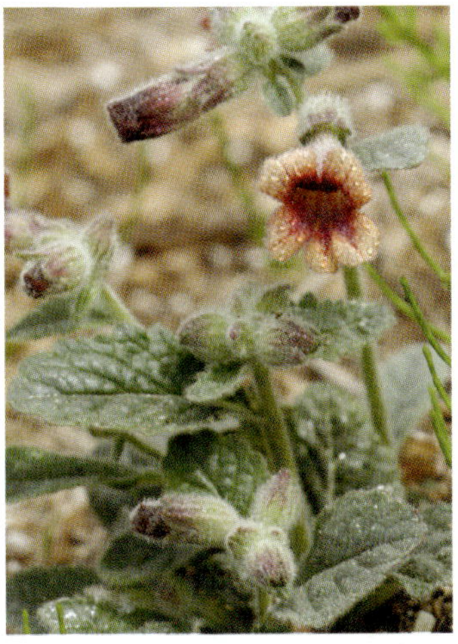

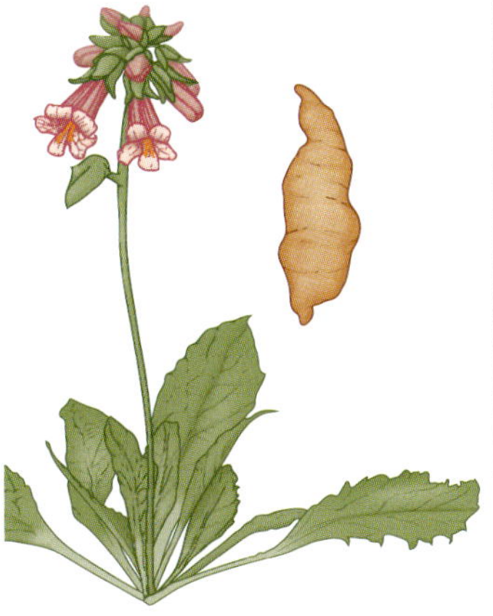

Rehmannia Root

- Common name: Rehmannia Root
- Latin name: *Rehmannia glutinosa*
- Family: Scrophulariaceae
- Part Used: Roots
- Habitat: Korea, China and Japan

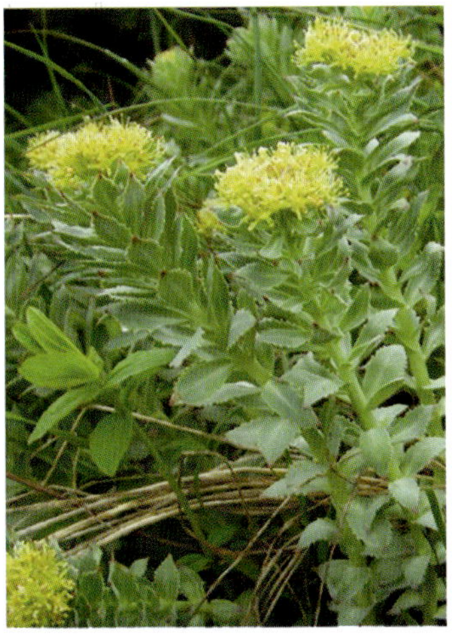

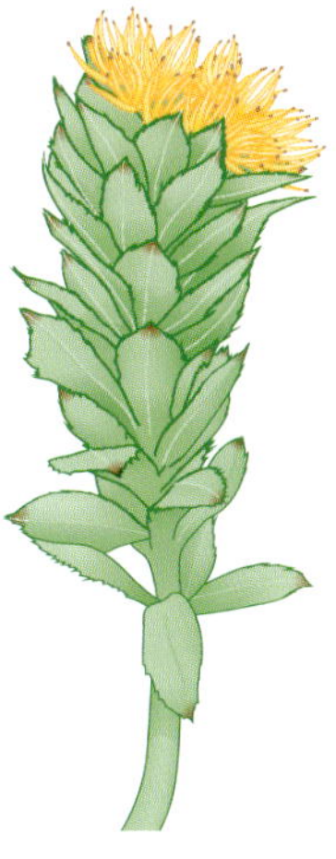

Rhodiola

- Common Names: Rhodiola, Golden root, Roseroot, Arctic root
- Latin Name: *Rhodiola rosea, Sedum roseum*
- Family: Crassulaceae
- Parts Used: Roots, Stems, Leaves, Flowers and Seeds
- Habitat: High elevations in Asia, Europe, and North America.

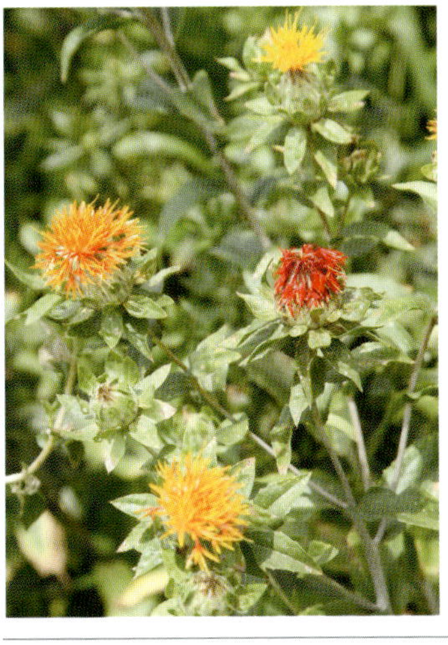

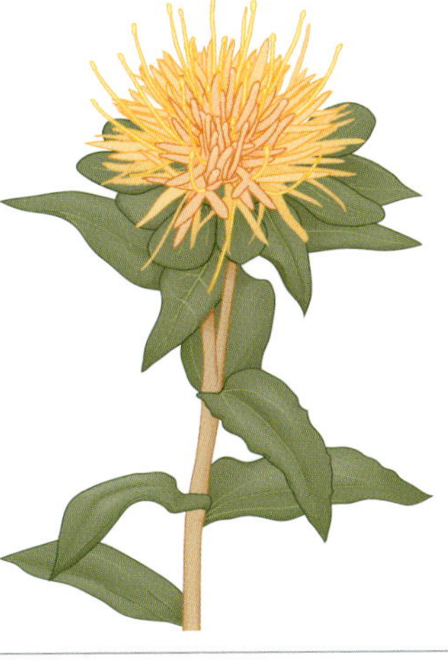

Safflower

- Common name: Safflower, Safflor, Bastard saffron
- Latin name: *Cathamus tinctorius*
- Family: Compositae
- Part Used: Flowers
- Habitat: China, India and in other parts of Asia

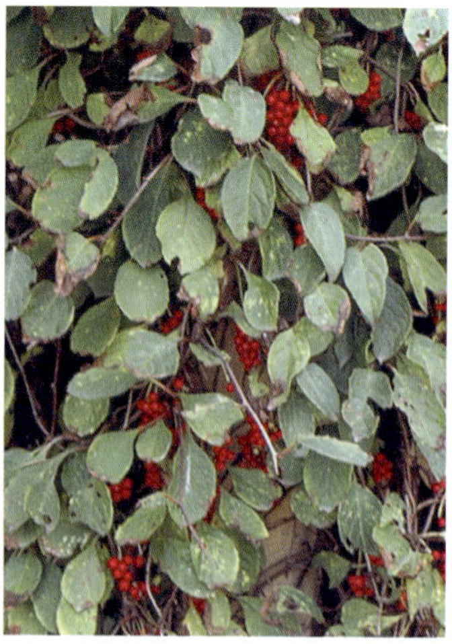

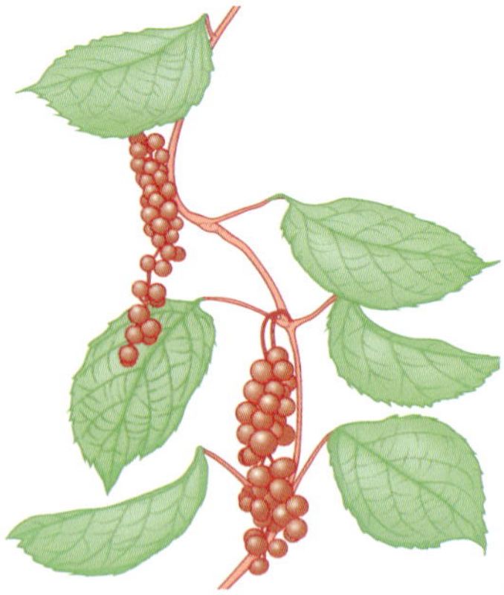

Schisandra

- Common Names: Schisandra, Magnolia vine, Star vine, Bay star vine, Wu wei zi.
- Latin Name: *Schisandra chinensis*
- Family: Schisandraceae
- Parts Used: Fruits, Berries and Leaves
- Habitat: Korea, China and Japan

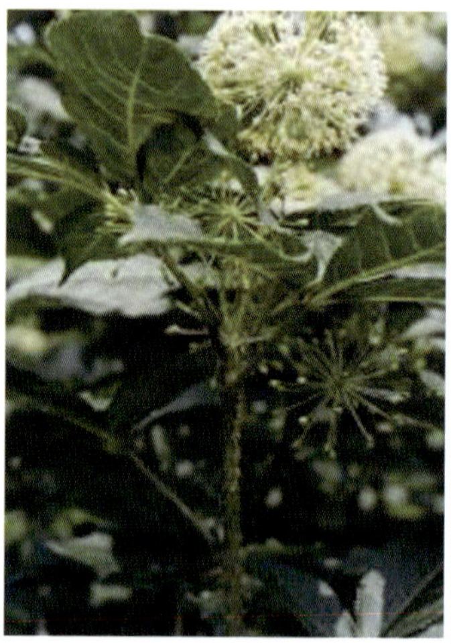

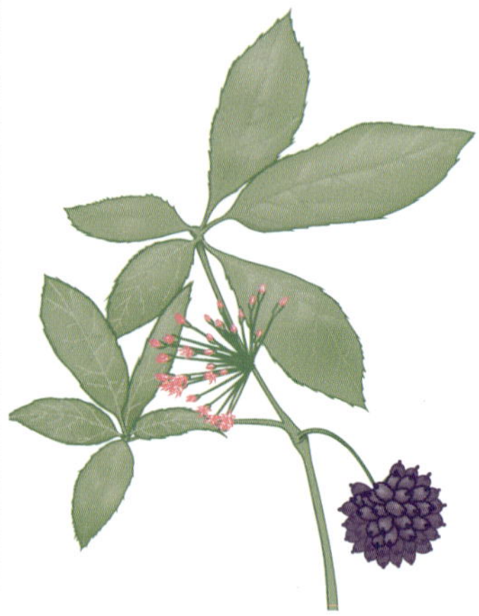

Siberian Ginseng

- Common Names: Siberian Ginseng, Eleuthero
- Latin Name: *Acanthopanax senticosus*
- Family: Araliaceae
- Parts Used: Roots, Rhizomes, Stems and Leaves
- Habitat: North parts of Korea, Eastern China, Japan and Eastern Russia

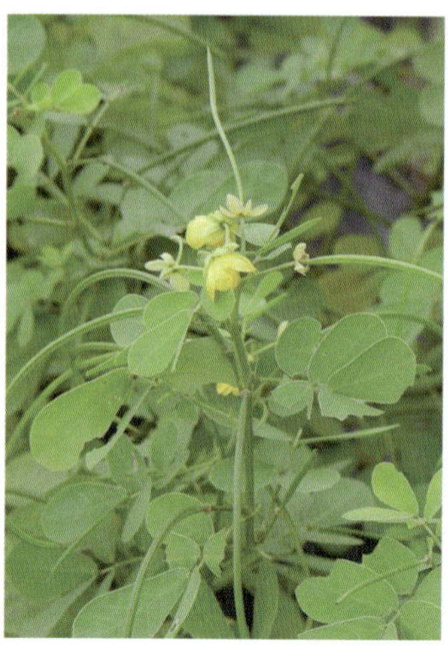

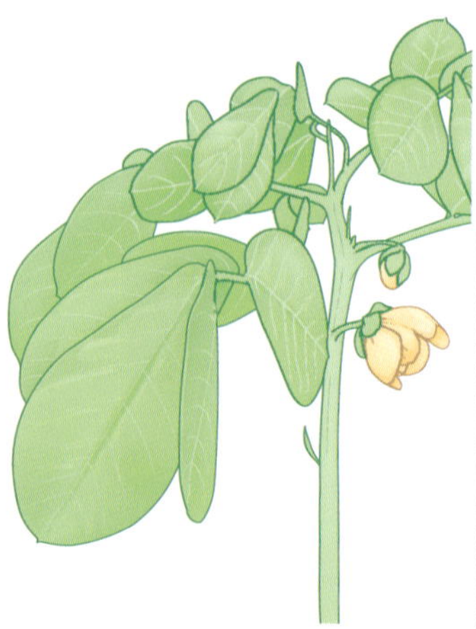

Sicklepod

- Common Names: Sicklepod
- Latin Name: *Cassia obtussifolia*
- Family: Leguminosae
- Parts Used: Seeds
- Habitat: Tropical parts of India

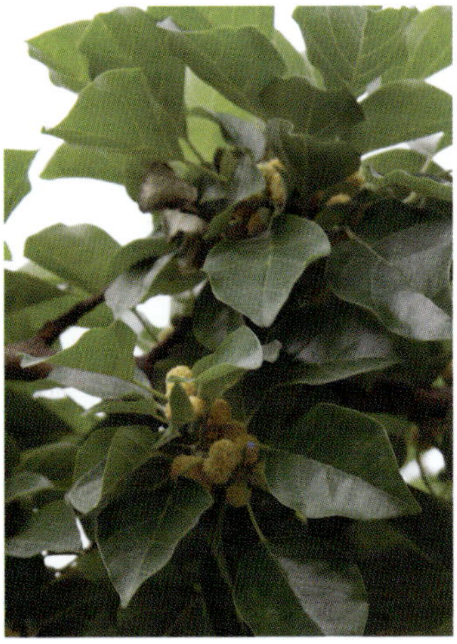

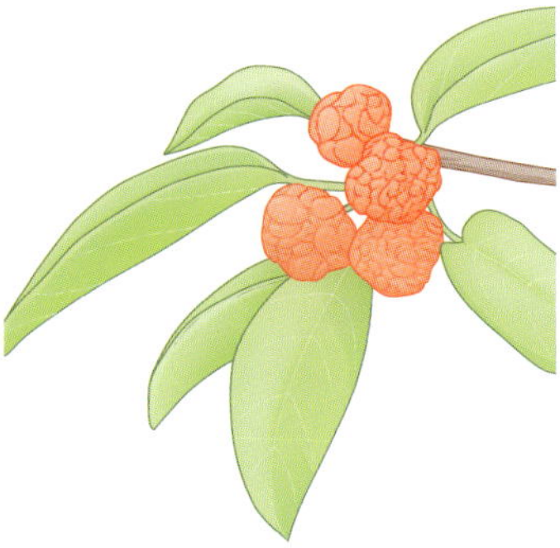

Silkworm Thorn

- Common Names: Silkworm Thorn
- Latin Name: *Cudrania tricuspidata*
- Family: Moraceae
- Parts Used: Fruits, Leaves and Stems
- Habitat: Korea, China and Japan

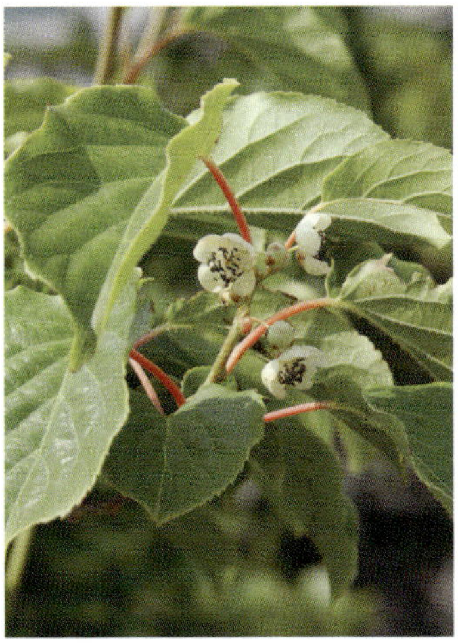

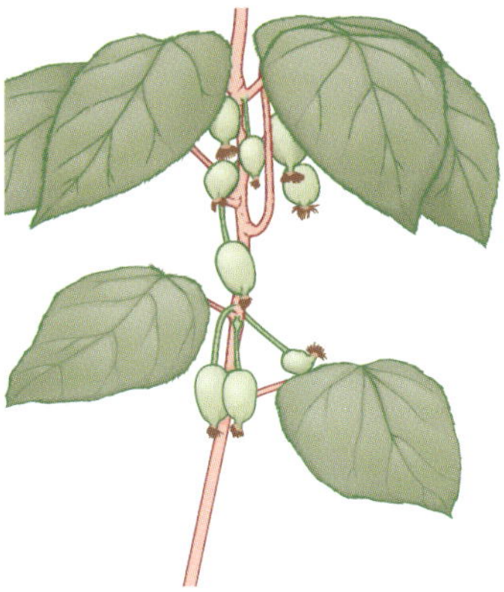

Silvervine

- Common name: Silvervine
- Latin name: *Actinidia polygama*
- Family: Actinidiaceae
- Part Used: Gall
- Habitat: Korea, China and Japan

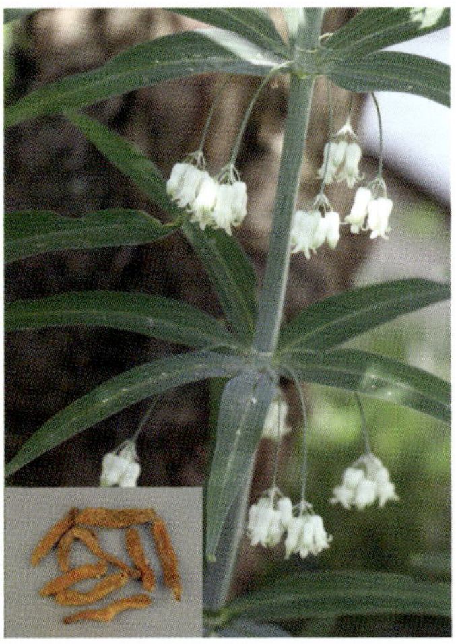

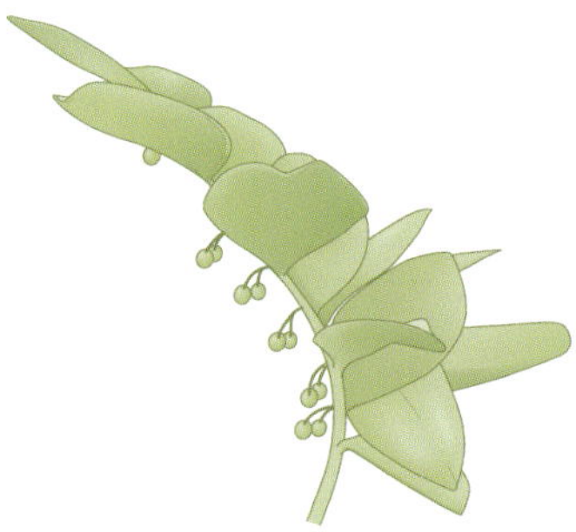

Solomonseal Rhizome

- Common name: Solomonseal Rhizome, Fragrant Solomonseal Rhizome
- Latin name: *Pdygonatum sibiricum*
- Family: Liliaceae
- Part Used: Roots
- Habitat: China

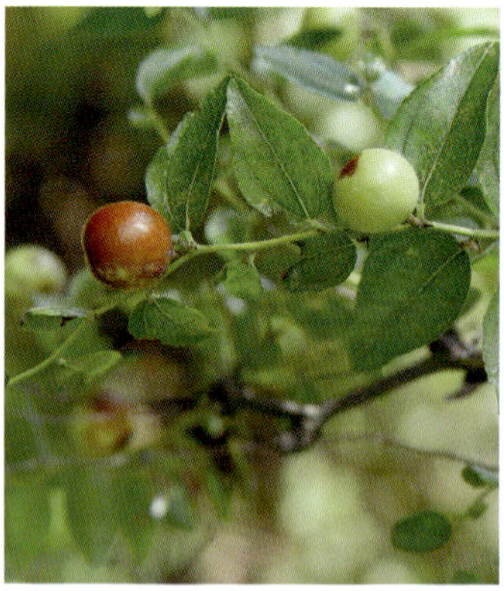

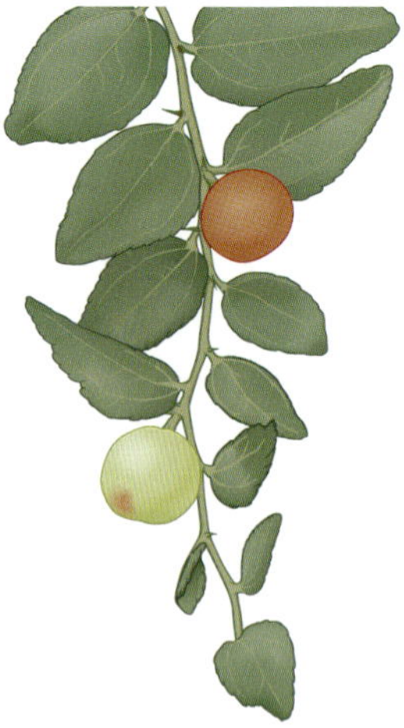

Spine Date Seed

- Common name: Spine Date Seed
- Latin name: *Zizyphus jujuba*
- Family: Rhamnaceae
- Part Used: Seeds
- Habitat: China, Mongolia and India

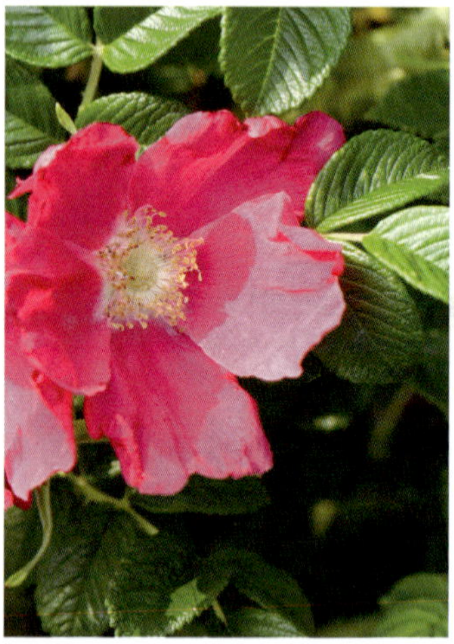

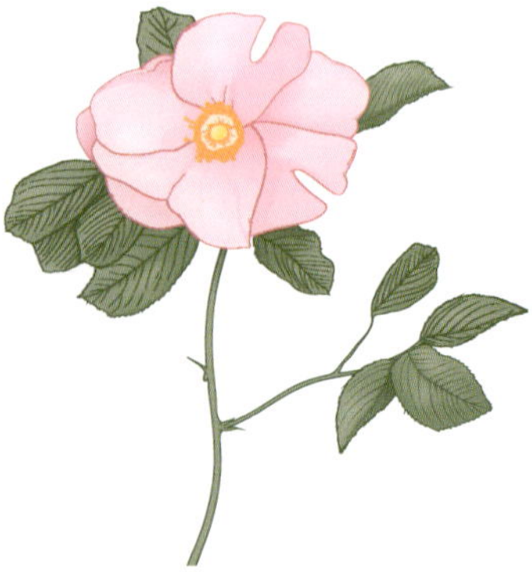

Sweetbrier

- Common Names: Sweetbrier
- Latin Name: *Rosa rugosa*
- Family: Rosaceae
- Parts Used: Flowers and Roots
- Habitat: Korea and Japan

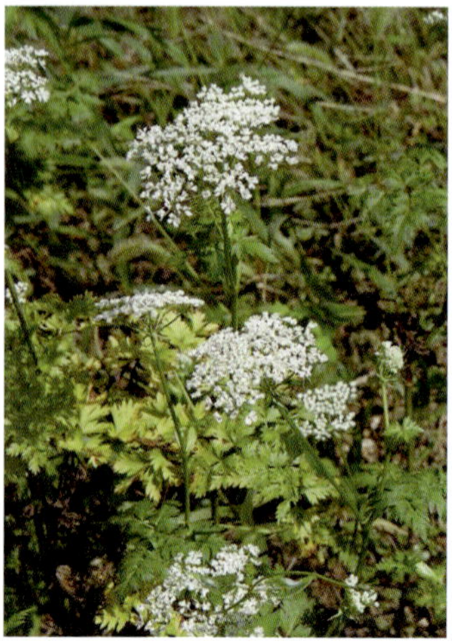

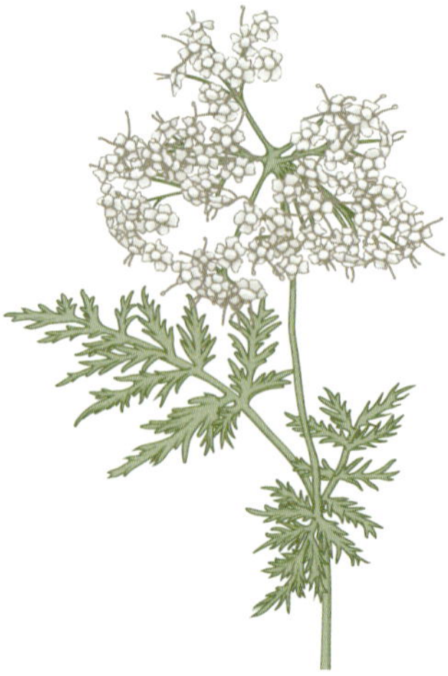

Szchwan Lovage Rhizome

- Common name: Szechwan Lovage Rhizome, Rhizoma Chuanxiong,
- Latin name: *Ligusticum chuanxiong*
- Family: Umbelliferae
- Part Used: Roots
- Habitat: China

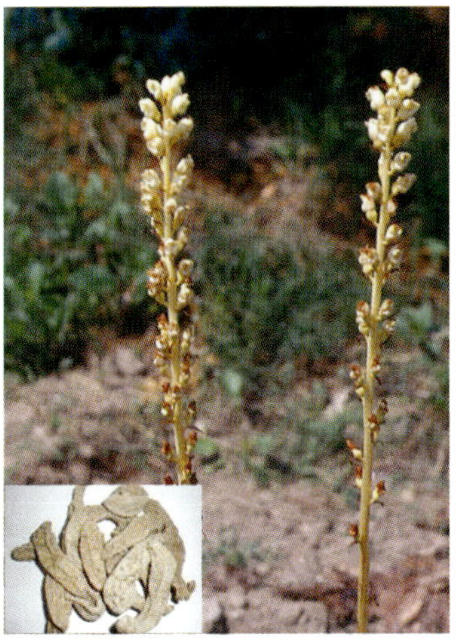

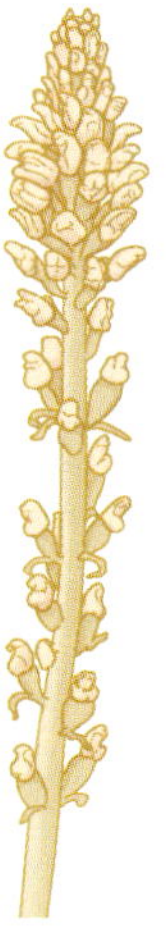

Tall Gastrodia Tuber

- Common name: Tall Gastrodia Tuber
- Latin name: *Gastrodia elata*
- Family: Orchidaceae
- Part Used: Tubers
- Habitat: Korea, China and Japan

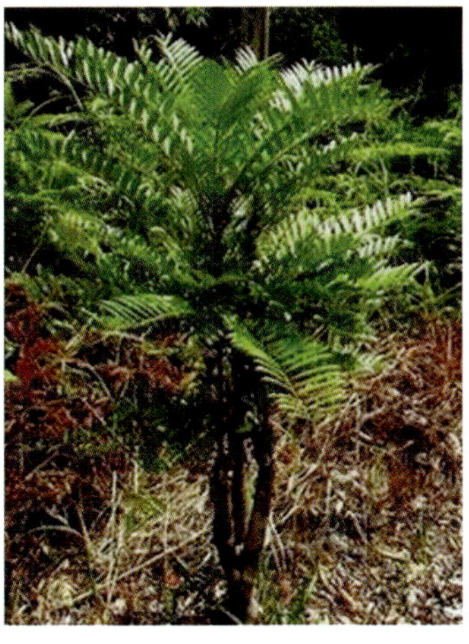

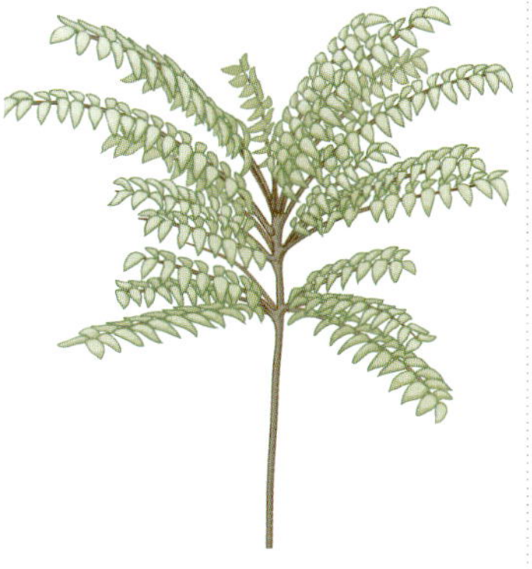

Tongkat Ali

- Common name: Tongkat Ali
- Latin name: *Eurycoma longifolia*
- Family: Simaroubaceae
- Part Used: Roots
- Habitat: Indonesia, Malay Peninsula, Thailand, Laos, Cambodia and Vietnam

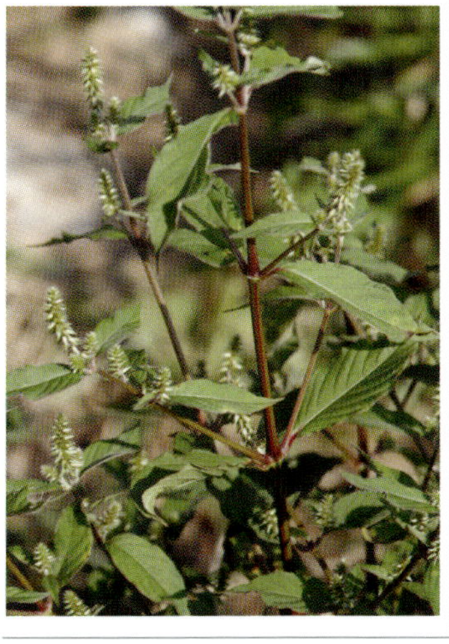

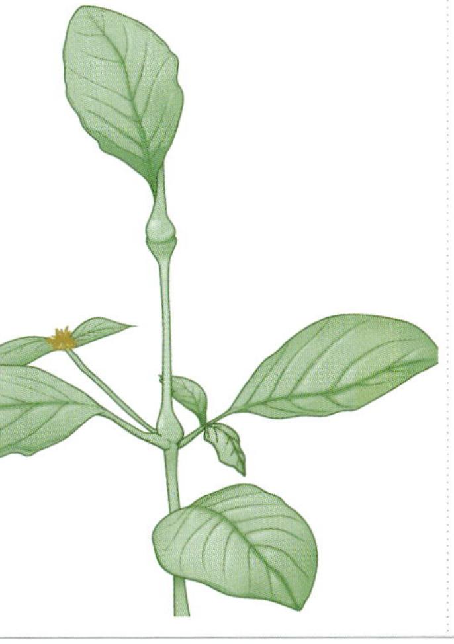

Twotoothed Achyranthes Roots

- Common name: Twotoothed Achyranthes Roots
- Latin name: *Achyranthes japonica*
- Family: Amaranthaceae
- Part Used: Roots
- Habitat: Korea, China and Japan

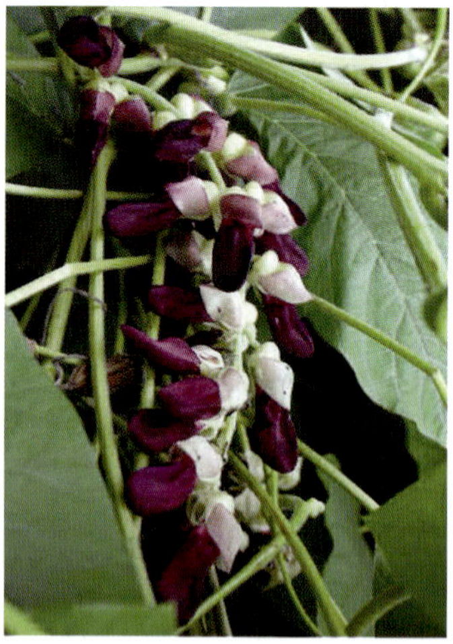

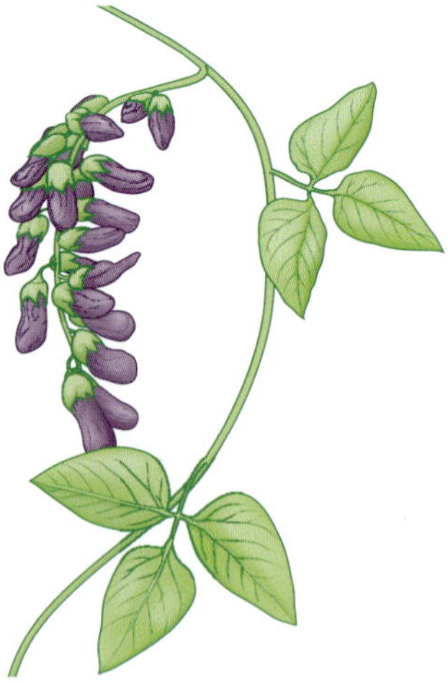

Velvet Bean

- Common Name:
  Velvet Bean, Cowitch, Common Cowitch, Konch
- Latin Name:
  Mucuna pruriens
- Family Name:
  Leguminosae
- Part Used:
  Roots, Seeds and Leaves
- Habitat: Southern Asia and Malaysia

Appendix

Literatures for Traditional Oriental Medicine

I. Literatures for Traditional Korean Medicine

No.	Title (Chines)	Year of Publication	Name of Author
1	Baekjesinjipbang (百濟新集方)	Baekje Era (AD18-660)	Unknown
2	Sillabeopsayugwanbimilyosulbang (新羅法師流觀秘密要術方)	Unified Shilla Era (654-935)	Unknown
3	Jejungiphyobang (濟衆立效方)	1147-1166	Kim Young-Seok (金永錫)
4	Sinjipeouichwalyobang (新集御醫撮要方)	1226	Choi Jong-Jun (崔宗峻)
5	Hyangyakgugeupbang (鄕藥救急方)	1236	Unknown
6	Hyangyakjipseongbang (鄕藥集成方)	1433	Yu Hyo-Tong (兪孝通) No Jung-Rye (盧重禮) Park Yoon-Deok (朴允德)
7	Taesanyorok (胎産要錄)	1434	No Jung-Rye (盧重禮)
8	Uibangyuchwi (醫方類聚)	1445	Kim Ye-Mong (金禮蒙) Yu Seong-Won (柳誠源)
9	Ganyibyeokonbang (簡易辟瘟方)	1525	Park Sae-Geo (朴世擧) Kim Sun-Mong (金順蒙) Yu Young-Jeong (劉永貞)
10	Uirimchwalyo (醫林撮要)	1567	Yang Ye-Su (楊禮壽)
*11	Donguibogam (東醫寶鑑)	1610	Heo Jun (許浚)
12	Eonhaetaesanjipyo (諺解胎産集要)	1608	Heo Jun (許浚)
13	Chimgugyeongheombang (鍼灸經驗方)	1644	Hoe Yim (許任)
14	Byeokonsinbang (辟瘟新方)	1653	An Gyeong-Chang (安景昌)
15	Geupyubang (及幼方)	1749	Jo Jeong-Jun (趙廷俊)
16	Uimunbogam (醫門寶鑑)	1724	Ju Myeong-Sin (周命新)
17	Gwangjebigeup (廣濟秘笈)	1790	Lee Gyeong-Hwa (李景華)
18	Magwahwaetong (麻科會通)	1798	Jeong Da-San (丁茶山)
19	Jejungsinpyeon (濟衆新編)	1799	Gang Myeong-Gil (康命吉)
20	Bangyakhappyeon (方藥合編)	1885	Hwang Do-Yeon (黃道淵)
21	Donguisusebowon (東醫壽世保元)	1894	Lee Je-Ma (李濟馬)

* "Donguibogam," or the "Principles and Practice of Eastern Medicine," was included in the UNESCO's Memor of the World Register on July 31. 2009.

II. Literatures for Traditional Chinese Medicine

No.	Title (Chines)	Year of Publication	Name of Author
1	Yellow Emperor's Internal Classic (黄帝内经)	BC(475-221)	Unknown
2	Shennong's Classic of Materia Medica (神农本草经)	AD 5	Unknown
3	Treatise on febrile and miscellaneous diseases (伤寒杂病论)	AD196-204	Zhang zhong-Jin (張仲景)
4	a handbook of prescriptions for emergencies (肘后备急方)	265-341	Ge Hong (葛洪)
5	Valuable Prescriptions for Emergency (备急千金要方)	581-682	Sun Si-Miao (孫思邈)
6	The Medical Secrets of an Official (外台秘要)	752	Wang Tao (王燾)
7	The Holy Benevolent Prescriptions (太平圣惠方)	982-992	Wang Huai-Yin (王懷隱)
8	Complete Record of Holy Benevolence (圣济总录)	1111-1117	co-edited by Medical Officers of Song dynasty (宋徽宗時由朝廷組織人員編纂)
9	Formularies of the Bureau of People's Welfare Pharmacies (太平惠民和剂局方)	1107	Chen Shi-Wen et al (陳師文等人)
10	Key to Therapeutics of Children's Diseases (小儿药证直决)	1119	Qian Yi (錢乙)
11	Jifeng's Formularies for Universal Relief (鸡峰普济方)	1133	Zhang Rui (張銳)
12	the Three Categories of Pathogenic Factors of Diseases on Slumber (三因极一病证方论)	1174	Chen Yan (陳言)
13	Confucians' Duties to Their Parents (儒门事亲)	1217-1221	Zhang Cong-Zheng (張從正)
14	Complete Effective Prescriptions for Diseases of Women (妇人大全良方)	1237	Chen Zi-Ming (陳自明)
15	Prescriptions for Succouring the Sick (济生方)	1253	Yan Yong-He (嚴用和)
16	Formulae Theory on Chickenpox and Measles in Children (小儿痘疹方论)	1254	Chen Wen-Zhong (陳文中)
17	Treatise on Spleen and Stomach (脾胃论)	1249	Li Gao (李杲)
18	Effective Formulas Handed Down for Generations (世医得效方)	1343	Wei Yi-Lin (危亦林)
19	Treatise on Ge Zhi (格致余论)	1347	Zhu Zheng-Heng (朱震亨)
20	Prescriptions for Universal Relief (普济方)	1406	Zhu Su (朱棣)
21	Compendium of Materia Medica (本草纲目)	1578	Li Shi-Zhen (李時珍)
22	Medical Formulae Investigations (医方考)	1584	Wu Kun (吳昆)
23	Jingyue's Complete Works (景岳全书)	1640	Zhang Jie-Bin (張介賓)
24	Variorum of Medical Recipes (医方集解)	1682	Wang Ang (汪昂)
25	Insights Into Medicine (医学心悟)	1732	Cheng Zhong-Ling (程钟龄)
26	Formulas of febrile diseases (伤寒类方)	1759	Xu D-Chun (徐大椿)
27	Feasible application of Set Prescriptions (成方切用)	1761	Wu Yi-Luo (吳儀洛)
28	Item Differentiation of Warm Febrile Diseases (温病条辨)	1798	Wu Tang (吴瑭)
29	Jiang's formulary of traumatology (江氏伤科方书)	1840	Jiang Kao-Qing (江考卿)
30	Medical Formulae Theory (医方论)	1865	Fei Bo-Xiong (費伯雄)

III. Literatures for Traditional Japanese Medicine

No.	Title (Chines)	Year of Publication	Author
1	Ishinpou (医心方)	984	Yasuyori-Tanba (丹波康頼)
2	Kissayoujouki (喫茶養生記)	1214	栄西 (Yousai)
3	Tonishou /Mananpou (頓医抄・萬安方)	1303	Shouzen-Kajiwara (梶原性全)
4	Shuuhoukiku (衆方規矩)	1626	Douzan-Manase (曲直瀬道三)
5	Wagohonzoukoumoku (和語本草綱目)	1698	Ippou-Okamoto (岡本一抱)
6	Ymatohonzou (大和本草)	1709	Ekiken-Kaibara (貝原益軒)
7	Youyakusuchi (用薬須知)	1726	Gentatu-Matuoka (松岡玄達)
8	Kokonhoui (古今方彙)	1747	Tuugen-kouga (甲賀通元)
9	Ruijuhou (類聚方)	1751	Toudou-Yoshimasu (吉益東洞)
10	Yakuchou (薬徴)	1771	Toudou-Yoshimasu (吉益東洞)
11	Kiketusuiyakuchou (気血水薬徴)	Unknown	Nangai-Yoshimasu (吉益南涯)
12	Kohoubinran (古方便覧)	1782	Sigetou-Rokkaku (六角重任)
13	Fukushoukiran (腹証奇覧)	1800	Bunrei-Inaba (稲葉文礼)
14	Juushuuhonzoukoumokukeimou (重修本草綱目啓蒙)	1802	Ranzan-Ono (小野蘭山)
15	Honzouzufu (本草図譜)	1828	Kanen-Iwasaki (岩崎灌園)
16	Ruijuhoukougi (類聚方広義)	1855	Youdou-Odai (尾台榕堂)
17	Naikahiroku (内科秘録)	1863	Souken-Honma (本間棗軒)
18	Futugoyakushituhoukankuketu (勿誤薬室方函口訣)	1878	Souhaku-Asada (浅田宗伯)
19	Ikainotettui (医界之鉄椎)	1910	Keijuurou-Wada (和田啓十朗)
20	Koukanigaku (皇漢医学)	1927	Kyushin-Yumoto (湯本求真)
21	Kanpousinryonojissai (漢方診療の実際)	1941	Keisetu-Otuka (大塚敬節)

INDEX

A

B

C

D

E

F

G

H

I

J

K

L

M

N

O

P

Q

R

S

T

U

V

W

X

Y

Z

Others